**Transfusion-Free
Medicine and
Surgery**

Transfusion-Free Medicine and Surgery

Second Edition

Edited by

Nicolas Jabbour, MD

Professor of Surgery
Chairman Service de Chirurgie et transplantation abdominale
Cliniques universitaires Saint-Luc
Bruxelles, Belgium

WILEY Blackwell

This edition first published 2014 © 2005, 2014 by John Wiley & Sons Ltd.

Registered office: John Wiley & Sons, Ltd, The Atrium, Southern Gate, Chichester, West Sussex, PO19 8SQ, UK

Editorial offices: 9600 Garsington Road, Oxford, OX4 2DQ, UK
   The Atrium, Southern Gate, Chichester, West Sussex, PO19 8SQ, UK
   111 River Street, Hoboken, NJ 07030-5774, USA

For details of our global editorial offices, for customer services and for information about how to apply for permission to reuse the copyright material in this book please see our website at www.wiley.com/wiley-blackwell

Library of Congress Cataloging-in-Publication Data

Transfusion-free medicine and surgery / edited by Nicolas Jabbour. – Second edition.
     p. ; cm.
  Includes bibliographical references and index.
  ISBN 978-0-470-67408-6 (cloth)
  I. Jabbour, Nicolas, editor of compilation.
  [DNLM: 1. Bloodless Medical and Surgical Procedures. 2. Blood Substitutes–therapeutic use. WH 450]
  RD33.35
  615′.39–dc23

                                                                                    2014004643

A catalogue record for this book is available from the British Library.

Wiley also publishes its books in a variety of electronic formats. Some content that appears in print may not be available in electronic books.

Cover image: iStock #11024906 © mediaphotos
Cover design by Garth Stewart

Typeset in 10/13pt Palatino LT std by Laserwords Private Limited, Chennai, India
Printed and bound in Malaysia by Vivar Printing Sdn Bhd

1   2014

To my family: Banu, Nicole and Jacques

Contents

Contributors

Katrina A. Bramstedt, PhD
Associate Professor
Medical Ethics and Professionalism
Bond University School of Medicine
Gold Coast, Queensland, Australia

Jason Bryant, MD
Staff Anesthesiologist
Department of Anesthesiology and
Pain Medicine
Nationwide Children's Hospital;
Department of Anesthesiology
The Ohio State University
Columbus, OH, USA

Fabrizio Di Benedettom, MD, PhD
Professor of Surgery
Hepato-pancreato-biliary Surgery and
Liver Transplantation Unit
University of Modena and Reggio Emilia
Modena, Italy

Elia Elia, MD
Clinical Associate Professor
Department of Anesthesiology
Thomas Jefferson University
Jefferson Medical College
Philadelphia, PA, USA

Shannon L. Farmer
Adjunct Research Fellow
School of Surgery, Faculty of Medicine
Dentistry and Health Sciences
University of Western Australia
Perth, Western, Australia;
Adjunct Senior Research Fellow
Centre for Population Health Research,
Curtin Health Innovation Research Institute
Curtin University, Perth, Western Australia

Lance W Griffin, MD
Instructor of General Surgery
University of Texas Medical Branch
Galveston, TX, USA

Randy Henderson
Program Director
Transfusion-Free Surgery and Patient Blood
Program Management
Keck Medical Center and
Keck Hospital of USC
University of Southern California
Los Angeles, CA, USA

James Isbister BSc(Med), MBBS,
FRACP, FRCPA
Clinical Professor of Medicine
University of Sydney, Sydney, Australia;
Adjunct Professor
University of Technology, Sydney;
Adjunct Professor
Monash University, Melbourne;
Conjoin Professor of Medicine
University of New South Wales
Sydney, Australia;
Emeritus Consultant
Haematology & Transfusion Medicine
Royal North Shore Hospital
Sydney, NSW, Australia

Nicolas Jabbour, MD
Professor of Surgery
Chairman Service de Chirurgie et
transplantation abdominale
Cliniques universitaires Saint-Luc
Bruxelles, Belgium

Mazyar Javidroozi, MD, PhD
Department of Anesthesiology and Critical
Care Medicine
Englewood Hospital and Medical Center
Englewood, NJ, USA

Yoogoo Kang, MD
Professor
Department of Anesthesiology
Thomas Jefferson University
Jefferson Medical College
Philadelphia, PA, USA

S. Kamran Hejazi Kenari, MD
Assistant Professor of Surgery
Division of Organ Transplantation
Department of Surgery
Rhode Island Hospital
Alpert Medical School of Brown University
Providence, RI, USA

Pamela J. Kling MD
Professor
Meriter Hospital and University of
Wisconsin
Madison School of Medicine and
Public Health
Madison, WI, USA

Senthil G. Krishna, MD
Staff Anesthesiologist
Department of Anesthesiology and
Pain Medicine
Nationwide Children's Hospital;
Department of Anesthesiology
The Ohio State University
Columbus, OH, USA

Michael F. Leahy, MB ChB, FRACP, FRCP, FRCPath.
Consultant Haematologist
Head of Department of Haematology
Fremantle Hospital and Health Service;
Clinical Professor in Medicine
School of Medicine and Pharmacology
University of Western Australia
Perth, WA, Australia

Irina Maramica, MD PhD
Associate Professor Health Sciences
Medical Director of Transfusion Medicine
Department of Pathology and Laboratory
Medicine
University of California Irvine
Medical Center
Orange, CA, USA

Seth Perelman, MD
Department of Anesthesiology and Critical
Care Medicine
Englewood Hospital and Medical Center
Englewood, NJ, USA

Reza F. Saidi, MD, FICS, FACS
Assistant Professor of Surgery
Division of Organ Transplantation
Department of Surgery
Rhode Island Hospital
Alpert Medical School of Brown University
Providence, RI, USA

Aryeh Shander, MD, FCCM, FCCP
Chief, Department of Anesthesiology,
Critical Care Medicine, Pain Management
and Hyperbaric Medicine
Englewood Hospital & Medical Center
Englewood, NJ

Shelly Sharma, MD
Clinical Research Fellow
Department of Radiation Oncology
St. Jude Children's Research Hospital
Memphis, TN, USA

Sharad Sharma, MD, MRCS
Assistant Professor
Department Of Transplant Surgery, UTMB
Galveston, TX, USA

Ira A. Shulman, MD
Vice Chair and Professor of Pathology
Keck School of Medicine at the University of
Southern California (USC)
Director of the USC Transfusion Medicine
Services Group
Los Angeles, CA, USA

Ahsan Syed, MD
Staff Anesthesiologist
Department of Anesthesiology and
Pain Medicine
Nationwide Children's Hospital;
Department of Anesthesiology
The Ohio State University
Columbus, OH, USA

Giuseppe Tarantino, MD
Hepato-pancreato-biliary Surgery and
Liver Transplantation Unit
University of Modena and Reggio Emilia
Modena, Italy

Joseph D. Tobias, MD
Chairman
Department of Anesthesiology and
Pain Medicine
Nationwide Children's Hospital;
Department of Anesthesiology
The Ohio State University
Columbus, OH, USA

Jean-Louis Vincent, MD, PhD
Professor of Intensive Care
Head, Department of Intensive Care
Erasme Hospital
Université libre de Bruxelles
Brussels, Belgium

Preface

This is the second edition of the book entitled *Transfusion-Free Medicine and Surgery*, which was first published in 2005.

Since its first publication, there have been some noticeable changes in the field.

1 As a result of more expended testing of blood donors, the blood has become safer; however, as mentioned in the first edition, blood will never be 100% safe because of the inherent risk of it's administration and storage such as clerical error. Therefore, the benefit of avoiding blood transfusion cannot be underestimated.

2 In most hospitals and in several services, we noticed that the notion of transfusion-free medicine and surgery is no longer limited to Jehovah's witness patients. The medical community pays more attention to blood utilization and has installed stricter criteria for blood transfusion both in and outside the operation room, in particular, in the intensive care unit.

3 In the area of artificial blood products, there is currently no real break-through, but ongoing research hopefully will lead to a product on the market in the near future.

4 Topical hemostasis has been more studied, and several new products were introduced in the operating room with measurable success in terms of control of bleeding and blood utilization.

5 Seemingly remote basic research in certain areas, such as reperfusion injury in organ transplantation, has contributed to the understanding of intraoperative bleeding.

The fact remains, however, that more than 50% of blood transfusion is prescribed by surgeons, and we as physicians in general and surgeons in particular have the responsibility of objectively assessing the risk, availability, and cost of blood products.

Blood conservation is still a measure of higher standard of care and has more room to grow.

CHAPTER 1

History of blood transfusion and patient blood management

Shannon L. Farmer[1], James Isbister[2], and Michael F. Leahy[3]

[1]School of Surgery, Faculty of Medicine, Dentistry and Health Sciences, University of Western Australia, Perth, Western Australia;
Centre for Population Health Research, Curtin Health Innovation Research Institute, Curtin University, Perth, Western Australia
[2]University of Sydney, Sydney, Australia;
University of Technology, Sydney, Australia;
Monash University, Melbourne, Australia;
University of New South Wales, Sydney, Australia;
Haematology & Transfusion Medicine, Royal North Shore Hospital, Sydney, Australia
[3]Department of Haematology, Fremantle Hospital and Health Service, Fremantle, Western Australia;
School of Medicine and Pharmacology, University of Western Australia, Perth, Western Australia

Introduction

For more than two decades authorities have been calling for a major change in transfusion practice [1]. This is now even more urgent as new challenges continue to emerge. These include supply difficulties due to a diminishing donor pool and an increasing aging and consuming population, spiraling costs of blood and ongoing safety issues. Knowledge of transfusion limitations continues to grow, while a burgeoning literature demonstrates a strong dose-dependent relationship between transfusion and adverse patient outcomes [2, 3]. These factors combine to now make change vital [4].

Historically, changing long-standing medical practice has been challenging – perhaps even more so in transfusion. Despite professional guidelines and educational initiatives, wide variations in transfusion practice exist between countries, institutions and even between individual clinicians within the same institution [5–8]. This suggests that much

Transfusion-Free Medicine and Surgery, Second Edition. Edited by Nicolas Jabbour.
© 2014 John Wiley & Sons, Ltd. Published 2014 by John Wiley & Sons, Ltd.

practice may be based on misconceptions, belief and habit rather than evidence.

It is not the first time strongly entrenched belief has been an impediment to scientific progress. Edwin Hubble's description of an expanding universe in 1929 has been hailed as one of the great intellectual revolutions of the twentieth century. However, it has been suggested that, because of knowledge of Newton's law of gravity, an expanding universe could have been predicted over two hundred years earlier [9]. What slowed scientific progress? The widely held belief in a static universe prevailed. The belief was so strong at the time that in 1915 Einstein even modified his theory of relativity to accommodate it [9].

A brief review of the history of transfusion provides some insights as to how a behavior-based practice developed in transfusion and therefore how change may be effected by a more patient-focused approach (Figure 1.1).

Blood: early beliefs and practice

Blood has always been viewed with awe and mysticism. It has been used in rituals, to seal treaties, as nourishment, a curative and poison – all based on the belief that blood had special power [10]. It appears that transfusion of blood was first conceived in Greek mythology where the sorceress Medea shows her ability to transfuse blood to give life to the dead and dying [11]. Athena, the goddess of wisdom, gave some of the blood of the slain Gorgon leader to Asclepius, the god of medicine. Hart notes,

> "This gift of blood became 'the gift of life' and empowered him to revive the dead" [12].

There are reports as early as the seventh century BC of physicians prescribing blood to be drunk to treat a variety of diseases. An ancient Assyrian physician wrote to the king and assured him that his son was *"doing better"* after giving him blood to drink [10]. First-century Greek physician Aretaeus of Cappadocia, describing treatments for epilepsy, wrote *"I have seen persons holding a cup below the wound of a man recently slaughtered, and drinking a draught of the blood!"* [13]. Historian Reay Tannahill reported that in 1483 dying Louis XI of France hoped to recover by swallowing blood from children [14].

Bloodletting was fundamental to the medical care of patients for over 2000 years [15]. It was one of the longest lasting medical practices in history. Yet its acceptance was based on a belief – that disease was caused by an imbalance of blood and other *"humors"* in the body. Bleeding was thought to restore balance. One seventeenth-century proponent of the

	DARK AGES Before 1900	ENLIGHTENMENT 1900s	ALTRUISM 1920s–1960s	MODERNISM 1960s–1980	POST-MODERNISM 1980s–1990s	BLOOD SUPPLY MANAGEMENT 1990s	RE-ENLIGHTENMENT 2001–2010	PATIENT BLOOD MANAGEMENT 2011 -
EVENTS	Trial and error in attempts to give transfusions in some cases with success and others ending in disaster	Discovery of ABO blood groups leading to the scientific basis for compatible red cell transfusions.	Commitment of clinicians and donors with anticoagulation and preservation of whole blood to develop blood banks	Improvements in the storage of whole blood, development of blood fractionation and involvement of industry in the blood sector	Increasing concern about transfusion-transmitted infections, hepatitis and ultimately the AIDS catastrophe	Increasing application of precautionary principle on safety of the blood supply resulting in exponential increases in costs	Recognition that transfusion of labile blood components did not have a good evidence base and transfusion per se is an independent risk factor for adverse clinical outcomes	Return to a patient focus with shared clinician/patient decision making with meaningful informed consent
FOCUS	**Patient focus** Treatment of mental disorders! attempts to help patients dying from hemorrhage	**Clinician patient/donor focus.** Direct vein-to-vein blood transfusion made possible	**Clinician patient/donor focus** Transfusions for bleeding or profound anemia	**Supply focus** Whole blood and blood products	**Product focus** Viral safety and sufficiency of the blood supply	**Bureaucratic & political economic focus** Blood supply	**Evidence-based medicine focus** Return to a focus on a patient's problem and clinical decision making	**Patient focus** Problem-oriented approach to management of hemopoietic deficiencies
CONCERNS	Why are some blood transfusions potentially lethal?	Saving lives of critically bleeding or anemic patients	Community awareness of the requirement for blood donors	Blood preservation and sufficiency of the blood supply	Blood sector, bureaucracy, politicians, clinicians and patients develop "conflicting" perspectives and agendas as to the quality and safety of blood supply	Product safety and increasing expenditure on the blood supply assuming all transfusions are appropriate	Questioning many long-held assumptions and dogmas about the efficacy and safety of blood transfusion	Ensuring that a patient's own blood is managed appropriately and allogeneic transfusion is only used with patient consent and when there are no other feasible options

Figure 1.1 Transfusion history timeline.

practice, Guy Patin, Dean of the Faculty of Medicine in Paris, wrote: *"There is no remedy in the world which works as many miracles as bleeding"* [16]. It was recommended in various medical texts to treat over 100 diverse ailments including pain, plague, fever, epilepsy, melancholy, liver disease, stroke, even broken bones and hemorrhage [15, 17]. It remained one of the most trusted procedures for treatment of sickness and maintenance of health until the mid-nineteenth century [15].

An example of its "life-saving" therapeutic reputation was reported in 1825 [18]. A French sergeant, who during combat sustained a stab wound through the chest, fainted from blood loss. He was taken to a local hospital where physicians immediately began bleeding him to prevent inflammation. Over the first 24 hours they bled over half his blood volume. Over subsequent days surgeons performed more bloodletting as well as applying leeches to the wound. The patient recovered and was discharged almost 3 months later. The sergeant's physician wrote,

> "by the large quantity of blood lost, amounting to 170 ounces [*almost eleven pints*], besides that drawn by the application of leeches, the life of the patient was preserved."

In this and other cases, physicians saw improvements in the patients' symptoms, reinforcing their belief in the practice. Of interest, Starr notes that bloodletting empowered physicians in the face of diseases they did not understand – finding comfort in the fact that they were doing something for the patient [16]. This practice reinforcement was echoed in the twentieth century by Dunphy in relation to the modern practice of transfusing blood *into* patients. He wrote,

> "Transfusion certainly makes the surgeon feel better, but it may not make the patient feel better. Perhaps we all have a tendency to transfuse to make ourselves more comfortable" [19].

Blood transfusion

The practice of transfusing blood was pioneered during a period of fierce competition between England and France for world ascendency in literature, arts, science and medicine. The quest to perform the first blood transfusion was part of this, and long-held beliefs about blood's qualities were its practice foundation. It was still held that disease was a result of imbalance of humors and that bleeding might *"draw out corruption."* It was also believed that blood carried characteristics and temperament. Thus the first transfusions into humans were performed to treat psychiatric illness, believing that the blood of a calm animal such as a lamb or calf would calm the *"phrensied"* person [10, 16, 20].

Transfusion with animal blood

Technical advances such as the description of the circulation by William Harvey in 1628 and the development of the "syringe" using a sharpened goose quill by Francis Potter in 1652 and Sir Christopher Wren in 1658 made injection of fluids into vessels possible. Members of the British Royal Society began experiments with injecting a variety of fluids including wine, beer, dye, opium and milk. Experiments with transfusing blood began between 1665 and 1668, with physicians believing it to be the most compatible fluid. The first were animal-to-animal transfusions, followed by animal-to-human transfusions [16, 21].

The English are credited with performing the first blood transfusion experiments. Beginning in 1665 scientist John Wilkins, surgeon Richard Lower and others made numerous attempts at transfusing blood from one dog to another [21]. The first successful animal-to-animal transfusion by Lower was reported in 1666. Speculation developed amongst colleagues as to what behavioral and physical changes transfusion might bring about in the recipient [16, 21]. In France physician Jean Baptiste Denis and colleagues claimed to have conceived the idea of transfusing humans almost 10 years earlier at a meeting in Paris, but only began their experiments in animal transfusions in 1667. They transfused dog blood into dogs, and then calf blood into dogs. They also reported that the transfusion of blood from a young dog into an elderly dog rejuvenated its vigor [21, 22].

These experiments led to the first human transfusion. The first is credited to Denis in June 1667 in which he transfused the blood of a lamb into a 16-year-old described as suffering a *"contumacious and violent fever,"* extreme lethargy and being possessed of an *"incredible stupidity"* [21, 23]. Denis' choice of *"mild"* animal blood for transfusion was based partly on his feeling that animal blood was more pure because *"debauchedness, envy, anger, melancholy and passions corrupted human blood"* [23]. He also reasoned that transfusion achieved the same effect as bleeding, without weakening the patient. They would draw out a quantity of blood and replace it with *"new and pure"* blood. Denis reported that physicians had for the past two months been obliged to bleed this patient 20 times *"to make for saving his life."* Denis first withdrew a further 3 ounces of the patient's blood and then transfused him with 9 ounces of the lamb's blood. The patient experienced a transfusion reaction described as *"heat along his arm"*, chills and *"soot black"* urine [24]. Yet Denis believed the lamb's blood worked as the patient's symptoms resolved after the treatment, he being described as *"cheerful,"* livelier and *"possessing a clear and smiling countenance."* Denis wrote,

> "that all these admirable effects undoubtedly proceed from that little Arterial blood of the Lamb, which having been mixt with the mass of his thick blood, was like a ferment to it, to rarifie and attenuate it more than ordinary."

The British, smarting at being beaten by the French, quickly followed this first animal-to-human transfusion with their own. Richard Lower and his colleague Edmund King paid one Arthur Coga 20 shillings to transfuse him with sheep's blood. He had been described as being *"a little frantic."* There appeared to be little adverse effects from the transfusion and a second was performed a week later because he still appeared to be *"a little cracked in the head"* [21, 25].

Rivalry intensified between the competitors, as did opposition from opponents of the practice [11, 21, 22]. The apparent good effects of the transfusion on some patients' symptoms fitted with its proponent's belief about blood and its character. This encouraged them to continue the practice despite its opponents and the yet-to-be-understood acute adverse effects of the transfusion they were observing. Denis continued his experiments with one patient dying and another with paralysis being viewed as cured. His most famous transfusion was in 1667 when he transfused calf's blood into Antoine Mauroy to treat his mania. The 34-year-old *"madman"* suffered *"phrensies"* during which he would swear and beat his wife, strip and run naked through the streets, setting fire to houses on the way. Denis and his assistants transfused Mauroy with *"mild"* calf blood in the hope of allaying *"the heat and ebullition"* of the patient's blood. The transfusion was stopped when Mauroy experienced a severe hemolytic reaction. The patient survived, and the next morning he appeared to be a much calmer man. Emboldened perhaps by the apparent success of the treatment, Denis performed a second and greater blood volume transfusion. After sixteen ounces of calf's blood was transfused the patient experienced an even more severe hemolytic reaction and the transfusion was stopped. The next morning he *"made a great glass full of urine, of a colour as black, as if it had been mixed with the soot of chimneys."* He survived, however, and it appeared he had been cured by the treatment. He was later calm, in great presence of mind and polite. Denis announced broadly the success of his treatment [11, 16, 20, 21].

Almost two months later Mauroy's mania returned and Denis was asked by the man's wife to carry out a third transfusion. The patient died the day after Denis' unsuccessful attempt to administer it. The death resulted in a charge of murder being brought against Denis, from which he was later acquitted with the court finding that Mauroy's wife had poisoned him. Recent reports suggest there may be greater intrigue surrounding this case [11].

The Faculty of Medicine in Paris subsequently proclaimed transfusion dangerous and scientifically unsound. In 1670, the French parliament banned the practice. After two more deaths from transfusions in Rome, the Pope banned transfusion in most parts of Europe, and England quietly discontinued the practice [21].

First human blood transfusion

The practice of transfusions remained almost dormant until the early 1800s. By this time advances had been made in understanding anatomy, physiology, blood and the dangers of hemorrhage. English obstetrician James Blundell, concerned about the high mortality associated with postpartum hemorrhage, saw blood transfusion as a means of replacing lost blood. After animal experiments he concluded that only human blood should be transfused into humans and only to treat blood loss, not madness. He performed the first human blood transfusion in 1818 to treat a man suffering internal hemorrhage. The patient did not survive. After three more failures he transfused a woman with postpartum hemorrhage who survived. Over 10 years Blundell performed 10 transfusions with 5 patients surviving [16, 26].

Although they gained popularity, transfusions remained problematic throughout the rest of the nineteenth century. With no knowledge of anticoagulation and storage, transfusions were performed direct from donor to recipient and blood clotting in the apparatus was common. Additionally, physicians had no understanding of blood types. Alfred Higginson, a surgeon from Liverpool, performed seven transfusions from 1847–1856. Although five of the seven patients died, Higginson concluded, *"transfusion may fairly be said to be of use"* [27]. Statistics compiled in 1873 found that mortality from transfusion was 56 per cent [16]. Starr reports that the pioneer of modern surgery, Theodor Billroth, and others *"denounced transfusion as a showpiece that brought attention to the clinic at the expense of the patient"* [16].

Karl Landsteiner to the twenty-first century

By the end of the nineteenth century progress had all but ceased and it seemed there was no way forward for transfusion as a medical therapy. Many clinicians probably questioned how blood transfusion could be "miraculously" life-saving in some cases, but lethal in others. The answer came at the dawn of the twentieth century with allogeneic blood transfusion moving out of the dark ages. In 1900 Karl Landsteiner outlined the background of his rediscovery of Mendelian genetics [28, 29]. To quote from the 1930 Nobel Prize award ceremony speech, *"Thirty years ago, in 1900, in the course of his serological studies Landsteiner observed that when, under normal physiological conditions, blood serum of a human was added to normal blood of another human the red corpuscles in some cases coalesced into larger or smaller clusters. This observation of Landsteiner was the starting-point of his discovery of the human blood groups"* [30].

A year later Landsteiner expanded on his observations, describing what is now recognized as the discovery of the ABO blood group system. It was some years before his landmark discovery resulted in the reinvigoration of interest in blood transfusion and its establishment as a therapy. To follow was the development of methods for the collection, anticoagulation, preservation and fractionation of allogeneic blood.

The history of modern transfusion had its origins at the bedside. In its early days the procedure centered on a patient and their clinical problem. The clinician responsible for diagnosing and managing the patient took the initiative in identifying the need for transfusion, for seeking out a blood donor, organizing the blood collection and performing the transfusion. This was usually by direct vein-to-vein transfer. In some respects there was, in today's terminology, a "conflict of interest," in that the clinician was responsible for both the donor and the recipient. There was thus a direct link between the donor and the recipient and overseen by the clinician.

Although citrate had been used as an *in vitro* anticoagulant in the late nineteenth century and in animal blood transfusions, it was not until 1914 that citrated blood transfusions in humans were first documented [31, 32]. It was during WWI that transfusion of citrated blood established its role in clinical practice and it was another Nobel prize winner of penicillin fame, Alexander Fleming, who published a large series of citrated blood transfusions for treating war casualties [33]. There was some debate at this time as to the best method for maintaining fluidity of donor blood following collection, and although a case was made for defibrination, citration became the accepted method. Logistically, defibrination was more difficult, but in retrospect it probably had the advantages of leucodepletion and better *in vitro* preservation [34].

With the development of effective methods for the anticoagulation, preservation and transport of blood, particularly during the Spanish civil war and WWII, the donor became separated from the recipient in time and place [35]. Vein-to-vein transfusions had been a lucrative procedure for surgeons of the day and they initially were reluctant to relinquish their control and vested interests in the supply side of blood transfusion [16]. However, the inevitable consequence was the evolution of large, centralized blood banks, involved in the mass collection and fractionation of blood. In many circumstances these developments resulted in the centralizing of blood transfusion expertise into blood banks geographically isolated from the clinical workface. Accordingly, most transfusion policy development has been determined by the central blood bankers, where the predominant concern was the recruitment of donors and the processing and distribution of blood. At first this was considered to be of little consequence, especially as the safety and interests of the donors were ensured. However, over the years a knowledge gap developed as expertise in blood transfusion was increasingly donor-related. Marshall McLuhan's aphorism *"the medium is the message"* found an analogy in modern blood transfusion. The initial emphasis on the why and when recipient-focus of blood transfusion was eclipsed by a what, how and how much donor-focus. Clinicians no longer had responsibilities in obtaining donor blood and were constantly assured by suppliers that transfusions were safe and effective.

For over two decades there have been references in the lay press alluding to the excessive focus on blood supply to the detriment of a patient focus as illustrated by the following: *"Blood services are a product of their past. They were born in crisis in the 1940's to help victims of war and conflict and depend on the altruism of donors to give blood for the benefit of others. It is the others, the patients, who may be forgotten by centralised services. It is time for blood transfusion services to focus on the people who receive blood as much as – if not more than – those who donate it."* Glennys Bell "Vein Glory" The Bulletin July 1991.

It was during the 1970s with the development of *in vivo* cell separators for the collection of blood components that bedside clinicians, generally clinical hematologists, again became interested and involved in transfusion medicine [36]. Additionally, there has been a rekindling of interest in the use of fresh whole blood as the impact of the storage lesion is increasingly being questioned, especially in the massive hemorrhage/transfusion setting [37, 38].

New transfusion issues emerge

Transfusion-transmitted hepatitis B had a devastating impact on US servicemen during WWII [39]. During the 1970s hepatitis C infected over

20% of multi-transfused patients in the United States [40]. However, the real shock did not occur until the 1980s when it was realized that acquired immunodeficiency syndrome (AIDS) was not restricted to gay men, drug addicts and Haitians, but that hemophiliacs were contracting it from their factor VIII therapy [41]. Although allogeneic blood transfusion has always been associated with recognized immunological, infective and other hazards, it was the appearance of AIDS that became the tipping point, stimulating a wide and in-depth analysis of the risk–benefit equation for blood transfusion.

The initial presumption that an infectious agent, for which there was no *in vitro* test, was responsible for AIDS meant the only possible strategies to minimize transfusion transmission were to avoid transfusion, exclude high risk donors or adopt available autologous blood transfusion techniques. With this, the concept of "alternatives" to blood transfusion began and has persisted. Although an understandable term the reality is that most "alternatives" are actually optimal medical management. However, at the time, an evidence base for many of the strategies was lacking, so action was predominantly taken on the basis of the precautionary principle.

There were assurances that, despite concerns, all was being done to make donor blood as "safe as it has always been" perpetuating complacency by clinicians, bureaucrats, and to a degree, patients.

> "Although the risk is extremely low the concern is great, and
> physicians can expect potential recipients to be anxious. Patients
> should be reassured that blood banks are taking all possible steps to
> provide for safe blood transfusion. In turn, physicians should use
> these products when, and only when, they are unquestionably
> indicated" [42].

A November 1983 article in the Wisconsin Medical Journal *"Is our blood supply safe?"* gave no hint of the AIDS tragedy that was to come [43].

> "The risk of developing AIDS from receiving a blood transfusion is
> minute. The health risk posed by a frantic, uninformed reaction to the
> AIDS mystery is great. Your informed cooperation is urgently
> requested."

Most clinicians insisted they had a good understanding and evidence-base for the indications and benefits of transfusions and were prepared to accept this "minute" risk and believed that any other risks were minimal. However, as one of the author's mentors used to say, *"it may well be a rare disease, but is very common for the person who has it."* Unfortunately, it was the patients accepting the risks and clinicians were, to a significant extent, confidently practicing in an "evidence-free zone." It was a tragedy that many patients in whom there was no valid and evidence-based indication for the transfusion contracted and died from transfusion-transmitted human immunodeficiency virus (HIV) infection.

Blood transfusion had grandfathered its way into medical therapeutics and become culturally imbedded into clinical practice, with benefit being assumed and risks regarded as minimal. However, there were repeated warnings as early as 1920 and during the 1940s from doyens of blood banking and transfusion medicine to the clinical community that transfusion remained and always will remain a potentially hazardous procedure for which the risks and benefits in terms of patient outcome need to be judiciously evaluated on an individual patient basis.

To quote from the archives:

> "At the beginning of the twentieth century, with the discovery of 'blood groups,' it was thought that all danger had been eliminated. At the present time the pendulum is swinging back again, and the problem of the complete elimination of danger is proving more complex than it was thought to be a few years ago."
>
> *(Keynes 1922) [44]*

> "Blood transfusion is ordinarily considered a simple and safe procedure .... but has caused the death of patients with relatively benign ailments from which they could have recovered if only left alone."
>
> *(Weiner 1949) [45]*

> "Clinicians would be less confident in the safety of blood, and therefore more eclectic in its use, if they kept in mind the many possibly weak links in the chain of its production. It has to be remembered that all reactions, and they are not as uncommon as they should be, increase the burden borne by the patient. Blood-transfusion has in recent years developed into a mass-produced remedy which daily presents fresh problems. In the hands of experts it is virtually safe, and very valuable; but there is little doubt that today, in this country as elsewhere, many deaths supposed to have occurred 'in spite of transfusion' have really been caused by it. Administration of fluids is not a duty that should be 'relegated' to inexperienced juniors. It is not just a problem of minor surgery. In fact, there are few risks in transfusion when the doctor fails to insert a needle or cannula into a vein; they begin to mount once he succeeds."
>
> *(Milner 1949) [46]*

It is only in recent years that there has been a concerted effort to establish a more sound evidence base for the benefits and hazards of transfusion in the wide range of clinical settings in which it is, may be, or is not, appropriate therapy. There has been a gradual awakening over the last 25 years throughout the blood sector, clinical practice, bureaucracies, governments, the community and the legal profession that, as Bob Dylan would have expressed, "the times they are a changin." There have been several drivers for change. The reassessment of the safety of transfusion in the context of questionable efficacy in improving clinical outcomes has been high on the agenda. Governments have become more focused on the blood sector leading to numerous national reviews, economic evaluations and, in some circumstances, criminal proceedings against individuals [47, 48]. The concerns about transfusion safety generally focus around transfusion-transmitted infections with increasing expenditure on ensuring infectious safety of the blood supply chain. Admirable as this may seem, the downside is the escalating costs, diversion of attention from the overall hazards of transfusion and the lack of an evidence base for improving clinical outcomes in many clinical settings [49].

There is no questioning the valuable and evidence-based role for fractionated plasma products in the management of many specific diseases, e.g. hemophilia, hypogammaglobulinemia, prevention of hemolytic disease of the newborn and others. However, the same cannot be said for the use of the labile blood components, i.e. red cells, platelets and plasma. Indeed the overwhelming accumulation of observational data implicates labile blood components as an independent risk factor for adverse clinical outcomes in hemodynamically stable patients [3].

It is rather ironic that, 100 years after the discovery of blood groups, the dawn of the twenty-first century saw the beginning of a re-analysis of why many patients were receiving transfusions that are exposing them to significant risk without evidence for meaningful clinical benefit. More and more expenditure is directed at the supply side to make products safer from infection transmission when on the demand side questions are being asked about transfusion efficacy [49]. There is unconvincing logic in making a therapeutic product safer and safer at great expense when evidence for efficacy is lacking. Few would doubt the role of transfusion in the management of hemorrhagic shock, critical life-threatening anemia, the development of major surgery procedures, the provision of blood-component therapy for specific cellular or plasma deficiencies and the development of hematological supportive care for the management of hematological malignancies. However, as the insatiable demand for allogeneic blood has continued, the usual response has been: "We need more donors, and more blood should be fractionated." The question, "Where is all the blood going, and are all the transfusions really necessary?" is less commonly addressed. Benchmarking studies in various patient populations have revealed major differences in red cell transfusion practices for comparable patient groups [5, 8, 50]. It is difficult to explain the significant variations in transfusion rates within individual countries and internationally.

When demand appears to be outstripping supply and cost-effectiveness is being questioned, concern has been expressed with regard to:

• excessive perioperative transfusion of blood during uncomplicated elective surgery with accumulating evidence that red cell transfusion adversely impacts on clinical outcome

• unnecessary compatibility testing of blood for elective surgery

• inappropriate use of blood components without a clear identification of the patient's hematological problem, and failure to consider more appropriate therapy, e.g. treating iron deficiency

• the lack of awareness of the numerous hazards of allogeneic blood transfusion, a therapy having the widest range of potential adverse consequences

• wastage of costly donated blood due to inappropriate transfusion and expiry.

When making decisions in transfusion there has been a tendency to ask the wrong question. Clinical practice guidelines, especially for blood component therapy, have been falling into the common trap of starting with an answer before the question has been clearly considered. This is a similar error to that which is commonly made in marketing when a business does not clearly identify the sector in which it is operating, known as marketing myopia. The point is emphasized and illustrated in the classic Harvard Business Review article by Levitt in 1960. In the early history of railroads the tycoons considered they were in the business of making railroads, when in fact they were in the transport business [51]. As a result they were not able to adapt appropriately when other means of transport became available. By analogy, transfusion medicine is in the business of improving clinical outcomes, not primarily blood banking to transfuse patients. Clinical outcomes are improved by evidence-based diagnosis and therapy of diseases in which blood component therapy may have a role to play and the risks are acceptable.

In this context, the primary responsibility of clinicians is to manage a patient's own blood as a precious and unique human resource that should not be wasted, and consider donor-sourced allogeneic blood components when there is no other option. This more recent concept of patient blood management is increasingly focusing on the patient and their clinical problems, as well as giving them a greater role and responsibility in their own clinical management. This shift towards a patient blood management philosophy in clinical practice is in contrast to behavior-based transfusion management as the main focus. Parallel to this paradigm shift is greater emphasis on clinical decision making based on sound scientific evidence and empowering of patients to be part of the process. Experiences with Jehovah's Witness patients in the early days of cardiac surgery sent a sobering message, challenging the dogma that it was impossible to operate without the use of blood transfusion. Most surgeons refused to take on such "high-risk" patients. It took the courage of Dr Denton Cooley, one of the fathers of cardiac surgery, to convince the medical community that major surgery could be undertaken on such patients if there was meticulous attention to preoperative, intraoperative and postoperative management of the patient's own blood [52]. His work, which became known as "bloodless surgery" or "transfusion-free surgery," was the foundation of patient blood management. Subsequently, there have been further observational studies on cardiac surgery in Jehovah's Witness patients confirming that, not only is surgery successful, but clinical outcomes in terms of adverse events may be better [53–55].

The history of blood transfusion is dotted with resistance to the implementation of new therapies and changes in clinical practices despite their being based on sound evidence. In many cases it is not new evidence that should have changed practice, but rather a reconsideration of the basic sciences and soundly based clinical decision making. Transfusion medicine has numerous examples of ironies, contradictions and resistance to change (Table 1.1).

The new paradigm

The "new" paradigm is a rebirth of the original. Evidence-based medicine and patient blood management should view a patient's own blood as a valuable and unique natural resource that should be conserved and managed appropriately. Altruistically donated blood is given in trust and is a valuable community resource. However, it is a costly resource with significant potential for harm. It should only be used as therapy with patient consent and when there is evidence for potential benefit, potential harm will be minimized, and there are no other feasible management options.

Paradigms shift suddenly or slowly depending on the "push-pull" factors which, as we have described in the case of blood, are numerous and complex. However, it is difficult to deny that the mission statement

Table 1.1 Ironies and contradictions in transfusion.

---

increasing expenditure on improving the safety of a therapeutic product when efficacy in
    many clinical settings has not been established; indeed in many of these circumstances
    the transfusion is an independent risk factor for adverse outcomes
labile blood products are the most widely used, yet have the highest potential for harm and
    a poor evidence base for their indication
Jehovah's Witness patients, who will not accept blood transfusion, have demonstrated that
    most major surgical procedures can be performed without the use of allogeneic blood
    transfusion
mechanistic evidence for adverse clinical outcomes from allogeneic transfusion not being
    acted upon until statistics-based research establishes level I evidence from randomized
    controlled trials (RCTs)
extreme application of the "precautionary principle" on blood supply side not based on any
    acceptable cost-benefit analysis, in contrast to application of the "assimilatory principle"
    on the demand side where cost-effectiveness can be justified
demands for "use by dates" for allogeneic blood for intravenous administration being
    established by *in vivo* human RCTs, in contrast to food for oral consumption being
    determined using *in vitro* mechanistic evidence, not RCTs
regarding minimizing bleeding and correction of treatable anemias as "alternatives" to
    allogeneic blood transfusion
perception that PBM is "an intervention" when in reality it is soundly based "good clinical
    medicine" in which a patient is diagnosed, treated, monitored and followed up
    appropriately
the concept that PBM is "appropriate transfusion practice" and "hemovigilance,"
    perpetuating the paradigm that transfusion medicine is donor/product-centric and not
    patient-centric
recruiting blood donors by marketing rather than behaviour-based research approaches
deterministic causation establishing the serious hazards of blood transfusion with product
    safety interventions rarely based on levels of evidence from statistic based research, as
    required by evidence-based medicine

---

of modern medicine is to make sick people better and keep well people
well. Whenever there are conflicting paradigms, as with any debate,
middle ground can be difficult to find and the language can be hijacked
by either side using words and terminology to mean what they want them
to mean. Transfusion alternatives, blood management, precautionary
principle, blood conservation and appropriate transfusions are examples
for which the meaning may be different from the blood supply and
demand perspectives.

The introduction of the term "blood management" and the formation of the Society for the Advancement of Blood Management
(www.sabm.org) were driven from the demand/patient perspective,
but blood bankers have regarded blood management as managing the
supply. At a Board Meeting of the Medical Society for Blood Management
(www.bloodmanagement.org) convened in Prague 2005, a Board member

and one of the authors (JI) advocated strongly that the problems of the language needed to be addressed to ensure that the direction for the new paradigm was towards the *patient*. From this time it was proposed that the terminology should be "Patient Blood Management." Consideration of other aspects of confusion with the language ensued, questioning the use of several of the above examples that implied a primary donor/supply focus for the blood sector rather than a patient focus.

Patient Blood Management is *not* an "intervention" per se. It is goal-oriented patient care based on sound evidence and cooperative inclusion and empowerment of patients when possible, with the aim of improving clinical outcomes [56, 57]. This book outlines how this concept can be effectively and safely incorporated into clinical practice.

References

1 Isbister JP. The paradigm shift in blood transfusion. Med J Aust. 1988 Mar 21; 148(6):306–8.

2 Hofmann A, Farmer S, Shander A. Five drivers shifting the paradigm from product-focused transfusion practice to patient blood management. The Oncologist. 2011;16 Suppl 3:3–11.

3 Isbister JP, Shander A, Spahn DR, Erhard J, Farmer SL, Hofmann A. Adverse blood transfusion outcomes: establishing causation. Transfus Med Rev. 2011 Apr;25(2):89–101.

4 Leahy MF, Muhktar S. From blood transfusion to patient blood management: a new paradigm for patient care and cost assessment of blood transfusion practice. Intern Med J. 2012 Mar;42(3):332–8.

5 Bennett-Guerrero E, Zhao Y, O'Brien SM, Ferguson TB, Jr., Peterson ED, Gammie JS, et al. Variation in use of blood transfusion in coronary artery bypass graft surgery. JAMA. 2010 Oct 13;304(14):1568–75.

6 Hofmann A, Farmer S, Towler SC. Strategies to preempt and reduce the use of blood products: an Australian perspective. Current Opinion in Anaesthesiology. 2012 Feb;25(1):66–73.

7 Gombotz H, Rehak PH, Shander A, Hofmann A. Blood use in elective surgery: the Austrian benchmark study. Transfusion. 2007 Aug;47(8):1468–80.

8 Rao SV, Chiswell K, Sun JL, Granger CB, Newby LK, Van de Werf F, et al. International variation in the use of blood transfusion in patients with non-ST-segment elevation acute coronary syndromes. Am J Cardiol. 2008 Jan 1;101(1):25–9.

9 Hawking SW. The illustrated A brief history of time. Updated and expanded ed. New York: Bantam Books; 1996.

10 Farmer S, Webb D. Your Body, Your Choice. Singapore: Media Masters; 2000.

11 Tucker H. Blood work : a tale of medicine and murder in the scientific revolution. 1st ed. New York: W.W. Norton; 2011.

12 Hart GD. Descriptions of blood and blood disorders before the advent of laboratory studies. British Journal of Haematology. [Historical Article Portraits]. 2001 Dec;115(4):719–28.

13 Aretaeus, AF. The extant works of Aretæus, The Cappadocian. London, 1856.
14 Tannahill R. Flesh and blood : a history of the cannibal complex. London: Hamilton; 1975.
15 Kuriyama S. Interpreting the history of bloodletting. J Hist Med Allied Sci. [Biography Historical Article]. 1995 Jan;50(1):11–46.
16 Starr DP. Blood: an epic history of medicine and commerce. 1st ed. New York: Alfred A. Knopf; 1998.
17 Blood-letting. British Medical Journal. 1871;a(533):283–91.
18 Delpech M. Case of a wound of the right carotid artery. Lancet. 1825;6:210–13.
19 Dunphy JE. Ethics in surgery: Going beyond good science. Bull Am Coll Surg. 1978;63(6):8–12.
20 Farr AD. The first human blood transfusion. Med Hist. [Biography Historical Article]. 1980 Apr;24(2):143–62.
21 Myhre BA. The first recorded blood transfusions: 1656 to 1668. Transfusion. 1990 May;30(4):358–62.
22 Walton MT. The first blood transfusion: French or English? Med Hist. [Historical Article]. 1974 Oct;18(4):360–4.
23 Denis J. A letter concerning a new way of curing sundry deseases by transfusion of blood, Written to Monsieur de Montmor, Counsellor to the French King and Master of Requests. Philos Trans R Sc Lond. 1667;2(27A):489–504.
24 Denis J. Report of transfusion. Le Journal des Scavans. 1667;1:272–84.
25 Samuel Pepys diary and correspondence. London: Beckers; 1876–1879.
26 Spiess BD, Spence R, Shander A, editors. Perioperative Transfusion Medicine. Philadelphia: Lippincott Williams & Wilkins; 2006.
27 Higginson A. Report of Seven Cases of Transfusion of Blood, with a Description of the Instrument by the Author. Liverpool Med Chir Journ. 1857;1:102–10.
28 Landsteiner K. Zur Kenntnis der antifermentativen, lytischen und agglutinierenden Wirkungen des Blutserums und der Lymphe. Zentbl. Bakt Orig. 1900;27:357–62.
29 Landsteiner K. Ueber Agglutinationserscheinungen normalen menschlichen Blutes. Wien Klin Wochenschr. 1901;14:1132–4.
30 Hedrén G. Award Ceremony Speech for Karl Landsteiner. http://www.nobelprize.org/nobel_prizes/medicine/laureates/1930/press.html. Accessed 29 Nov 2013.
31 Hustin A. Note sur une nouvelle meÂthode de transfusion. Annales et Bulletin des SeÂances: SocieÂteÂ des Sciences MeÂdicales et Naturelles de Bruxelles. 1914(72e AnneÂe):104–11.
32 Agote L. Nuevo procedimiento para la transfusion del sangre. Anales Del Instituto Modelo de Clinica MeÂdica. 1915;1:24–31.
33 Fleming AF, Porteus AB. Blood transfusion by the citrated method. Lancet. 1919 June 7:973–5.
34 Platt R. Blood Transfusion: A plea for the defibrination method. Lancet. 1926 Jan 23:173–5.
35 D'Alessandro A, Liumbruno G, Grazzini G, Zolla L. Red blood cell storage: the story so far. Blood Transfus. 2010 Apr;8(2):82–8.
36 Isbister JP. Cytapheresis: the first 25 years. Ther Apher. 1997 Feb;1(1):17–21.
37 Kaufman R. A fresh take on whole blood. Transfusion. 2011 Feb;51(2):230–3.

38 Wang D, Sun J, Solomon SB, Klein HG, Natanson C. Transfusion of older stored blood and risk of death: a meta-analysis. Transfusion. 2012 Jun;52(6):1184–95.

39 Seeff LB. Transfusion-associated hepatitis B: past and present. Transfus Med Rev. 1988 Dec;2(4):204–14.

40 Alter HJ, Klein HG. The hazards of blood transfusion in historical perspective. Blood. [Historical Article Review]. 2008 Oct 1;112(7):2617–26.

41 Evatt BL. The tragic history of AIDS in the hemophilia population, 1982–1984. Journal of Thrombosis and Haemostasis: JTH. [Historical Article Review]. 2006 Nov;4(11):2295–301.

42 Bove JR. Transfusion-associated AIDS–a cause for concern. N Engl J Med. 1984 Jan 12;310(2):115–6.

43 Fritz RD, Menitove JE. Is our blood supply safe? Wisconsin Medical Journal. 1983 Nov;82(11):26–7.

44 Keynes G. Blood Transfusion: Dangers of Blood Transfusion. Oxford Medical Publications. 1922;Chapter 4:67.

45 Weiner AJ. Foolproof Blood Transfusions. The Lancet. 1949 June 18; 253(6564):1073–4.

46 Milner IH. Foolproof blood transfusions. The Lancet. 1949 July 30; 254(6570):217.

47 Wilson K. The Krever Commission–10 years later. CMAJ. 2007 Nov 20;177(11): 1387–9.

48 Simons M. Courtroom anguish as France tries 4 over tainted blood. The New York Times. [News Newspaper Article]. 1992 Jul 31:A1, A6.

49 Shander A, Fink A, Javidroozi M, Erhard J, Farmer SL, Corwin H, et al. Appropriateness of allogeneic red blood cell transfusion: the international consensus conference on transfusion outcomes. Transfus Med Rev. 2011 Jul;25(3):232–46 e53.

50 Gombotz H, Rehak P, Shander A, Hofmann A. Blood use in elective surgery: the Austrian benchmark study. Transfusion. 2007;47(8):1468–80.

51 Levitt T. Marketing Myopia. Harvard Business Review. 1960(July–August):45–56.

52 Ott DA, Cooley DA. Cardiovascular surgery in Jehovah's Witnesses. Report of 542 operations without blood transfusion. Jama. 1977 Sep 19;238(12):1256–8.

53 Emmert MY, Salzberg SP, Theusinger OM, Felix C, Plass A, Hoerstrup SP, et al. How good patient blood management leads to excellent outcomes in Jehovah's witness patients undergoing cardiac surgery. Interact Cardiovasc Thorac Surg. 2011 Feb;12(2):183–8.

54 Reyes G, Nuche JM, Sarraj A, Cobiella J, Orts M, Martin G, et al. Bloodless cardiac surgery in Jehovah's witnesses: outcomes compared with a control group. Rev Esp Cardiol. 2007 Jul;60(7):727–31.

55 Pattakos G, Koch CG, Brizzio ME, et al. Outcome of patients who refuse transfusion after cardiac surgery: a natural experiment with severe blood conservation. Archives of internal medicine 2012;172:1154–60.

56 Bardes CL. Defining "patient-centered medicine". N Engl J Med. 2012 Mar; 366(9):782–3.

57 Barry MJ, Edgman-Levitan S. Shared decision making–pinnacle of patient-centered care. N Engl J Med. 2012 Mar;366(9):780–1.

CHAPTER 2

The ethical complexities of transfusion-free medicine, surgery and research

Katrina A. Bramstedt

Medical Ethics and Professionalism, Bond University School of Medicine, Queensland, Australia

Introduction

Ethical issues associated with transfusion-free medicine and surgery have been around since the inception of the concept of this clinical practice. For example, in the 1800s, intravenous milk was attempted as a substitute for blood transfusion but it often had tragic consequences [1]. Blood is always a limited resource: limited in supply and limited in terms of shelf-life. Additionally, while blood can be a lifesaver, there is always the risk of infectious transmission, transfusion reaction, and sensitization. Medical and surgery teams are becoming more aware that "bloodless surgery" isn't just for Jehovah's Witnesses [2], but rather, many approach their doctors with clinical and or philosophical concerns about transfusion. The commonly known Jehovah's Witness tenet of blood refusal is now just one of many reasons to pursue transfusion-free medicine and surgery.

For clinicians, ethical concern and outright moral distress can arise in many situations. While the shared goal between doctor and patient might be transfusion-free clinical practices, the physician is always making mental calculations that attempt to balance the need for tissue oxygenation against the need for human blood transfusion. At some point, the clinical need for such transfusion might be urgent so as to prevent irreversible ischemia or death. Without human blood, substitutes, or other measures, science and the community must recognize the limits imposed and accept the negative consequences (or choose to accept transfusion). This is the underpinning of informed consent.

Transfusion-Free Medicine and Surgery, Second Edition. Edited by Nicolas Jabbour.
© 2014 John Wiley & Sons, Ltd. Published 2014 by John Wiley & Sons, Ltd.

Ethics and informed consent

The field of medical ethics has long opined that adults with decision-making capacity must be allowed to refuse any medical intervention, including those which are life saving (e.g., blood transfusion, artificial nutrition and hydration, artificial ventilation, dialysis). In fact, adults are encouraged to write a Living Will/Advance Directive which expressly indicates which therapies are wanted and not wanted so that medical teams and surrogate decision-makers devise care plans that respect and honor the patient's values [3]. Even lacking a written declaration such as these, verbal declarations are valid and must direct care planning. Adults with decision-making capacity can give an informed refusal for blood transfusion via their Living Will/Advance Directive or via a separate and distinct informed refusal form which can be provided by hospitals, surgery centers, and other entities. Whatever the mechanism, their informed refusal must be honored.

What is an informed refusal? These are refusals of a specific medical intervention made after the patient has been given information about the nature of the intervention, how the intervention applies to his/her specific medical situation, and the risks and benefits of receiving and not receiving the intervention. The patient must then analyze this information, along with their personal value system, and formulate and express a choice about whether to accept or reject the intervention offered.

In situations of verbal or written refusal, care should be taken to verify, whenever possible, that the refusal is indeed informed and still desired. For patients who have decision-making capacity, they should be approached to validate their understanding of the risks and benefits of abstaining from whole blood/blood products. An attempt should also be made to validate that the patient is making the decision objectively and without coercion. These patient interviews and capacity assessments should be done in private without the patient's friends or family present so as to minimize external influences. If a foreign language translator is needed, a medical translator should be used (e.g., hospital employee, translation vendor service), not a friend or relative of the patient, so as to ensure the integrity of the conversation. Indeed, sometimes peoples' values change due to their personal life experiences and situations. The purpose of these discussions is never to coerce a decision, but rather to validate a voluntary choice.

For patients who presently lack decision-making capacity but had expressed their wishes prior (before losing cognitive function), these wishes should be honored unless there is serious doubt as to the voluntariness or cognitive capacity of the patient at the time they expressed their choice. In these situations an ethics consultation should be sought to gain clarity. Professional medical ethicists are on staff at most academic medical centers, as well as throughout the community in independent clinical practice [4].

For adult patients who never expressed their wishes and who presently cannot due to lack of decision-making capacity, surrogates should be queried about the patient's values. The legal and ethical duty of the surrogate decision-maker is to speak the values of the patient when these are known, even if these values conflict with those of the surrogate. If the patient's values are unknown, decision-making should proceed according to what is determined to be in the patient's best interest. This takes into account the standards of medical practice and the patient's unique clinical features. This is especially important in emergency situations when time is limited and interventions must be quickly administered or the consequences can be severe and irreversible [5].

Children, assent, and consent

In the United States, children (those under age 18 years) are unable to give "informed consent" (or informed refusal) because the legal system does not recognize them as adults. The term "assent" is generally under-stood to be a child giving permission, rather than consent, because children legally do not meet the standard for medical decision-making. In general, US courts have generally upheld the rights of children to receive stan-dard medical care and they are not subject to the personal, religious, or philosophical views of their parents/guardians in terms of clinical prac-tices [6]. Young children don't have the cognitive capacity to analyze com-plex medical information or to form belief systems for guiding medical decision-making thus they are legally and ethically bound to receive the standard of care as determined by the medical profession.

As children mature, some develop the ability to make their own medical decisions before becoming legal adults. For example, in the United States, some teenagers are able to make their own medical decisions with regard to certain types of clinical care and this is supported by state legal statutes as well as the Code of Ethics of the American Medical Association [7, 8]. In extreme cases, some teenagers are recognized as legal adults if they have been living independently as adults, if they are married, or if they have joined the military [9]. Whenever clinicians have concern about these matters they should seek legal counsel from a licensed attorney. The state or local professional medical society, as well as medical ethicists can also provide general guidance on these matters.

Professionalism and transfusion-free practices

Currently there are two professional societies that educate and advocate for transfusion-free medicine and surgery: Society for the Advancement of Blood Management (http://www.sabm.org) and Network for the Advancement of Transfusion Alternatives (www.nataonline.com). Both offer educational resources such as conferences and reading materials, but neither have an Ethics Committee nor a Code of Ethics for their members. Because of the ethical issues inherent to this subspecialty it seems both would be critical resources for those who work in this field. A professional society Ethics Committee can be helpful in matters of clinical and research ethics consultation, as well as formulating position statements on matters of ethical import. A Code of Ethics can guide ethical behavior of professionals and be informative with regard to ethically appropriate and inappropriate conduct, the responsibilities of the clinician to the patient, and even denote sanctions for ethical breaches. Additionally, patients and the community look to professional societies for objective advice and guidance so it is important for these entities to have their efforts backed up by strong ethical values and principles.

Clinicians who work in the field of transfusion-free medicine and surgery are like other clinicians in that they are free to choose their patients; unless it is an emergency (patients cannot be abandoned in clinical crisis). If a clinician has personal moral distress about a case, he/she should seek counsel from colleagues and/or a medical ethicist and potentially sign off the case. The ethical duty is to honor informed refusals rather than transfuse against the wishes of an informed patient. The latter can result in legal liability [10]. If a doctor decides to end the doctor–patient relationship rather than accede to the patient's wishes, the patient should be given reasonable notice, and preferably, a referral to another clinician or to the referral service of the local professional medical society [11, 12].

Jehovah's witnesses

As mentioned earlier, an express tenet of the Jehovah's Witness denomination is abstinence from human blood. According to their official website, "taking blood into body through mouth or veins violates God's laws" [2]. This tenet stems from literal interpretation of several Biblical texts including Genesis 9:3, 4 and Leviticus 17:14. For those who don't adhere to this belief, they risk ostracizing and even ex-communication from church membership. The only exceptions are blood transfusions received without their knowledge or express consent, or confession and repentance after willful consent to the procedure.

While this "blood abstinence" tenet is interconnected with the Jehovah's Witness denomination it is a mistake to assume that everyone who calls themselves a Jehovah's Witness adheres to this church tenet. Amid the belief system of blood abstinence there are many variations of values rather than a uniformity of belief. Some members will accept blood components, fractions, recombinant erythropoietin, or even whole blood. While donation of one's own blood for personal use is also forbidden by the Jehovah's Witness church, some members do pursue this route. Similarly, some may find the use of cell-saver technology acceptable depending on the length of the circuit and priming arrangements. Having said this, it is important to note that some members are fearful of their friends or pastor knowing their personal values when these conflict with the strict tenet of blood abstinence. Because of this, all adults should be asked about their health care treatment preferences to ensure they are provided with the interventions they desire and can benefit from. Some church members who desire transfusion may ask for extra measures such as privacy during the transfusion process so that there is no visual evidence of the procedure. These privacy matters are ethically important because it is known that members of Jehovah's Witness hospital liaison committees sometimes coerce patients to refuse blood/blood products [13, 14].

Organ transplantation

Several transplant centers around the world have developed expertise in "bloodless" organ transplantation surgery. These efforts are praiseworthy in their attempt to be good stewards of scarce human blood, but they are not without ethical controversy. Firstly, donor organs are in scarce supply and care must be taken so as not to increase the risk of graft failure or patient death. Ischemia is a key word in the field of transplantation thus anything that has a negative effect on this parameter must be avoided. Secondly, while some may view "bloodless" transplant surgery as a mechanism to facilitate lifesaving transplants to Jehovah's Witnesses or others who refuse blood/blood products, the fact remains that the need for transfusion may arise after successful transplant surgery and failure to accept this clinical resource can result in preventable graft loss [15]. The donor family who provided the graft to the recipient patient expects the patient to be compliant with all medical therapies that promote graft health and thus refusal of blood/blood products *after* transplant is a serious ethical problem.

Two mechanisms to address this potential dilemma are as follows: 1) requiring transfusion contracts for Jehovah's Witnesses which permit doctors to give blood/blood products to these patients; and 2) providing Jehovah's Witnesses with grafts from fellow Jehovah's Witnesses who share their value system about blood abstinence [15]. At the University of Pisa (Italy), transfusion contracts are required for patients receiving kidney and/or pancreas transplants [16]. Logistically, rescue transfusion could apply to operative and postoperative settings. Ethically, transfusion contracts are no different than other behavior contracts used in the field of transplantation but they are not a guaranteed method of ensuring transfusion because patients can revoke their consent at any time after receiving their lifesaving organ. In fact, vulnerable patients awaiting transplant might likely consent to a myriad of prerequisites as mere "hoops" to jump through in order to receive an organ. Transfusion contracts are not legal documents and thus not legally enforceable. If a patient subsequently refuses transfusion after an organ transplant and is found to need re-transplant, there would be ethical justification to deny re-transplantation due to contract non-compliance (unless a Jehovah's Witness donor could be found – see below).

While deceased donations from fellow Jehovah's Witnesses would allow this group their own playing field with regard to transplant, a foundational construct which is medicoreligious has generally *not* been accepted as an ethically permissible justification to permit a private playing field for transplant for any group. The exception to this is if a deceased donation is from one identified Jehovah's Witness directly to another identified Jehovah's Witness patient [17]. If these individuals were *living* donors, however, the medicoreligious allocation argument would have ethical grounding because the shared medicoreligious value justifies the risk to the donor in a setting where the recipient will knowingly refuse transfusion – risking graft loss and death.

Research ethics

The search for human blood substitutes is ongoing and the process is difficult for many reasons, including the ethical complexity of clinical trials [18]. Currently, there are only two products approved for human use. Synthetic hemoglobin-based oxygen carrier, Hemopure (HBOC-201, OPK Biotech, Cambridge, Massachusetts) is a modified lactated Ringer's solution containing polymerized bovine hemoglobin. It works as a red cell alternative in the management of acute surgical anemia, as well as a volume expander for the treatment of patients suffering from acute surgical hypovolemia. The product has been available for use in South Africa since 2001 but physicians in other countries can petition for compassionate use access in emergency situations [19]. South Africa has a very limited supply of donor blood so it is imperative that options such as this be available [20]. Perfloran is a perfluorocarbon-based blood substitute approved for human use in Mexico and Russia [21].

In 2006, Northfield Laboratories conducted a highly controversial phase III clinical trial of Polyheme, an investigational hemoglobin-based oxygen carrier. Individuals in hemorrhagic shock received either the standard of care or Polyheme in both the pre-hospital (e.g., ambulance) and hospital (emergency department) settings. This was ethically problematic because only standard of care, not investigational therapy, should have been administered once the patients arrived at the hospital according to the research regulations of the US Food and Drug Administration [22]. Specifically, the waiver of informed consent allowed Polyheme to be administered in pre-hospital settings but not at the hospital because hospitals have the ability to provide the standard of care (blood transfusions) to all patients. Legally and ethically, the investigational therapy could have been used in the hospital setting only if the standard of care was not available (but, in fact, it was). Other ethical problems with the trial included the complexity of educating the public about the trial and its option of non-participation, as well as other matters [23].

The US military is expected to start human clinical trials of "pharmed blood" [24]. This O-negative blood is made from human umbilical cord hematopoietic cells using a technology called NANEX™ which uses a bio-functional nanofiber-based 3D scaffold to rapidly *ex-vivo* produce large volumes of red blood cells [25]. Each umbilical cord can potentially provide approximately 20 units of blood (grown over the course of three days) for transfusion to patients of any blood type. Also, the risks of transfusion are lowered because recipients can potentially receive their transfusion(s) from one batch of blood rather than several different lots.

A key ethical issue with all clinical trials involving blood substitutes is the vulnerability of the research subject. Because these technologies are intended for lifesaving situations, the people receiving these investigational products are in life-threatening conditions. Under these conditions, they may not have the ability to give informed consent because they are unconscious, in shock, or otherwise physically and emotionally compromised. Family members who might provide surrogate consent are also likely emotionally compromised and their capacity to understand complex information about investigational blood substitute technology and research protocols during a time of tense crisis is suspect. Additionally, a prime target for these products is the battlefield due to the potential for hemorrhaging injuries and the inadequate supply of donor blood. This battlefield setting places military personnel directly in the hands of clinical investigators who are looking for research subjects for clinical trial enrolment. Not only is there a power differential between a soldier and the commanding officer, but there can be an implied notion of soldiers losing their autonomy (and thus ability to give informed consent) because of the fact their bodies belong to the military. Soldiers should not be forced to participate in military clinical research just because they are members of the military. Soldiers may feel a duty to participate in clinical research and they may also fear repercussions if they opt out. Similar ethical concerns have been raised in the setting of astronauts participating in research during space travel sponsored by their employer (the government) [26].

Notwithstanding these concerns, the challenge to find blood substitutes must continue. Human blood is a scarce resource, and transfusion risks remain, as does violent crime, traumatic injury and other conditions which clinically indicate the continued need for tissue oxygenation. Medical and surgical teams have a lot of variables in their clinical calculations, including ethical and legal matters, making transfusion-free medicine and surgery a complex yet worthwhile challenge.

References

1 Jennings CE. The intravenous injection of milk. Br Med J. 1885;1(1275):1147–9.
2 Jehovah's Witnesses – Who Are They? What Do They Believe? http://www.watch tower.org/e/jt/index.htm Accessed May 9, 2011.
3 Bramstedt KA. Living Will Template. http://www.transplantethics.com/living willadvdirective.html. Accessed May 9, 2011.
4 American Society for Bioethics and Humanities. http://www.asbh.org. Accessed May 9, 2011.
5 Estate of Dorone. 535 A.2d 452 (Pa 1987).
6 Cain J. Refusal of blood transfusion. In Elkins T. *Exploring Medical-Legal Issues in Obstetrics and Gynecology.* Washington, DC: Association of Professors of OB/GYN, 1994:62–64.
7 California Family Code Section 6926.
8 American Medical Association. Opinion 10.016: Pediatric Decision-Making. November 2007. http://www.ama-assn.org/ama/pub/physician-resources/med ical-ethics/code-medical-ethics/opinion10016.page. Accessed May 9, 2011.
9 California Family Code Section 7000–7002.
10 Malette v. Shulman, et al. (1991). 2 Med LR 162 (Ont CA), 1991.

11 American Medical Association. Opinion 10.05 - Potential Patients. November 2007. http://www.ama-assn.org/ama/pub/physician-resources/medical-ethics/code-medical-ethics/opinion1005.page? Accessed May 10, 2011.

12 American Medical Association. Opinion E-8.115 Termination of the Physician-Patient Relationship. June 1996. http://www.ama-assn.org/ama/pub/physician-resources/medical-ethics/code-medical-ethics/opinion8115.page? Accessed May 10, 2011.

13 Muramoto O. Medical confidentiality and the protection of Jehovah's Witnesses' autonomous refusal of blood. J Med Ethics. 2000;26(5):381−6.

14 Muramoto O. Bioethics of the refusal of blood by Jehovah's Witnesses: Part 3. A proposal for a don't-ask-don't-tell policy. J Med Ethics. 1999;25(6):463−8.

15 Bramstedt KA. Transfusion contracts for Jehovah's Witnesses receiving organ transplants: ethical necessity or coercive pact? J Med Ethics. 2006;32(4):193−5.

16 Boggi U, Vistoli F, Del Chiaro M, et al. Kidney and pancreas transplants in Jehovah's Witnesses: ethical and practical implications. Transplant Proc. 2004;36:601−2.

17 Code of Federal Regulations Title 42 Part 121 Section 121.8 (Allocation of Organs), item 2(h): Directed Donation. 1999.

18 U.S. Food and Drug Administration Center for Biologics Evaluation and Research. December 9, 2010 Transcript: Product Development Program for Interventions in Patients with Severe Bleeding Due to Trauma or Other Causes, p 355−72. http://www.fda.gov/BiologicsBloodVaccines/NewsEvents/WorkshopsMeetings Conferences/ucm241912.htm#p355. Accessed May 10, 2011.

19 Fitzgerald MC, Chan JY, Ross AW, Liew SM, Butt WW, Baguley D, et al. A synthetic haemoglobin-based oxygen carrier and the reversal of cardiac hypoxia secondary to severe anaemia following trauma. Med J Aust. 2011;194(9):471−3.

20 Aaron M. Speech by the Minister of Health on the launch of the South African Transfusion Medicine Training Centre. February 22, 2010. http://www.doh.gov.za/docs/sp/2010/sp0222.html. Accessed May 10, 2011.

21 Neelam S, Semwal BC, Krishna M, Ruqsana K, Shravan P. Artificial blood: A tool for survival of humans. Intl Res J Pharm 2012;3(5):119−123.

22 Food and Drug Administration. Part 50- Protection of human subjects Subpart B- informed consent of human subjects Sec 50.24 Exception from informed consent requirements for emergency research. 1996. http://www.accessdata.fda.gov/scripts/cdrh/cfdocs/cfcfr/CFRSearch.cfm?fr=50.2. Accessed May 10, 2011.

23 Apte SS. Blood substitutes- the polyheme trials. Mcgill J Med. 2008;11(1):59−65.

24 Drummond K. Darpa's Lab-Grown Blood Starts Pumping. July 9, 2010. http://www.wired.com/dangerroom/2010/07/darpas-blood-makers-start-pum ping/. Accessed May 10, 2011.

25 Arteriocyte. Arteriocyte Announces the Launch of NANEX™ Stem Cell Expansion System at the upcoming American Society of Cell Biology Meeting. December 2, 2010. http://www.arteriocyte.com/Press%20releases/Arteriocyte%20NANEX %20Press%20Release.pdf. Accessed May 10, 2010.

26 Institute of Medicine. Exploring the Ethics of Space Medicine. In: Ball Jr and Evans CH, eds. *Safe Passage: Astronaut Care for Exploration Missions*. Washington, DC: National Academy Press; 2001, 183.

CHAPTER 3

Transfusion therapy – Balancing the risks and benefits

Irina Maramica[1] and Ira A. Shulman[2]

[1]Department of Pathology and Laboratory Medicine, University of California Irvine Medical Center, Orange, CA, USA
[2]Keck School of Medicine at the University of Southern California (USC), USC Transfusion Medicine Services Group, Los Angeles, CA, USA

Introduction/overview

Dr. James Blundell performed the first transfusion of human blood to a patient on December 22, 1818 in London, England [1]. This followed a one hundred and fifty years ban on blood transfusion that was imposed in several European countries in response to numerous bad outcomes resulting from transfusion of animal blood to humans. In some cases, blood was given to patients for dubious indications, a practice that continues to this day. One reason for a transfusion to be administered for questionable indication is the perception that the benefits of the treatment outweigh the known risks. Modern transfusion therapy is safer today than ever in the past. To make transfusions safer for patients, three hurdles had to be overcome. First, the safety of transfusions had to be improved to avoid hemolytic transfusion reactions. This required the introduction of donor and recipient testing for ABO group, so that transfusions could be ABO compatible. Dr. Karl Landsteiner worked at the Institute of Pathological Anatomy in Vienna in 1900 when he discovered the ABO blood group system, which remains the most important for safe matching of donor red cells for transfusion of recipients. With the introduction of crossmatching of donor red cells with recipient serum/plasma by Dr. Ottenberg, the number of patients experiencing post-transfusion hemolytic reactions due to non-ABO antibodies decreased dramatically. At the same time, efforts were made to improve transfusion methods by the introduction of various transfusion equipment and cooling methods used to prevent

Transfusion-Free Medicine and Surgery, Second Edition. Edited by Nicolas Jabbour.
© 2014 John Wiley & Sons, Ltd. Published 2014 by John Wiley & Sons, Ltd.

blood clotting. The development of anti-coagulation methods using citrate by Dr. Lewisohn in 1915, made transfusions practical and allowed collection of blood in glass jars from which blood was transfused directly to the patient using the attached rubber tubing with the hollow needle for accessing patient's veins.

These seminal discoveries allowed for the development of blood donor recruitment programs, the first of which was the "Greater London Red Cross Blood Transfusion Service". This was the world's first municipal panel, organized by Dr. Oliver in the 1920s, and comprised of only volunteer donors.Dr. Fantus at the Cook County Hospital of Chicago organized the first blood bank that stored citrated blood collected in glass jars in 1937. Through the heroic efforts and determination of many physicians it became possible to transport stored blood to remote locations, which saved the lives of numerous soldiers in World War II. Wartime was also a time of rapid growth of the transfusion medicine field. Methods were developed to separate whole blood into components. Methods for industrial processing of plasma were developed by Dr. Drew and plasma fractionation by Dr. Cohn. These changed the face of transfusion medicine and led to the development of the blood industry.

Currently in the United States most of the donated blood collected by phlebotomy is processed into components. Whole blood is rarely used in the United States or other developed countries, except occasionally for pediatric cardiovascular surgery or exchange transfusions of neonates. Whole blood is used by the United States Armed Forces to resuscitate injured soldiers in areas of military conflict. Today, blood products are also being collected by apheresis methods, which allow targeted collections of red blood cells (RBCs), platelets, plasma, granulocytes and other products used in cellular therapy.

During 2008, Americans donated an estimated 17 286 000 units of whole blood and apheresis RBCs, over 2 million adult doses of apheresis platelets, nearly 6 million units of plasma, and 1.5 million units of cryoprecipitate [2]. About 5.8 million Americans received transfusion therapy of RBC products, and each day approximately 47 000 units of this product are transfused in the United States. While the use of transfusion therapy has grown dramatically over the decades to accommodate advances in medical and surgical treatments and practices – and clearly has afforded life-saving treatment to millions of patients – its use comes at a cost. When considering a transfusion in patients it is imperative to keep in mind that all blood products carry risk! Many of these risks are well known and the majority can be prevented by the appropriate transfusion practice; however, there are many potential risks that are not well understood, some related to known or unknown pathogens. With that in mind, each clinician should carefully balance the risks and benefits of transfusion therapy in the context of the patient's clinical situation. Transfusing patients only when medically necessary can improve patient outcomes by decreasing transfusion reactions and exposure to infections, including post-operative infections.

To be able to make responsible decisions regarding the transfusion therapy, physicians have to be aware of new insights into risks, benefits and ways to reduce known risks of this therapy, as well as the availability of alternative therapies.

The clinical utility of transfusion therapy

Red blood cell transfusion

RBC transfusion therapy is administered to correct tissue hypoxia, which develops as a result of inadequate oxygen delivery to meet the metabolic demands of the tissues. Oxygen delivery normally exceeds oxygen consumption by several-fold [86]. However, decrease in hemoglobin (Hgb) concentration (anemic hypoxia), cardiac output (stagnant hypoxia), or Hgb saturation (hypoxic hypoxia), can decrease oxygen delivery to tissues, which becomes critical when it falls to the level of oxygen consumption, at which point metabolism shifts from aerobic to anaerobic.

When anemia develops over an extended period of time, the patient adjusts to lower Hgb levels by compensatory mechanisms, which depend on the etiology, speed of onset and chronicity of anemia. In euvolemic anemia, compensatory changes include increased cardiac output through increased stroke volume and myocardial contractility with variable contribution of increased heart rate; decreased peripheral vascular resistance; decreased blood viscosity; rightward shift in oxyhemoglobin dissociation curve and subsequent increase in oxygen off-loading to tissue due to elevation in red cell 2,3-diphosphoglycerate (2,3-DPG) levels. High baseline oxygen extraction ratios limit compensation via this mechanism in the myocardium and brain, which instead rely on increased blood flow diverted away from the splanchnic circulation [5]. Overall, age, cardiovascular status, and clinical circumstances determine the extent to which compensation is possible. Beyond a certain Hgb and HCT and/or ability for adequate compensation, demand outpaces supply heralding ischemia and infarction. Increased cardiac output begins at a Hgb <10 g/dl, though significant increases begin only with the Hgb <7 g/dl [6, 7]. With worsening anemia, cardiac output increases steeply, peaking at 180% of normal at the Hgb value of 6–7 g/dl. Below the Hgb of 3-5 g/dl, shifts in coronary blood flow from endocardium to epicardium signal imminent danger in the otherwise healthy patient [7–9]. Coexistence of coronary vascular stenosis changes this threshold to 7–10 g/dl [10]. The importance of coexisting cardiac disease when determining the tolerance to anemia is further highlighted in studies showing increased morbidity and mortality in anemic patients undergoing percutaneous coronary interventions [11] or with congestive heart failure [12], presumably due to greater burden of the compensatory increase in cardiac output. Other disease processes, such as sepsis, can impair red cell deformability and adaptive mechanisms at the level of microcirculation thereby decreasing tissue oxygen delivery [86].

Despite current evidence and best practice guidelines, clinical practice regarding when to transfuse RBCs varies among physicians and institutions. Even though most would agree that RBCs should only be given when the benefits outweigh the harm, this decision is often difficult to make due to a limited number of randomized clinical trials demonstrating the beneficial effect of RBC transfusions. RBCs are the blood component of choice in patients with symptomatic anemia. Signs and symptoms of anemia that would trigger symptomatic-driven RBC transfusions include palpitations, anxiety, tinnitus, dizziness, tingling, anorexia, nausea, headaches, and scotomata. As the anemia worsens, dyspnea, tachycardia, fatigue, and malaise become manifest, though many previously and otherwise healthy patients may remain apparently asymptomatic even with profound anemia. Dyspnea at rest, if present, is an ominous finding in any patient with diminished RBC mass and requires immediate transfusion therapy [42]. Patients with significant underlying cerebral, coronary, or peripheral atherosclerosis (especially the elderly) may instead complain of claudication, angina, syncope, or transient ischemic attacks [6]. RBCs should not be used for treatment of asymptomatic compensated chronic anemia that can be corrected with pharmacologic agents (vitamin B12, folic acid, recombinant erythropoietin or iron therapy). RBCs should also not be used specifically for blood volume expansion, to increase oncotic pressure, to improve wound healing, or merely to improve a person's sense of wellbeing [3].

Two concepts form the basis for the use of hemoglobin-driven blood transfusions – the optimal Hgb and minimally acceptable Hgb. The optimal Hgb level is difficult to define in anemic patients other than young and otherwise healthy patients due to large number of factors interfering with compensatory mechanisms. The minimally acceptable Hgb level for sustained tissue life was defined in the 1930s by Carrel and Lindberg as approximately 3 g/dL, which corresponds to the critical delivery of oxygen that coincides with the metabolic shift from aerobic to anaerobic

[4, 131]. An analysis of case reports of patients who refused blood for religious reasons concluded that nearly all deaths due to anemia occurred in patients with Hgb levels less than 5 g/dL [13–14]. Asymptomatic electrocardiographic changes can be detected in young, healthy human volunteers who underwent isovolemic Hgb reduction with Hgb levels between 5 and 7 g/dL [136]. A retrospective study of nearly two thousand Jehovah's Witness patients found that the risk of death increases with decreasing Hgb below 10 g/dL in all patients, but this increase is more dramatic in patients with cardiovascular disease than in patients without [10]. In identifying and predicting surgical patients at risk from anemia, operative blood loss must be evaluated in concert with the initial and subsequent Hgb and/or HCT values. Thus, in the group of Jehovah's Witness patients undergoing elective surgery, there was no mortality found at Hgb levels as low as 6 g/dL as long as blood loss was kept below 500 mL [15]. The odds of death increase 2.5 times (95% CI, 1.9–3.2) for each gram decrease in Hgb level [16].

Given all these considerations, it is paramount to make rational transfusion decisions using results of randomized controlled trials as a basis for evidence-based decisions regarding transfusion triggers. Some of these studies are pointing to the fact that transfusions may actually worsen outcomes of non-bleeding euvolemic ICU patients, the majority of whom are anemic after more than three days' stay in ICU. Meta-analysis [86] of clinical trials evaluating the impact of using restrictive versus liberal transfusion triggers confirmed the initial finding of the TRICC trial, the only adequately powered study to evaluate clinically important outcomes. Specifically, non-surgical, critically ill patients maintained at Hgb levels of 7–9 g/dl (restrictive) versus 10–12 g/dl (liberal) seem to have no increase in mortality or morbidity [17] unless there is underlying coronary atherosclerotic disease [18–22]. Further subgroup analysis [17], however, found that mortality rates were lower with the restrictive transfusion strategy among younger, less acutely ill patients. The total number of RBC transfusions a patient received was independently associated with the longer ICU and hospital stay and increase in mortality [23]. Surprisingly, among critically ill patients, transfusions may also increase morbidity in euvolemic non-bleeding patients with acute myocardial infarction or unstable angina [18]. In this patient subgroup of ICU patients, liberal transfusion showed no advantage in survival, but patients with more transfusions had higher incidence of multiorgan failure, which was also found to be increased by transfusion of non-leukoreduced RBCs [24]. In summary, although a restrictive RBC transfusion strategy generally appears to be safe in most critically ill euvolemic patients with cardiovascular disease, the appropriate transfusion trigger in most anemic patients with cardiovascular disease is unknown. It is certain, however, that patients undergoing cardiovascular surgery should be transfused with leukoreduced blood.

The "transfusion trigger" has evolved over time, and has been influenced most by an understanding of risks associated with anemia, and has been particularly critically evaluated following HIV crisis [131]. Pending additional clinical trials, the best data suggest that a restrictive transfusion trigger of 7 g/dL be used for euvolemic anemic patients [25–32]. However, the literature also emphasizes the importance of evaluation of each patient's individual need, guided by both laboratory findings and clinical assessment, which takes into consideration patient history, acuteness of developing anemia, symptoms and physical findings [6, 13, 33–41]. In patients with acute bleeding, Hgb measurements are usually an imprecise measure of tissue oxygenation. Therefore, patients with critical bleeding should be transfused with RBCs irrespective of measured Hgb and HCT, as should most patients with Hgb <6 g/dl, especially if anemia has developed acutely [3]. However, some clinical conditions such as medically stable patients with sickle cell disease may permit even lower Hgb triggers than 6 g/dl, and these patients should not be transfused to Hgb>10 g/dl. In fact, in many patients with sickle cell disease RBC transfusions may do more harm than good [43]. Specifically, in sickle cell hemolytic transfusion reaction syndrome, even phenotypically matched RBCs are hemolyzed, possibly by bystander hemolytic mechanism, resulting in worsening anemia [135]. In these cases withholding of RBC transfusions, despite profound anemia, results in cessation of hemolysis and reconstitution of bone marrow erythropoesis [133, 134]. Several clinical situations warrant RBC transfusion therapy in patients with Hgb values between 6 and 10 g/dl. In these patients the decision to transfuse should be based on the ongoing indication of organ ischemia, potential or actual ongoing bleeding, the patient's intravascular volume status and the patient's risk for complications of inadequate oxygenation due to low cardiovascular reserve and high O_2 consumption. Thus, patients with acute blood loss >30% of blood volume, or anemic patients with anticipation of acute bleeding or presence of ischemic cardiovascular or CNS disease should be transfused at these Hgb values. Other examples include exchange transfusion or red cell exchange in diseases such as hemolytic disease of the fetus and newborn or acute chest syndrome in sickle cell disease or transfusion-dependent patients with severe thalassemia [3, 44]. Red blood cell transfusions are usually not indicated for Hgb >10 g/dl.

Based on all these considerations, it behooves clinicians to administer transfusions only when clinically necessary and in a minimally effective

dose. In an effort to avoid inappropriate over- or under-transfusion institutional blood transfusion guidelines should be developed and followed.
Blood management programs are advocating a unit-by-unit approach to
RBC transfusions, whereby in the absence of acute hemorrhage RBC transfusion should be given as single units with Hgb increments determined
between each unit given. Interestingly, a simple measure of challenging
clinicians to justify post-transfusion hemoglobin levels greater than 11
resulted in an increase in single-unit transfusions from 5% to 20% [45].
We now understand better the link between anemia and an increased
post-operative morbidity and mortality and decreased quality of life in
surgery patients. Here, the principle that an ounce of prevention is worth
a pound of cure applies well. The practice of timely pre-operative testing
for anemia in patients undergoing major blood loss surgeries is now
considered to be optimal management at many institutions so that anemic
patients can receive diagnosis and treatment of their anemia (such as
with iron with or without erythropoietin) in advance of their scheduled
surgery [46, 151]. Furthermore, techniques to reduce blood loss during
surgery should be used whenever possible.

Clinical outcomes and efficacy of transfusion are also to be influenced by
RBC "storage lesion" due to progressive biochemical and biomechanical
changes in red blood cells that occur after 2 to 3 weeks of storage. These
changes are mediated by a decrease in red cell pH, 2,3-DPG and nitric
oxide levels, as well as decreased red cell deformability due to a decrease
in ATP content and resultant spherocyte formation. With storage, there is
also an increase in potassium and free Hgb, microparticle formation and
accumulation of pro-inflammatory substances. Although these changes
are reversible within 24–48 hours, they are thought to be translated into
physiological effects of decreased oxygen delivery, increased mortality
and infection rates [47–54]. Indeed, an independent association of transfusion of more than five units of RBCs of increased storage age (greater
than 28 days) with increased in-hospital mortality was observed for
critically ill trauma patients transfused similar total amounts of RBCs.
Furthermore, the rate of deep vein thrombosis and death as a result of
multiorgan failure were increased and ICU-free days were decreased for
patients transfused RBCs of increased age [55]. Similarly, an increased
number of complications were observed after cardiac surgery in patients
given older RBC units, including increased mortality, renal failure and
sepsis [56, 132]. Further investigation of the association of RBC storage
age and clinical outcomes is required before any systematic changes are
proposed in current transfusion practices.

Platelet transfusions

The main function of platelets is to maintain hemostasis and endothelial integrity. Platelets accumulate at sites of vascular injury and form hemostatic plugs. Platelets adhere to the exposed endothelium and they aggregate through an interaction of adhesive glycoproteins vWF and fibrinogen to their respective receptors on activated platelets, GpIb/IX/V and GpIIb/IIIa. In 1910, Duke demonstrated the clinical effectiveness of platelet transfusions, but it took fifty years to make platelets available for transfusion as a blood component [57]. Today, platelet concentrates are the third most frequently used blood component (after RBCs and plasma) with more than 2 million doses transfused annually in the United States.

Platelets are transfused prophylactically, to prevent bleeding, or therapeutically, to treat an ongoing bleeding. One indication for platelets is the treatment of thrombocytopenia due to decreased platelet production associated with chemotherapy, irradiation or aplastic anemia. Indeed, use of platelet transfusion therapy has revolutionized the treatment of hematopoetic malignant disorders and today is the mainstay of treatment of numerous malignant disorders requiring ablative chemotherapy. Thrombocytopenia can also be caused by increased destruction of activated platelets in disseminated intravascular coagulation, thrombotic thrombocytopenic purpura, cavernous hemangioma, or immune processes such as autoimmune thrombocytopenia (ITP), drug-induced immune thrombocytopenia, or neonatal immune thrombocytopenia. Platelets are increasingly being used for the management of massively transfused patients who develop thrombocytopenias due to dilutional consumption and impaired platelet function related to hypothermia. Implementation of massive transfusion protocols in which one dose of platelets is given following a pre-set number of RBCs and plasma has been shown to be associated with improved outcomes in massively transfused trauma patients, although it remains for randomized controlled clinical trials to prove a causal relationship [58, 83]. Other indications for platelet transfusions include non-immune mediated platelet inhibition due to exposure to certain drugs (aspirin, ticlopidine, clopidrogel, prasugrel, abciximab, to name the few) or uremia. Platelet transfusions might also be required to treat dysfunctional thrombocytopenias related to congenital platelet defects or the damage caused by the exposure to extracorporeal devices. Platelets are not indicated for the treatment of bleeding due to anatomic defects only, or to control bleeding that can be controllable with local measures. Immune thrombocytopenias such as ITP or PTP represent relative contraindications to platelet transfusions due to the clearance of transfused platelets by antibodies, rendering platelet transfusions ineffective. On the other hand, except in cases of life-threatening hemorrhage, platelet transfusions should be withheld in patients with TTP (prior to the initiation of therapeutic apheresis) or heparin-induced thrombocytopenia (HIT) due to potential harm to the patient by aggravation of the thrombotic process.

Studies evaluating the relationship between platelet count and bleeding risk in thrombocytopenic patients have helped define transfusion guidelines currently in use. As with RBC transfusions, studies involving Jehovah's Witness patients provided useful information regarding the absolute minimum platelet count sufficient to prevent life-threatening hemorrhage and suggested that therapeutic-only versus prophylactic platelet transfusion did not result in increased hemorrhagic morbidity or mortality. In this group of patients no significant bleeding occurred as long as platelet counts were greater than 5000/υl. One patient died due to CNS bleeding when their platelet count dropped to 2000/υl. None of 33 other patients being treated with chemotherapy or autologous stem cell transplant had severe bleeding in spite of receiving no blood products [59–61]. However, randomized controlled trials comparing hemorrhagic episodes in patients receiving prophylactic versus therapeutic platelet transfusions demonstrated a significant difference in the incidence of cerebral bleeding, two of which were fatal, in the therapeutic arm, suggesting that a therapeutic transfusion strategy may not be as safe in some patients as a prophylactic strategy [62, 63]. To further define prophylactic platelet transfusion triggers, two studies evaluated the hemorrhagic risk in thrombocytopenic patients not being supported by platelet transfusions. Remarkably, with platelet counts between 5000/υl and 20 000/υl gross bleeding occurred only on 3% of days [64]. Similarly, stool blood measured with chromium 51-labeled red cells, was markedly increased only at platelet counts of less than 5000/υl [65, 66].

Given that serious bleeding occurs only with platelet counts of <10 000/υl and fatal bleeding is unlikely to occur at platelet counts of >5000/υl, the threshold for *prophylactic* platelet transfusions in uncomplicated patients is established as 10 000/υl, with the target platelet count of >20 000/υl. The recommended threshold for *therapeutic* platelet transfusions for bleeding due to thrombocytopenia is <50 000/υl and due to platelet dysfunction, platelets should be transfused irrespective of the platelet count. As profound thrombocytopenia represents an independent risk-factor for procedure-related bleeding [67] platelet transfusions are also recommended before an invasive procedure if platelet count is <50 000/υl or <100 000/υl for CNS or retinal procedures [3]. There has been suggestion in the literature that further reduction in the risk of hemorrhage in thrombocytopenic patients can be achieved through avoiding low hematocrit by transfusing RBCs [137, 138]. As is the case with RBC transfusions, the decision whether to transfuse platelets should be based on the patient's complete clinical picture, and not on the basis of quantitative criteria only. Despite these well-established guidelines for platelet transfusions, there has been no improvement in the wide variability of transfusion rates for platelets [68]. For example, in the recent Transfusion Requirements After Cardiac surgery (TRAC) study, platelet use for patients undergoing isolated primary coronary artery bypass graft surgery ranged from 0.4% to 90.4% at 408 hospitals [69].

Another question is what the most appropriate dose is for patients who require platelet transfusion. The optimal prophylactic dose is a subject of examination in several studies [70, 71]. Evaluating an increment in post-transfusion platelet count to a level sufficient to prevent spontaneous, thrombocytopenic bleeding is a common way to assess the response to prophylactic platelet transfusions. The increase in platelet count 10–60 minutes post transfusion determines platelet recovery, and 18–24 hours post transfusion determines platelet survival. However, before refractoriness is diagnosed, a calculation of the corrected count increment (CCI), which takes into account patient's size and the number of platelets transfused, should be performed. Platelet refractoriness is defined as a poor response to platelet transfusions on at least two occasions, expressed as an increment of less than 10 000/unit of apheresis platelets or the CCI of less than 5000 platelets $\times$ m^2 per υL [72].

Evaluating platelet recovery and survival can help distinguish immune from non-immune refractoriness. Immune refractoriness is mediated by anti-HLA class I or anti-platelet glycoprotein antibodies and is characterized by rapid clearance of transfused platelets. This is the most common cause of platelet refractoriness in chronically transfused hematology–oncology patients or multifarious women. The best approach to providing platelet support to patients with immune refractoriness due to anti-HLA antibody of known specificity is with HLA antigen-negative (phenotype safe) or HLA-matched platelets. If the specificity is unknown, or the patient has anti-platelet glycoprotein antibodies, cross-match compatible platelets are an appropriate choice. As ABO antigens are present on platelets and can influence their survival, ABO-identical platelets are preferred for transfusion of refractory patients. Non-immune refractoriness is caused by delayed platelet clearance in patients with fever, sepsis, DIC, splenomegaly or drugs such as vancomycin, amphotericin B or heparin. Judicious use of platelets, especially in chronically transfused patients is the best way to prevent development of refractoriness to platelet transfusions.

In the United States, platelet transfusion therapy is currently accomplished using two types of platelet components – whole blood derived platelets and platelet pheresis. Since the introduction of plateletpheresis methods in the early 1970s [73–75], there has been an increased reliance, especially within the last 10 years, on platelets collected by apheresis from single donors. To achieve the adequate therapeutic dose of 3.0×10^{11} platelets, 5–6 units of whole blood derived platelets have to be pooled. Each type of platelet product has advantages and disadvantages. Advantages of platelet pheresis products over whole blood derived platelets include single donor exposure, matching potential for the management of alloimmunized patients, and low red cell and white cell content. Platelet transfusions are associated with adverse events, including transfusion-transmitted bacterial and viral infections, hemolytic transfusion reactions due to ABO incompatibility and Transfusion Related Acute Lung Injury (TRALI).

Plasma component therapy

Plasma is the fluid portion of blood and is composed of over 90% water, 6–8% protein, including coagulation factors, as well as lipids and carbohydrates. Coagulation factors are present in plasma at a concentration of 1 international unit (IU) per ml of undiluted plasma. Some of these coagulation factors, including Factors V and VIII, are labile and will degrade with storage without freezing. Plasma for therapeutic use may be prepared from whole blood or by apheresis collection. Depending on the handling during manufacture, a plasma product will be labeled as either Fresh Frozen Plasma (FFP), which is frozen within 8 hours, or Plasma Frozen Within 24 Hours After Phlebotomy (FP24). FP24 can safely be used in place of FFP for most indications, including in patients with liver disease or for management of warfarin reversal [76]. Plasma products are stored frozen and have to be thawed for 30 minutes prior to use. Thawed plasma products are instantly available and can be stored for 5 days, with a negligible decline in Factors V and VIII [77–79]. Plasma collected by apheresis is also used for the large scale fractionation in the production of factor concentrates, albumin or immunoglobulin preparations.

The goal of plasma component therapy is the management (or prevention) of coagulopathy or the treatment of TTP. To guide plasma component therapy, laboratory assessment of coagulopathy should be performed in concert with transfusing plasma components, although many institutions that employ a massive transfusion protocol initiate plasma transfusions based on the number of red cell units used for resuscitation, rather than waiting for laboratory results of the patient's coagulation status to be reported. A therapeutic dose of plasma components is 10–20 mL/kg body weight. Each 100 mL of plasma raises coagulation factors in an average size adult by 2–3%.

Most commonly, plasma is administered to correct elevated INR, with the threshold usually determined by institutional guidelines. There are only a few clear indications for plasma administration and those include massive transfusion with critical or coagulopathic bleeding, replacement of multiple coagulation factor deficiencies with associated severe bleeding and/or DIC, replacement of inherited single coagulation factor deficiencies for which no virus-safe fractionated product exists, replacement of specific protein deficiencies (e.g. C-1 esterase inhibitor), emergent reversal of warfarin effect when severe bleeding is present or anticipated, anti-thrombin III deficiency in patient requiring heparin, and as a component of plasma exchange for TTP/HUS [3, 80]. However, based on a systematic review and meta-analysis of the literature by the AABB task force, only two indications are evidence-based: massive transfusion with coagulopathic bleeding and patients with warfarin anticoagulation-related intracranial hemorrhage [81]. Higher plasma to RBC ratio was found to be an independent predictor of survival in massively transfused patients and aggressive early use of plasma may improve outcome in patients with early trauma induced coagulopathy, although it remains for randomized controlled clinical trials to prove a causal relationship [82, 83].

Approximately 4.5 million units of plasma were transfused during 2008 in the United States. The use of plasma has increased significantly within last two decades and is much higher, relative to RBCs, compared to other countries with similar healthcare level [84]. Up to 30% of plasma transfusions in the United States are not administered according to the published guidelines. The most common reason for prescribing plasma found in the hospital-based survey [85] was to normalize an elevated pre-procedural INR, despite numerous studies that have not shown a correlation between the risk of bleeding and mild-to-moderate test abnormalities or the lack of correlation between prophylactic plasma transfusion and decrease in bleeding events [67, 87, 88]. Not surprisingly, legal considerations are reported as a major factor in the decision to transfuse plasma. We now understand that the degree of INR normalization with plasma depends on the extent of pre-transfusion test abnormality and that plasma is ineffective for correcting minimally elevated INRs [89, 90]. Comparing changes in recipients' INR after transfusion of therapeutic dose of plasma within therapeutic guidelines (INR > 1.6) to transfusions of plasma outside of guidelines (INR < 1.6) revealed inadequate response to transfusions in later group, with mean change in INR of −0.03/unit transfused. The reason for this apparent lack of plasma efficacy in correcting minimally elevated INRs is most likely due to the wide variability in INRs (0.9 to 1.3) of plasma units collected from healthy donors. Another reason for inappropriate response to plasma transfusion is the administration of inappropriate dose (<10 ml/kg body weight). Given the known toxicity of plasma, clinicians should carefully evaluate the risk to benefit ratio when transfusing this product outside of established guidelines and in an inadequate therapeutic dose.

Cryoprecipitate

Cryoprecipitated AHF (Cryoprecipitate) is made up of cold insoluble proteins from FFP. Each bag of cryoprecipitate contains 5–20 mL of plasma and (at least) 150 mg fibrinogen, 80–120 units of Factor VIII:C (depending on the blood type) 50–80 units of factor XIII and variable amount of vWF. Main indication for cryoprecipitate is replacement of fibrinogen in either congenital or acquired fibrinogen deficiency. However, an FDA approved human-derived and virally inactivated fibrinogen concentrate is now considered first line treatment for congenital fibrinogen deficiency [91]. In the absence of consumption, one bag of cryoprecipitate raises fibrinogen level of an average size adult by approximately 7 mg/dL and the transfused fibrinogen has a half-life of approximately 4 days in the circulation. The common starting dose is 1 bag per 10 kg body weight. Cryoprecipitate is used as a second line therapy in vWD only if virus-inactivated factor VIII concentrate that contains vWF is not available or desmopressin is either ineffective or contraindicated. Cryoprecipitate is also used to treat isolated Factor XIII deficiency in patients who cannot tolerate the volume of plasma transfusions or as a second line therapy for coagulopathy associated with uremia [3, 92, 93].

Transfusion-related adverse reactions

It is widely accepted that the blood supply is safer today than at any time in history [94]. In 2008, an estimated 60 000 transfusion-related adverse reactions were reported in the United States (occurrence rate of 0.25%) and the FDA received 184 reports of transfusion-related fatalities between 2008 and 2010 [2]. Owing to the focusing of tremendous efforts and resources within the last three decades towards the prevention of HIV and hepatitis transmission by transfusion, the incidence of infectious complications has long been surpassed by non-infectious complications [95, 96]. Table 3.1 summarizes the adverse effects of transfusion therapy.

Table 3.1 Adverse effects of transfusion therapy.

Type of Risk	Estimated Frequency (per unit)	Comment
Hemolytic Transfusion Reactions • Acute (due to ABO) • Acute (due to other causes) • Delayed • Transfusion to the wrong patient	• 1:606 978* • 1:164 936* • 1:28 887* • 1:14 000–1:19 000	Fatality from acute hemolytic reactions occurs in about 1 in 1 800 000 RBC transfusions. About 1/3rd of fatal acute hemolytic reactions are due to ABO incompatibility, and 2/3^{rds} of fatal acute hemolytic reactions are due to other alloantibodies. Severe hemolysis and death have occurred due to infusion of ABO incompatible plasma. Focus on prevention of medical errors, ABO incompatible considered a hospital-acquired condition.
Febrile Non-hemolytic Transfusion Reactions	1:816*	Rise in temperature >1 °C not explained by patient's underlying disease. Fever might be absent in premedicated patients. Mediated by antibodies or storage-generated biologic response modifiers. Decreased rate is seen with the use of prestorage leuko-reduced products.
Allergic Reactions • Urticaria • Severe allergic reactions • Anaphylaxis	• 1:50–100 • 1:3611* • 1:20 000–50 000	Most are type I hypersensitivity reactions, mediated by IgE. Anaphylaxis caused by class-specific anti-IgA in patients with complete IgA deficiency, or antibodies to haptoglobin or C3 and C4. Transfusion recommendations: premedication for allergic reactions; washing of blood products for moderate-severe reactions; IgA-deficient products for IgA deficient patients with documented anti-IgA.
Transfusion-transmitted viral infections • Hepatitis B virus • Hepatitis C virus • HIV • HTLV-I/II	• 1:100 000–200 000 • 1:1–2 million • 1:2–3 million • 1:641 000	Transfusion-transmitted viral infections represent significant problem in the underdeveloped world, and account for 5–10% of new HIV cases. Emerging infections (West Nile Virus, Chikungunya virus) represent global threat to transfusion safety. CMV transmission reduced by leukoreduction.

(*continued overleaf*)

Table 3.1 (*continued*)

Type of Risk	Estimated Frequency (per unit)	Comment
Post-transfusion sepsis	1:738 437*	Major risk with platelet transfusions.
Transfusion-transmitted parasitic infections • Malaria • Babesia • Chagas	 • 1:4 million • 1:617 RBCs (Connecticut) • 1:21 000 (aggregate donor prevalence)	More than 50 cases of transfusion-transmitted babesiosis reported in Northeast and Upper Midwest regions of US. Blood centers implementing Chagas' screening.
Transfusion-Related Acute Lung Injury (TRALI)	1:51 443*	Leading cause of FDA reported fatalities. Highest risk with transfusion of plasma and platelets donated by multiparous females. Both immune and non-immune mechanism proposed. Significant risk reduction achieved by transfusion of male-only plasma.
Transfusion-Associated Graft-vs-Host Disease (TAGVHD)	Very rare, incidence unknown	Mediated by viable transfused T lymphocytes; risk determined by HLA mismatch between donor and recipient and immune status of the recipient. High fatality rate due to development of marrow aplasia. Prevented by gamma irradiation of cellular blood components.
Hypotensive Transfusion Reactions	1:20 757*	Mediated by vasoactive kinins generated by the activation of contact system. Seen with use of negatively charged bedside leukocyte filters in patients on ACE inhibitors receiving platelets or with therapeutic apheresis and hemodyalisis. ACE inhibitors should be discontinued prior to these procedures.
Post-transfusion Purpura	1:47 993*	Severe, self-limiting thrombocytopenia that develops 5–10 days post-transfusion. Mediated by platelet-specific antibodies. Treated with IGIV, good prognosis.

Table 3.1 (*continued*)

Type of Risk	Estimated Frequency (per unit)	Comment
Transfusion Associated Circulatory Overload (TACO)	1:16 706*	Cardiogenic pulmonary edema, in patients who cannot tolerate the volume or rate of transfusion. Manifests with dyspnea, hypertension, tachycardia. Elevated BNP or post/pre BNP ratio. Responds to diuretics and supportive care. Slow transfusion in susceptible patients. Should be differentiated from TRALI and anaphylaxis.
Immuno-modulatory (TRIM) and proinflammatory effect of blood transfusion	Incidence unknown	Immune function alterations documented in association with transfusion. Mechanism may involve soluble HLA peptides, WBCs and mononuclear cells. Proven beneficial effect in renal transplantation; detrimental clinical effects need confirmation.

*[2] The 2009 National Blood Collection and Utilization Survey Report

Thus, most of the reactions reported to the Transfusion Service today are due to febrile non-hemolytic, allergic or delayed hemolytic transfusion reactions or transfusion-associated circulatory overload (TACO). In 2012, TRALI remained the most common cause of transfusion-related fatalities reported to the FDA (45%), followed by TACO (21%) and hemolytic transfusion reactions (21% for both non-ABO and ABO). Though significant efforts continue to be invested in the prevention of infectious disease transmission, including bacterial infections, there is an increasing awareness within the last decade of the morbidity and mortality associated with non-infectious transfusion-related complications.

Hemolytic transfusion reactions
Hemolytic Transfusion Reactions are potentially serious (and in some cases life-threatening) reactions, which are typically caused by the transfusion of immunologically incompatible red cells (and rarely ABO-incompatible plasma). Hemolytic transfusion reactions can be acute or delayed. Acute reactions typically occur within minutes to hours of the inciting transfusion, while delayed reactions typically occur days later.

Acute hemolytic reactions are much more likely to be clinically serious than delayed reactions.

The great majority of acute hemolytic transfusion reactions (including those caused by ABO incompatible transfusion) are not fatal [144]. When ABO incompatibility causes a serious hemolytic reaction, clerical or systems errors typically predispose to the hemolytic event [145–147].

Based on fatalities reported to FDA following transfusion [94], the most common cause of fatal ABO incompatible transfusion is misidentification of the blood recipient, which may occur at any of the following steps:
- drawing the recipient's crossmatch specimen
- labeling the recipient's blood specimen
- performing pre-transfusion testing in the transfusion service
- issuing the donor blood from the transfusion service
- identifying patient and donor unit immediately prior to transfusion.

Thus, it should not be surprising that The Joint Commission's national patient safety goal #1 specifically addresses the need to properly identify each patient and to eliminate transfusion errors related to patient misidentification.

Goal 1 – Improve the accuracy of patient ID
   – Use at least two patient identifiers and label specimen containers in the presence of the patient (NPSG.01.01.01)
   – Eliminate Transfusion Errors related to patient misidentification (NPSG.01.03.01).

Furthermore, beginning in 2011, as a financial incentive to eliminate ABO incompatible hemolytic transfusion reactions, the Centers for Medicare/Medicaid Services (CMS) replaced Hospital Acquired Condition of ICD-9-CM code 999.6 with a new subcategory of 999.6 to identify new diagnoses relating to ABO incompatibility reaction due to transfusion of blood or blood products [148].

The new subcategories include …

999.60 – ABO incompatibility reaction, unspecified;
999.61 – ABO incompatibility with hemolytic transfusion reaction not specified as acute or delayed;
999.62 – ABO incompatibility with acute hemolytic transfusion reaction;
999.63 – ABO incompatibility with delayed hemolytic transfusion reaction;
999.69 – Other ABO incompatibility reaction.

With the above new codes, ABO incompatible transfusion has become a hospital acquired condition for which CMS has reformed payment of inpatient facility services for which Medicare no longer pays the additional costs associated with the complication if they are considered preventable.

The incidence of acute hemolytic reactions varies with location and when data were gathered. Estimates varying between 1:12 500 units and 1:40 000 units. About one third of fatal acute hemolytic reactions are due to ABO incompatibility and two thirds are due to other alloantibodies [94, 149, 150].

Preventing hemolytic transfusion reactions from incompatible red cell transfusions depends on proper patient identification and labeling of samples and blood components in each and every step, from sample collection to blood administration.

Hemolytic transfusion reactions due to infusion of donor antibodies are usually considered to be low risk events due to the small volume of plasma in most blood components. However, because plasma and apheresis platelets have 200 or more milliliters per unit, these products are much more likely to cause hemolytic reactions in group A, group B and group AB patients if the donor product is group O. In fact, FDA fatality reports show that severe life-threatening hemolytic transfusion reactions and death have occurred, presumably due to the infusion of high titer anti-A or anti-B. Thus, it is prudent to limit the volume of infused ABO incompatible plasma and/or to restrict the use of high titer ABO antibody containing products for group O patients.

When an acute hemolytic reaction occurs, signs and symptoms may appear within minutes after the transfusion is started but can occur anytime during the transfusion. They may include (but are not limited to):
- fever (temperature increase of more than 1C)
- chills
- rigors
- nausea and vomiting
- anxiety
- malaise
- hypotension
- tachycardia
- burning along site of infusion
- skin flushing
- chest pain
- dyspnea, wheezing
- severe low back pain
- hemoglobinemia
- hemoglobinuria
- oliguria/anuria
- uncontrolled bleeding.

In the anesthetized patient, the only signs may be unexplained bleeding due to disseminated intravascular coagulation (DIC), falling blood pressure, and/or fever.

Treatment varies with the clinical condition of each patient and focuses on providing cardiovascular support with IV fluids and vasopressors. Care should be taken to avoid fluid overload in patients with impaired cardiac or renal function. If present, disseminated intravascular hemolysis and hypotension must be treated early to limit renal damage. If possible, further transfusions should not be given until the transfusion service has completed its serologic investigation and determined the cause of the reaction.

The majority of acute hemolytic reactions could probably be avoided if healthcare providers always accurately identified each patient and specimen collected at the time of phlebotomy, and always accurately identified each recipient and blood product at the time of blood product administration.

Delayed Hemolytic Transfusion Reactions are typically not as severe as acute hemolytic transfusion reactions. These reactions involve the destruction of transfused red blood cells after an interval of time, usually 3 to 21 days following transfusion, with most occurring about 7 days post-transfusion. Delayed hemolytic reactions typically occur when weak alloantibodies that are undetected in pre-transfusion antibody screening tests increase in strength following a secondary (anamnestic) antibody response to transfused donor red cells possessing the corresponding antigen. Such antibodies occur in persons originally sensitized by exposure to RBCs through previous transfusions and/or pregnancies. Antibodies of several blood group systems may cause delayed hemolytic reactions, with antibodies in the Rh (anti-c, -E), Kidd (anti-Jka), Kell (anti-K), and Duffy (anti-Fya) systems often being implicated.

The reported incidences of delayed hemolytic reactions vary with the patient population under study, the degree of surveillance, the length of time following the transfusion over which data is collected, the criteria used to define the reactions, and the sensitivity of antibody detection methods. In studies performed since the 1980s, the incidence of delayed hemolytic transfusion reactions includes rates ranging from about one in every 2500 to 10 000 red cell units transfused.

Delayed hemolytic transfusion reactions may go undetected, as the symptoms may be mild and subclinical. Red cell destruction is usually by extravascular hemolysis. When present, typical signs and symptoms include: fever with or without chills, unexplained drop in hemoglobin and hematocrit and transient jaundice due to elevated serum bilirubin.

Treatment of a delayed hemolytic transfusion reaction is usually support-ive. Some patients may require additional transfusion if anemia is severe enough to require treatment. If possible, transfusion should be avoided.

Preventing delayed hemolytic reactions may be impossible if the patient's antibody is too weak to be detected by routine antibody detection methods. However there are many standard procedures and protocols that transfusion services can use to minimize this complication. Some examples include:

• Performing a history check to identify patients who are known to have existing antibodies that may have become weaker over time.

• Using sensitive antibody detection methods such as column agglutina-tion or solid phase based methodologies.

• Using antibody screen cells from donors who have a homozygous expression of key antigens, so that those antigens are expressed more strongly on the reagent red cell (i.e., show a "dosage effect"). This is particularly important for detection of Kidd and Rh antibodies.

• For patients who have been transfused or pregnant in the last three months, using pre-transfusion specimens that are no older than three days (where the date of collection is day zero).

• For patients who have (or had in the past) clinically significant anti-bodies, using antigen phenotyped donors who lack the corresponding alloantigen, even when the antibody (antibodies) are not currently detectable.

• Employing a testing scheme that assures the detection of additional alloantibodies in patients who are already alloimmunized.

TRALI

TRALI was first recognized as a clinical entity in 1983, three decades following initial reports of transfusion-associated non-cardiogenic pulmonary edema [97–99]. Most centers today rely on the Canadian Consensus Conference criteria and the NHLBI working group definition for diagnosis of TRALI [100–102]. TRALI is a new acute lung injury (ALI) that presents as an acute onset hypoxemia ($PaO_2/FiO_2 \leq 300$ mmHg or O_2 saturation $\leq 90\%$ on room air). Symptoms of respiratory distress occur within 6 hours of transfusion, coinciding with the appearance of bilateral pulmonary infiltrates on frontal chest radiograph (CXR) with no evidence of left atrial hypertension. To make the diagnosis of TRALI, there should be no preexisting acute lung injury before transfusions and no temporal relationship to an alternate risk factor for ALI. TRALI should be differentiated from other pulmonary transfusion reactions, including allergic/anaphylactic, TACO, bacterial contamination and hemolysis. It might be challenging to distinguish TRALI from TACO due to limitations imposed by the incomplete patient data set, difficulty in determining the patient's volume status, decreasing use of PA lines, low sensitivity of CXR as a test for pulmonary edema and the co-existence of TRALI and TACO in the same patient [103, 104]. Laboratory findings that support diagnosis of TRALI include transient leucopenia, hypocomplementemia and brain natriuretic peptide measurement to rule out circulatory overload [105–107].

Actual incidence of TRALI is not known and the most cited is 1 in 5000 transfused components. Two recent studies reported incidence of 1 in 2400 and 1 in 1271 transfused components. In each study, the computer screening system was used to identify patients with post-transfusion hypoxemia or ventilator support requirement, which were then evaluated for TRALI using consensus criteria [108, 109]. Most cases of TRALI are self-limited and patients usually recover within 72 hours. Mortality of TRALI is approximately 5%; it is estimated that TRALI contributes to mortality in 1 in 200 000 transfusion recipients, and accounted for 37% of transfusion-related fatalities reported to FDA from 2008 through 2012 [94, 110]. Although the pathophysiology of TRALI is not fully understood, the discovery of leukocyte antibodies in up to 90% of implicated donors, the cognate antigen on neutrophils of > 50% of recipients, or antibodies in 6% of recipients (inverse TRALI), points to the immune nature of TRALI [99]. Implicated antibodies include anti-HLA (class II and to a lesser degree class I), -neutrophil and -monocyte antibodies [99, 111, 112]. However, since not every case of TRALI is associated with the donor or recipient antibodies, the non-immune mechanism was proposed [113, 114]. Thus, according to the two-hit hypothesis, the underlying medical condition of the patient leads to the priming of neutrophils, with their subsequent agglutination and activation in the patient's lungs by antibodies, biologic response modifiers accumulated during a blood product storage, biologically active lipids or soluble CD40 ligand [115, 116]. Complement activation and elastase release from activated neutrophils lead to pulmonary edema development. Cardiopulmonary bypass surgery and induction therapy for hematological malignancy are common pre-existing conditions in patients with TRALI [117]. Furthermore, liver surgery, chronic alcohol abuse, shock, higher peak airway pressure while being mechanically ventilated, current smoking, and positive fluid balance are recipient risk factors identified by multivariate analysis [152]. Any blood product containing more than 50 ml of plasma can cause TRALI, but the risk, including fatal TRALI cases, was found to be significantly higher with plasma or platelets, donated by a previously pregnant female [118].

The link between donor history of pregnancy and the risk of TRALI is through an increased risk of HLA alloimmunization with each pregnancy, from less than 1% in never pregnant women to 31% in women with more than three pregnancies [119]. To this end, several strategies have been proposed or implemented to reduce the risk of TRALI [120–122]. One such measure, limiting plasma transfusions from female donors, was found to be concurrent with reduced TRALI incidence: 2.57 in 2006 versus 0.81 in 2009 per 10 000 transfused units [152]. However, it is currently impossible to eliminate the risk of TRALI with a single strategy. Therefore, a restrictive transfusion practice for high plasma volume components that does not compromise patient outcomes is the most effective TRALI risk-reduction strategy.

Sepsis

Sepsis is a serious consequence of the transfusion of bacterially contaminated blood components. Due to the successful risk reduction of viral pathogen transmission, bacterial pathogens are currently the greatest threat of transfusion-transmitted disease, with an estimated risk of transfusion-related septic reactions of <1:15 000 to 1:100 000 transfusions [139]. Currently, septic transfusion reactions are the third leading cause of transfusion-related fatalities (after TRALI and hemolysis), accounting for 11% of fatalities reported to the FDA over the last six fiscal years [94]. Of the implicated organisms, babesiosis accounted for 31% of fatalities, mostly RBC product deaths, followed by Staphylococcus aureus, which accounted for 20%. Most (61%) of the 35 reported fatalities are attributed to the transfusion of bacterially contaminated platelet products.

Most patients experiencing septic transfusion reactions develop fever during or within 4 hours of the transfusion. Fever associated with sepsis is usually ≥39 °C or represents ≥2 °C increase from pre-transfusion value; it might be accompanied by rigors, tachycardia, dyspnea, and nausea or vomiting. Fatal cases of sepsis are usually associated with the infusion of a unit contaminated with Gram-negative organisms that produce high levels of endotoxin. A high index of suspicion for sepsis may be necessary in patients who are already on antipyretics, are in the operating room or are immunosupressed so the fever can be attributed to other causes. Thus, sepsis associated with the transfusion of contaminated platelet products is underreported if only passive surveillance methods are used.

There is a significant variability in the prevalence data reported for bacterial contamination of individual blood products, with the overall estimated prevalence reported for blood products of 32.4 per 100 000 units [140]. The rate of bacterial contamination of RBCs and platelets differs, owing to the different temperature requirement for their storage. Red blood cells are stored at 1 to 6 °C, and are less likely to grow bacteria than platelets, which are stored at room temperature. Septic reactions due to transfusion of contaminated RBCs occur at an estimated rate of 1 in 250 000 units transfused, and are caused by psychrophilic bacteria that can grow at cold temperatures. These septic reactions are usually severe and rapid in onset, and are associated with Gram-negative bacteria, including Yersinia enterocolitica, Pseudomonas species, and Serratia species. Most common source of Yersinia is asymptomatic donor with transient bacteremia and of Serratia contaminated collection packs. Pseudomonas species have been cultured from plasma and cryoprecipitate thawed in contaminated water baths [141].

Bacterial contamination of platelets remains a significant problem, with an estimated 1 in 4000 doses contaminated by bacteria [123], although the rate differs for different platelet components, and is higher for whole blood derived platelets [143]. Platelet contamination occurs more commonly with Gram-positive bacteria, often found on the donor skin. These bacteria are capable of rapid proliferation at room temperature, and include Staphylococcus epidermidis, Staphylococcus aureus and Bacillus species. Significant improvement in bacterial safety of platelet products has been achieved through an improved skin preparation, diversion of the initial volume of collected blood, culturing apheresis platelets 24 hours after the collection and limiting platelet shelf life to only five days [124]. As a result, there has been an overall decrease since 2001 in the number of bacterial infections, especially caused by Gram-negative bacteria, associated with apheresis platelets [94]. Based on passive surveillance, it is estimated that the residual risk of sepsis due to transfusion of bacterially contaminated apheresis platelets is 1 in 108 000 and of fatality 1:500 000 distributed products [142]. However, up to 70% of contaminated products are missed by day-1 culture, mostly related to false-negative cultures due to a very low level of bacterial contamination at the time of sampling. Current efforts are focused on an improved detection of bacterial contamination, development and implementation of pathogen reduction methodology and optimization of the storage temperature for blood products, for example by elucidating the mechanism of rapid clearance of transfused platelets that were stored at cold temperatures [125–130, 152]. Finally, reducing the risk of transfusion-associated sepsis can be achieved by limiting recipient exposure to blood donors through a preferential use of apheresis platelets and the judicious use of blood products.

Summary and conclusions

Great leaps forward have been made in our understanding of both the benefits and risks of blood transfusion. We know today that patients can be harmed by either the omission or the delay of transfusion when transfusion is medically indicated. Furthermore, some patients experience harm from receipt of inappropriately administered transfusion therapy, or suffer adverse consequences inadvertently from appropriately administered transfusion therapy. This concern over appropriateness of blood transfusions, and the effect it has on the quality of patient care has given rise to the field of blood management that is being introduced to an increasing number of hospitals in the United States. The guiding principle of blood management is that patients should receive all the blood they need and none they don't. This approach is driven by patient outcomes, limited blood supply and the cost of blood. In other words, the five R's could summarize blood management: the right patient receives the right donor unit at the right time, for the right medical reason and the right way.

The authors would like to thank Drs. Yomtovian and Downes for their contributions to the previous edition of this chapter, on which this work was based.

References

1 Starr D. Blood: An Epic History of Medicine and Commerce; Pete Moore. Blood and Justice. Chichester: John Wiley and Sons; 2003.
2 The 2009 National Blood Collection and Utilization Survey Report. http://www.aabb.org/programs/biovigilance/nbcus/Documents/09-nbcus-report.pdf
3 A compendium of transfusion practice guidelines American Red Cross First Edition; 2010.
4 Spence RK and Mintz PD. Transfusion in Surgery, Trauma and Critical Care. In: Mintz PD, ed. Transfusion Therapy: Clinical Principles and Practice, 2nd ed. Bethesda, MD: AABB Press, 2005: 203–41.
5 Tuchschmidt J, Oblitas D, Fried JC. Oxygen consumption in sepsis and septic shock. Critical Care Medicine. 1991;19:664–70.
6 Stehling, L. The red blood cell transfusion trigger. Physiology and clinical studies. Archives of Pathology and Laboratory Medicine. 1994 Apr;118(4):429–34.
7 Crosby, ET. Perioperative haemotherapy: I. Indications for blood component transfusion. Canadian Journal of Anesthesiology. 1992;39:695–707.
8 American Society of Anesthesiologists Task Force on Blood Component Therapy. Practice Guidelines for Blood Component Therapy. Anesthesiology. 1996;84:732–47.
9 Welch HG, Meehan KR, Goodnough LT. Prudent strategies for elective red blood cell transfusion. Annals of Internal Medicine. 1992;116:393–402.

10 Carson JL, Duff A, Poses RM, Berlin JA, Spence RK, Trout R, Noveck H, Strom BL. Effect of anaemia and cardiovascular disease on surgical mortality and morbidity. Lancet. 1996;348:1055–60.

11 Reinecke H, Trey T, Wellman J, Heidrich J, Fobker M, Wichter T, Walter M, Breithardt G, Schaefer RM. Haemoglobin-related mortality in patients undergoing percutaneous coronary interventions. Eur Heart J. 2003;24:2142–50.

12 Szachniewicz J, Petruk-Kowalcyzk J, Majda J, Kaczmarek A, Reczuch I, Kalra PR, Piepoli MF, Anker SD, Banasiak W, Ponikowski P. Anaemia is an independent predictor of poor outcome in patients with chronic heart failure. Int J Cardiol. 2003;90:303–8.

13 Pearlman ES, Ballas SK. When to transfuse blood in sickle cell disease? Lessons learned from Jehovah's Witnesses. Annals of Clinical Laboratory Science. 1994;24:396–400.

14 Viele, MK. What can we learn about the need for transfusion from patients who refuse blood? The experience with Jehovah's Witnesses. Transfusion. 1994;34:396–401.

15 Carson JL, Poses RM, Spence RK, Bonavita G. Severity of anaemia and operative mortality and morbidity. Lancet. 1988;1(8588):727–9.

16 Carson JL, Noveck H, Berlin JA, Gould SA. Mortality and morbidity in patients with very low postoperative Hgb levels who decline blood transfusion. Transfusion. 2002;42:812–8.

17 Hebert PC, Wells G, Blajchman MA, Marshall J, Martin C, Pagliarello G, Tweeddale M, Schweitzer I, Yetisir E. A multicenter, randomized, controlled clinical trial of transfusion requirements in critical care. NEJM. 1999;340:409–7.

18 Hebert PC, Yetisir E, Martin C, Blajchman MA, Wells G, Marshall J, Tweeddale M, Pagliarello G, Schweitzer I. Is a low transfusion threshold safe in critically ill patients with cardiovascular diseases? Crit Care Med. 2001;29:227–34.

19 Freudenberger RS, Carson JL. Is there an optimal hemoglobin value in the cardiac intensive care unit? Curr Opin Crit Care. 2003 Oct;9(5):356–61.

20 Mangano DT, Hollenberg M, Fegert G, Meyer ML, London MJ, Tubau JF, Krupski WC. Perioperative myocardial ischemia in patients undergoing noncardiac surgery–I: Incidence and severity during the 4 day perioperative period. The Study of Perioperative Ischemia (SPI) Research Group. J Am Coll Cardiol. 1991 Mar 15;17(4):843–50.

21 Hogue CW Jr, Goodnough LT, Monk TG. Perioperative myocardial ischemic episodes are related to hematocrit level in patients undergoing radical prostatectomy. Transfusion. 1998 Oct;38(10):924–31.

22 Nelson AH, Fleisher LA, Rosenbaum SH. Relationship between postoperative anemia and cardiac morbidity in high-risk vascular patients in the intensive care unit. Crit Care Med. 1993 Jun;21(6):860–6.

23 Corwin HL, Gettinger A, Pearl RG, et al. The CRIT Study: Anemia and blood transfusion in the critically ill-current clinical practice in the United States. Crit Care Med. 2004;32:39–52.

24 van de Watering LMG, Hermans J, Houbieris JGA, et al. Beneficial effects of Lekocyte depletion of transfused blood on postoperative complications in

patients undergoing cardiac surgery. A randomized clinical trial. Circulation. 1998;97:562–8.

25 Spiess BD, Ley C, Body SC, et al. Hematocrit value on intensive care unit entry influences the frequency of Q-wave myocardial infarction after coronary artery bypass grafting. The Institutions of the Multicenter Study of perioperative Ischemia (McSPI) Research Group. J Thorac Cardiovasc Surg. 1998;116:460–7.

26 Blair SD, Janvrin SB, McCollum CN, et al. Effect of early blood transfusion on gastrointestinal hemorrhage. Br J Surg. 1986;73:783–5.

27 Bracey AW, Radovancevic R, Riggs SA, et al. Lowering the hemoglobin threshold for transfusion in coronary artery bypass procedures: effect on patient outcome. Transfusion. 1999;39:1070–7.

28 Bush RL, Pevec WC, Holcroft JWA. Prospective, randomized trial limiting perioperative red blood cell transfusions in vascular patients. Am J Surg. 1997;174:143–8.

29 Carson JL, Terrin ML, Barton FB, et al. A pilot randomized trial comparing symptomatic vs. hemoglobin-level-driven red blood cell transfusions following hip fracture. Transfusion. 1998;38:522–9.

30 Furtune JB, Feustel PJ, Saifi J, et al. Influence of hematocrit on cardiopulmonary function after acute hemorrhage. J Trauma. 1987;27:243–9.

31 Hebert PC, Wells G, Marshall J, et al. Transfusion requirements in critical care. A pilot study. Canadian Critical Care Trials Group (published erratum appears in JAMA 1995:274:944). JAMA. 1995;273:1439–44.

32 Johnson RG, Thurer RL, Kruskall MS, et al: Comparison of two transfusion strategies after elective operations for myocardial revascularization. J Thorac Cardiovasc Surg. 1992 Aug;104(2):307–14.

33 Weiskopf RB. Do we know when to transfuse red cell to treat anemia? Transfusion. 1998;38:517–21.

34 McLellan SA, McClelland DB, Walsh TS. Anaemia and red blood cell transfusion in the critically ill patient. Blood Rev. 2003;17:195–208.

35 Petrides M. Red cell transfusion "trigger": a review. South Med J. 2003;96:664–7.

36 Crosby E. Re-evaluating the transfusion trigger: how low is safe? Amer J Ther. 2002;9:411–6.

37 Carson JL, Hill S, Carless P, Hebert P, Henry D. Transfusion triggers: a systematic review of the literature. Transfus Med Rev. 2002;16:187–99.

38 Carson JL, Chen AY. In search of the transfusion trigger. Clin Orthop. 1998;357:30–5.

39 Hill SR, Carless PA, Henry DA, Carson JL, Hebert PC, McClelland DB, Henderson KM. Transfusion thresholds and other strategies for guiding allogeneic red blood cell transfusion. Cochrane Database Syst Rev. 2002;(2):CD002042.

40 Lundsgaard-Hansen P. Safe hemoglobin or hematocrit levels in surgical patients. World J Surg. 1996 Nov–Dec;20(9):1182–8.

41 Engelfriet CP, Reesink HW, McCullough J, Hebert PC, McIntyre LA, Carson JL, Ferreira G, Thurer RL, Brock H, Boyce N, Jones J, Wulf H, Lukasewitz P, Kretschmer V, Walsh TS, McClelland B. Perioperative triggers for red cell transfusions. Vox Sang. 2002;82:215–26.

42 Carson JL, Duff A, Berlin JA, Lawrence VA, Poses RM, Huber EC, O'Hara DA, Noveck H, Strom BS. Perioperative blood transfusion and postoperative mortality. JAMA. 1998;279:199–205.

43 Josephson CD, Su LL, Hillyer KL, Hillyer CD. Transfusion in the patient with sickle cell disease: a critical review of the literature and transfusion guidelines. Transf Med Rev. 2007;21:118–33.

44 Practice guidelines for perioperative blood transfusion and adjuvant therapies: an updated report by the American Society of Anesthesiologists Task Force on Perioperative Blood Transfusion and Adjuvant Therapies. Anesthesiology. 2006;105:198–208.

45 Garrioch M, Sandbach J, Pirie E, Morrison A, Todd A, Green R. Reducing red cell transfusion by audit, education and a new guideline in a large teaching hospital. Transf Med. 2004;14:25–31.

46 Ferraris VA, Ferraris SP, Saha SP, et al. Perioperative blood transfusion and blood conservation in cardiac surgery: The Society of Thoracic Surgeons and the Society of Cardiovascular Anesthesiologists Clinical Practice Guideline. Ann Thorac Surg. 2007;83:S27–86.

47 Carson JL, Armas-Loughran B. Blood transfusion: Less is more? Crit Care Med. 2003;31:2409–10.

48 Fitzgerald RD, Martin CM, Dietz GE. Transfusing red blood cells stored in citrate phosphate dextrose adenine-1 for 28 days fails to improve tissue oxygenation in rats. Crit Care Med. 1997;25:726–32.

49 Marik PE, Sibbald WJ. AC Burton. Effect of stored-blood transfusion on oxygen delivery in patients with sepsis. JAMA. 1993;269:3024–9.

50 Zallen G, Offner PJ, Moore EE, Blackwell J, Ciesla DJ, Gabriel J, Denny C, Silliman CC. Age of transfused blood is an independent risk factor for postinjury multiple organ failure. Am J Surg. 1999;178:570–2.

51 Purdy FR, Tweeddale MG, Merrick PM. Association of mortality with age of blood transfused in septic ICU patients. Can J. Anaesth. 1997;44:1256–61.

52 Mynster T, Nielsen HJ. The impact of storage time of transfused blood on postoperative infectious complications in rectal cancer surgery. Danish RANX05 Colorectal Cancer Study. Scand J Gastroenterol. 2000;35:212–7.

53 McMahon TJ, Moon RE, Luschinger BP, Carraway MS, Stone AE, Stolp BW, Gow AJ, Pawloski JR, Watke P, Singel DJ, Piantadosi, Stamler JS. Nitric oxide in the human respiratory cycle. Nature Med. 2002;8:711–17.

54 Lane P, Gross S. Hemoglobin as a chariot for NO bioactivity. Nature Med. 2002;8:657–8.

55 Spinella PC, Carroll CL, Staff I, Gross R, Mc Quay J, Keibel L, Wade CE, Holcomb JB. Duration of red blood cell storage is associated with increased incidence of deep vein thrombosis and in hospital mortality in patients with traumatic injuries. Critical Care. 2009;13:R151.

56 Koch CG, Li L, Sessler DI, Figueroa P, Hoeltge GA, Mihaljevic T, Blackstone EH. Duration of red cell storage and complications after cardiac surgery. N Engl J Med. 2008;358:1229–39.

57 Duke WW. The relation of blood platelets to hemorrhagic disease. JAMA. 1910;60:1185–92.

58 Dente CJ, Shaz BH, Nicholas JM, et al. Improvements in early mortality and coagulopathy are sustained better in patients with blunt trauma after institution of a massive transfusion protocol in a civilian level I trauma center. J. Trauma 2009:66(6);1616–24.

59 Ballen KK, Becker PS, Yeap BY, et al. Autologous stem cell transplantation can be performed safely without the use of blood product support. J. Clin Oncol. 2004;22:4087–94.

60 Mazza P, Prudenzano A, Amurri B, et al. Myeloablative therapy and bone marrow transplantation in Jehovah's Witnesses with malignancies; single center experience. Bone Marrow Transplant. 2003;32:433–6.

61 Mazza P, Palazzo G, Amurri B, et al. Acute leukemia in Jehovah's Witnesses: a challenge for hematologists. Haematologica. 2000;85:1221–2.

62 Wandt H, Schaefer-Eckart K, Pilz B, et al. Experience with a therapeutic platelet transfusion strategy in acute myeloid leukemia: preliminary results of a randomized multicenter study after enrollment of 175 patients (abstract #20). Blood. 2009;114 (22 Suppl):14.

63 Stanworth SJ, Dyer C, Choo L, Bakrania, L, et al. for the TOPS Study Group. Do all patients with hematological malignancies and severe thrombocytopenia need prophylactic platelet transfusions? background, rationale, and design of a clinical trial (trial of platelet prophylaxis to assess the effectiveness of prophylactic platelet transfusions. Transf Med Rev. 2010;24:163–71.

64 Gaydos LA, Freireich EJ, Mantel N. The quantitative relation between platelet count and hemorrhage in patients with acute leukemia. N Engl J Med. 1962; 266:905–9.

65 Slichter SJ, Harker LA. Thrombcytopenia: mechanism and management of defects in platelet production. Clin Haematol. 1978;7:523–39.

66 Slichter SJ. Controversies in platelet transfusion therapy. Ann Rev Med. 1980; 31:509–40.

67 Dzik WH. Component Therapy Before Bedside Procedures. In: Mintz PD, ed. Transfusion Therapy: Principles and Practice, 2nd ed. Bethesda, MD:AABB Press:1–26.

68 Whitaker BI, Green J, King MR, et al. Blood supply and utilization report. United States Department of Health and Human Services. http://www.hhs .gov/ash/bloodsafet/2007nbcus_survey.pdf.

69 Hajjar LA, Vincent JL, Galas FR, et al. Transfusion requirements after cardiac surgery: the TRACS randomized controlled trial. JAMA. 2010;394:1559–67.

70 Estcourt LJ, Stanworth SJ, Murphy MF. Platelet transfusions for patients with haematological malignancies: who needs them? Br J Haematol. 2011;154(4):425.

71 Slichter SJ. New thoughts on the correct dosing of prophylactic platelet transfusions to prevent bleeding. Curr Opin Hematol. 2011;18:427–35.

72 Benson K. Criteria for diagnosing refractoriness to platlet transfusions. In: Kickler TS, Herman JH, eds. Current issues in platelet transfusion therapy and platelet alloimmunity. Bethesda, MD: AABB Press, 1999:33–61.

73 Tullis JL, Eberle WG, II, Baudenza P, Tinch R. Platelet-pheresis. Description of a new technic. Transfusion. 1968;8:154.

74 Tullis JL, Tinch RJ, Baudanza P, Gibson II, JG, DiForte S, Connelly G, Murthy K. Plateletpheresis in a disposable system. Transfusion. 1971;11:368–77.

75 Szymanski IO, Patty K, Kliman I. Efficacy of the latham blood processor to perform plateletpheresis. Transfusion. 1973;13:405–11.

76 O'Neill EM, Rowley J, Hansson-Wicher M, McCarter S, et al. Effect of 24-hour whole-blood storage on plasma clotting factors. Transfusion. 1999;39:488–91.

77 Downes KA, Wilson E, Yomtovian R, Sarode R. Serial measurement of clotting factors in thawed plasma stored for 5 days. Transfusion. 2001;41:570.

78 Yazer MH, Cortese-Hassett A, Triulzi DJ. Coagulation factor levels in plasma frozen within 24 hours of phlebotomy over 5 days of storage at 1 to 6 °C. Transfusion. 2008;48:2525–30.

79 Nilsson L, Hedner IU, Nillson IM, Robertson B. Shelf-life of banked blood and stored plasma with special reference to coagulation factors. Transfusion. 1983;23(5):377–81.

80 Kor DJ, Stubbs JR, Gajic O. Perioperative coagulation management-fresh frozen plasma. Best Pract Res Clin Anesthesiol. 2010;24:51–64; Practice Guidelines, Anesthesiology. 2006;105:198–208.

81 Roback JD, Caldwell S, Carson J, et al. Evidence-based practice guidelines for plasma transfusion. Transfusion. 2010;50:1227–39.

82 Teixeira PG, Inaba KM, Shulman I, Salim A, Demetriades D, et al. Impact of plasma transfusion in massively transfused patients. J Trauma. 2009;63:693.

83 Shaz BH, Dente CJ, Nicholas J, MacLeod JB, MacLeod JB, Young AN, et al. Increased number of coagulation products in relationship to red blood cell products transfused improves mortality in trauma patients. Transfusion. 2010; 50:493–500.

84 Wallis JP, Dzik S. Is fresh frozen plasma overtransfused in the United States? Transfusion. 2004;44:1674–5.

85 Dzik W, Rao A. Why do physicians transfuse fresh frozen plasma? Transfusion. 2004;44:1393–4.

86 Carson JL, Hebert P. Anemia and Red Blood Cell Transfusion. In: Simon TL, Snyder EL, Solheim BG, Stowell CP, Strauss RG, Petrides M, eds. Rossi's Principles of Transfusion Medicine. 4th ed. AABB published by Blackwell Publishing, 2009: 131–148.

87 Abdel-Wahab OI, Healey B, Dzik WH. Effect of fresh-frozen plasma transfusion on prothrombin time and bleeding in patients with mild coagulation abnormalities. Transfusion. 2006;46:1479–85.

88 Segal JB, Dzik WH. Paucity of studies to support that abnormal coagulation test results predict bleeding in the setting of invasive procedures: an evidence-based review. Transfusion. 2005;45:1413–25.

89 Holland LL, Foster TM, Marlar RA, Brooks JP. Fresh frozen plasma is ineffective for correcting minimally elevated international normalized ratios. Transfusion. 2005;45:1234–5.

90 Holland LL, Brooks JP. Toward rational fresh frozen plasma transfusion: The effect of plasma transfusion on coagulation test results. Am J Clin Pathol. 2006;126: 1–7.

91 Kreuz W, Meili E, Peter-Salonen K, et al. Efficacy and tolerability of a pasteurized human fibrinogen concentrate in patients with congenital fibrinogen deficiency. Transfus Apher Sci. 2005;32:247–53.

92 Callum JL, Karkouti K, Lin Y. Cryoprecipitate: the current state of knowledge. Transfus Med Rev. 2009;23:177–88.

93 Hedges SJ, Dehoney SB, Hooper JS, Amanzadeh J, Busti, AJ. Evidence-based treatment recommendations for uremic bleeding. Nat Clin Pract Nephrol. 2007;3:138–53.

94 Center for Biologics Evaluation and Research, Food and Drug administration, U.S. Department of Health and Human Services. Fatalities reported to FDA Following Blood Collection and Transfusion: Annual Summary for the FiscalYear 2012. http://www.fda.gov/BiologicsBloodVaccines/SafetyAvailability/Reporta Problem/TransfusionDonationFatalities/ucm346639.htm. Accessed 12/08/2003.

95 Zhou S, Mousavi F, Notari EP, Stramer SL, Dodd RY. Prevalence, incidence, and residual risk of major blood-borne infections among apheresis collections to the American Red Cross Blood Services, 2004 through 2008. Transfusion. 2010;50:1487–94.

96 Zou S, Dorsey KA, Notari EP, Foster GA, Krysztof DE, Musavi F, Dodd RY, Stramer SL. Prevalence, incidence, and residual risk of human immunodeficiency virus and hepatitis C virus infections among United States blood donors since the introduction of nucleic acid testing. Transfusion. 2010;50:1495–504.

97 Barnard RD. Indiscriminate transfusion: A critique of case reports illustrating hypersensitivity reactions. NY State J Med. 1951;51:2399–402.

98 Popovsky MA, Abel MD, Moore SB. Transfusion-related acute lung injury associated with passive transfer of antileukocyte antibodies. Am Rev Res Dis. 1983;128:185–9.

99 Popovsky MA, Moore SB. Diagnostic and pathogenetic considerations in transfusion-related acute lung injury. Transfusion.1985;25:573–7.

100 Kleinman S, Caulfield T, Chan P, et al. Toward an understanding of transfusion-related acute lung injury: Statement of a consensus panel. Transfusion. 2004;44:1774–89.

101 Toy P, Popovsky MA, Abraham E, et al. Transfusion-related acute lung injury: Definition and review. Crit Care Med. 2005;33:721–6.

102 Kopko PM, Popovsky MA. Transfusion-related acute lung injury. In: Popovsky MA, ed. Transfusion reactions. 3rd ed. Bethesda, MD: AABB Press; 2007, pp. 207–8.

103 Ware LB, Matthay MA. Clinical practice. Acute pulmonary edema. N Engl J Med. 2005 Dec 29;353(26):2788–96.

104 Ichimura H, Parthasarathi K, Issekutz AC, Bhattacharya J. Pressure-induced leukocyte margination in lung postcapillary venules. Am J Physiol Lung Cell Mol Physiol. 2005 Sep;289(3):L407–12.

105 Looney MR, Gropper MA, Matthay MA. Transfusion-related acute lung injury: a review. Chest. 2004 Jul;126(1):249–58.

106 Zhou L, Giacherio D, Cooling L, Davenport RD. Use of B-natriuretic peptide as a diagnostic marker in the differential diagnosis of transfusion-associated circulatory overload. Transfusion. 2005 Jul;45(7):1056–63.

107 Rana R, Vlahakis NE, Daniels CE, Jaffe AS, Klee GG, Hubmayr RD, Gajic O. B-type natriuretic peptide in the assessment of acute lung injury and cardiogenic pulmonary edema. Crit Care Med. 2006 Jul;34:1941–6.

108 Finlay HE, Cassorla L, Feiner J, Toy P. Designing and testing a computer-based screening system for transfusion-related acute lung injury. Am. J Clin Pathol. 2005;124(4):601–9.

109 Rana R, Fernández-Pérez ER, Khan SA, Rana S, Winters JL, Lesnick TG, Moore SB, Gajic O. Transfusion-related acute lung injury and pulmonary edema in critically ill patients: a retrospective study. Transfusion. 2006 Sep;46(9):1478–83.

110 Kleinman S. A perspective on transfusion-related acute lung injury two years after the Canadian Consensus Conference. Transfusion. 2006 Sep;46(9):1465–8.

111 Popovsky MA, Haley NR. Further characterization of transfusion-related acute lung injury: demographics, clinical and laboratory features, and morbidity. Immunohematology. 2000;16(4):157–9.

112 Kopko PM, Paglieroni TG, Popovsky MA, Muto KN, MacKenzie MR, Holland PV. TRALI: correlation of antigen-antibody and monocyte activation in donor-recipient pairs. Transfusion. 2003 Feb;43(2):177–84.

113 Triulzi DJ. Transfusion-related acute lung injury: an update. Hematology Am Soc Hematol Educ Program. 2006:497–501.

114 Toy P, Hollis-Perry KM, Jun J, Nakagawa M. Recipients of blood from a donor with multiple HLA antibodies: a lookback study of transfusion-related acute lung injury. Transfusion. 2004;44(12):1683–8.

115 Silliman CC, Ambruso DR, Boshkov LK. Transfusion-related acute lung injury. Blood. 2005 Mar 15;105(6):2266–73.

116 Bux J, Sachs UJ. The pathogenesis of transfusion-related acute lung injury (TRALI). Br J Haematol. 2007 Mar;136(6):788–99.

117 Silliman CC, Boshkov LK, Mehdizadehkashi Z, Elzi DJ, Dickey WO, Podlosky L, Clarke G, Ambruso DR. Transfusion-related acute lung injury: epidemiology and a prospective analysis of etiologic factors. Blood. 2003 Jan 15;101(2):454–62.

118 Eder AF, Herron, R, Strupp A, Dy B, Notari EP, Chambers LA, Dodd RY, Benjamin, RJ. Transfusion-related acute lung injury surveillance (2003-2005) and the potential impact of the selective use of plasma from male donors in the American Red Cross. Transfusion. 2007;47:599–607.

119 Triulzi DJ, Kleinman S, Kakaiya RM, Norris PJ, Steele WR, Glynn SA, et al. The effects of previous pregnancy and transfusion on HLA alloimmunization in blood donors: implications for a transfusion-related acute lung injury risk reduction strategy. Transfusion. 2009;49:1825.

120 Kopko P, Silva M, Shulman I, Kleinman S. AABB survey of transfusion-related acute lung injury policies and practices in the United States. Transfusion. 2007 Sep;47(9):1679–85.

121 Kleinman S, Grossman B, Kopko P. A national survey of transfusion-related acute lung injury risk reduction policies for platelets and plasma in the United States. Transfusion. 2010 Jun;50(6):1312–21.

122 Eder AF, Herron RM Jr, Strupp A, Dy B, White J, Notari EP, Dodd RY, Benjamin RJ. Effective reduction of transfusion-related acute lung injury risk with

male-predominant plasma strategy in the American Red Cross (2006–2008). Transfusion. 2010;50:1732–42.

123 Dodd R, Kurt RW, Ashford P, et al. Transfusion Medicine and safety. Biologicals. 2009;37:62–70.

124 Eder AF, Kennedy JM, Dy BA, et al. Limiting and detecting bacterial contamination of apheresis platelets: inlet-line diversion and increased culture volume improve component safety. Transfusion. 2009;49:1554–63.

125 Smith D, Heaton WA, Zantek ND, Good CE. PGD Study Group. Detection of bacterial contamination in prestorage culture-negative aphereiss platelets on day of issue with the Pan Genera Detection test. Transfusion. 2011;51:2573–82.

126 Pathogen Inactivation: The Penultimate Paradigm Shift. AuBuchon JP and Prowse CV, eds. Bethesda, MD: AABB Press, 2010: 1–278.

127 Murphy S, Gardner FH. Effect of storage temperature on maintenance of platelet viability–deleterious effect of refrigerated storage. N Engl J Med. 1969;280: 1094.

128 Hoffmeister KM, Felbinger TW, Falet H, et al. The clearance mechanism of chilled blood platelets. Cell. 2003;112:87.

129 Hoffmeister KM, Josefsson EC, Isaac NA, et al. Glycosylation restores survival of chilled blood platelets. Science. 2003;301:1531.

130 Spiess BD. Risks of transfusion: outcome focus. Transfusion. 44;2004:4S–14S.

131 Sanders J, Patel S, Cooper J, Berryman J, Farrar D, et al. Red blood cell storage is associated with length of stay and renal complications after cardiac surgery. Transfusion. 2011;51:2287–94.

132 Petz LD, Calhoun L, Shulman I, Johnson C, Herron R. The sickle cell haemolytic transfusion reaction syndrome. Transfusion. 1997;37:382–92.

133 Win N, Doughty H, Telfer P, Wild B, Pearson T. Hyperhaemolytic transfusion reaction in sickle cell disease. Transfusion. 2001;1:323–8.

134 Petz LD, Garratty G. Bystander immune hemolysis immune hemolytic anemias. 2nd ed. Philadelphia (PA): Churchill Livingstone; 2004, pp. 358–64.

135 Leung J, Weiskopf RB, Feiner J, et al. Electrocardiographic ST-segment changes during acute, severe isovolemic hemodilution in humans. Anesthesiology. 2000;93:1004–10.

136 Livio M, Marchesi D, Remuzzi G, et al. Uraemic blleeding: role of anaemia and beneficial effect of red cell transfusions. Lancet. 1982;320:1013–5.

137 Valeri CR, Cassidy G, Pivacek LE, et al. Anemia-induced increase in the bleeding time: implications for treatment of non-surgical blood loss. Transfusion. 2001;41:977–83.

138 Eder AF, Goldman M. How do I investigate septic transfusion reactions and blood donors with culture-positive platelet donations? Transfusion. 2011;51:1662–8.

139 Hyllyer CD, Josephson CD, Blajchman MA, Vostal JG, et al. Bacterial contamination of blood components: risks, startegies, and regulation. Hematology. 2003:575–89.

140 Park YA, Brecher ME. Bacterial contamination of blood products. In: Simon TL, Snyder EL, Solheim BG, Stowell CP, Strauss RG, Petrides M, eds. Rossi's Principles of Transfusion Medicine. 4th ed., AABB Press, Bethesda, 2009, Chapter 49; pp. 773–790.

141 Eder AF, Kennedy JM, Dy BA Notari, Ep et al. Bacterial screening of apheresis platelets and the residual risk of septic transfusion reactions: the American Red Cross experience (2004–2006). Transfusion. 2007;47:1134–42.

142 Benjamin RJ, Kline L, Dy BA, Kennedy J, Pisciotto P, et al. Bacterial contamination of whole blood-derived platelets: the introduction of sample diversion and prestorage pooling with culture testing in the American Red Cross. Transfusion. 2008;48:2348–55.

143 Linden JV, Wagner K, Voytovich E, Sheehan J. Transfusion errors in New York state: an analysis of 10 years' experience. Transfusion. 1990;40:1207–13.

144 http://www.fda.gov/BiologicsBloodVaccines/SafetyAvailability/Reporta Problem/TransfusionDonationFatalities/ucm113649.htm

145 http://www.fda.gov/downloads/BiologicsBloodVaccines/SafetyAvailability/ ReportaProblem/TransfusionDonationFatalities/UCM205620.pdf

146 http://www.fda.gov/BiologicsBloodVaccines/SafetyAvailability/Reporta Problem/TransfusionDonationFatalities/ucm254802.htm

147 http://www.medicine.uic.edu/UserFiles/Servers/Server_442934/File/2011%20 ICD-9%20Code%20Changes.pdf

148 Kleinman S, Chan P, Robillard P. Risks associated with transfusion of cellular blood components in Canada. Transfus Med Rev. 2003 Apr;17(2):120–62.

149 AABB Technical Manual 17th Edition 2011 editor, John D. Roback.

150 Goodnough LT, Shander A. Blood management. Arch Pathol Lab Med. 2007; 131:695–701.

151 Jacobs MR, Smith D, Heaton WA, Zantek ND, Good CE, PGD Study Group. Detection of bacterial contamination in prestorage culture-negative apheresis platelets on day of issue with the Pan Genera Detection test. Transfusion. 2011 Dec; 51(12):2573–82.

152 Toy P, Gajic O, Bacchetti P, et al. Transfusion-related acute lung injury: incidence and risk factors. Blood. 2012;119(7):1757–1767.

CHAPTER 4

The physiology of anemia and the threshold for blood transfusion

Senthil G. Krishna, Ahsan Syed, Jason Bryant, and Joseph D. Tobias

Department of Anesthesiology and Pain Medicine, Nationwide Children's Hospital and Department of Anesthesiology, The Ohio State University, Columbus, OH, USA

Introduction

Oxygen is the key component necessary for all aerobic processes. During the evolutionary process, as unicellular and multicellular organisms progressed to more complex forms, the process of diffusion became an ineffective means of delivering oxygen to the tissues due to the constraints of time and distance. Although simple diffusion still functions at the gas–blood interface in the lungs and the blood–tissue interface at the capillary level, a functioning cardiovascular system with a fluid capable of delivering oxygen to the tissues is needed. Since oxygen is poorly soluble in water, the process of evolution in most organisms has resulted in a compound capable of binding oxygen thereby increasing its solubility in the fluid milieu. In mammalian species, this compound is hemoglobin and it is contained in the red blood cells (RBC) or erythrocytes.

In humans and other mammalian species, the production of RBCs, otherwise known as erythropoiesis, is regulated to match the natural loss of RBCs as they age and are removed from the system in addition to any abnormal losses that occur due to hemorrhage or hemolysis. The process of erythropoiesis is regulated by erythropoietin, a glycoprotein hormone produced by the peritubular cells of the renal cortex and the liver [1]. The primary stimulus for the production and release of erythropoietin is tissue hypoxia and a decrease in oxygen delivery to the tissue beds related either to anemia or a decreased oxygen saturation [2]. This need for oxygen is sensed by a heme-containing protein which then triggers the synthesis of erythropoietin and its release into the bloodstream. The action

Transfusion-Free Medicine and Surgery, Second Edition. Edited by Nicolas Jabbour.
© 2014 John Wiley & Sons, Ltd. Published 2014 by John Wiley & Sons, Ltd.

of erythropoietin depends upon the presence of an adequate number of responsive progenitor cells, availability of sufficient iron and cofactors (folate and vitamin B_{12}) to support heme and globin synthesis, and an appropriate microenvironment to support erythrocyte development. Erythropoietin concentrations can increase up to 1000-fold in the presence of hypoxia and increase exponentially as the hemoglobin concentration decreases. However, in chronic disease states or during critical illness, the erythropoietin response may be blunted thereby making it inadequate to maintain a normal hemoglobin concentration.

Etiologies of anemia

In a general sense, anemia can be defined as a decrease in the amount of hemoglobin or a reduction of the total circulating red cell mass below normal limits. Anemia reduces the oxygen-carrying capacity of the blood and can lead to tissue hypoxia. Generally accepted values defining anemia include a hemoglobin concentration less than 13 grams/dL or a hematocrit less than 39% in an adult male and a hemoglobin concentration less than 12 grams/dL or a hematocrit less than 36% in an adult female [3]. Although these parameters are generally accepted, they should not be confused with or automatically become the "transfusion trigger" – the hemoglobin and hematocrit values at or below which packed red cells are usually ordered for transfusion. Additionally, although hemoglobin and hematocrit values are helpful in determining the presence or absence of anemia and the need for blood component therapy, factors such as the patient's ability to increase oxygen delivery to the tissues by increasing cardiac output or by increasing the oxygen extraction ratio and the status of the peripheral vascular system will affect the ultimate transfusion trigger.

The absolute hemoglobin or hematocrit value can also be affected by various pathologic processes which may mask the presence of anemia. An acutely exsanguinating patient may have normal hemoglobin and hematocrit if intravenous fluids have not been administered to replace the lost blood. Alternatively, the hemoglobin concentration may be low in a patient with a normal red cell mass who has received excessive intravenous fluids or the hemoglobin concentration may be normal when the anemia is masked by the concomitant association of dehydration. Although the measurement of the red blood cell mass is technically feasible, it requires the use of radio-labeled red blood cells [4]. As such, it is time consuming and expensive, thereby eliminating it from the clinical arena.

The etiologies of a decreased red blood cell mass or anemia can be separated into three broad categories: 1) increased losses, 2) decreased survival time or increased destruction, and 3) decreased production. Another classification, based on red cell morphology, can point to the etiology and includes: 1) microcytic, hypochromic anemias which are the result of disorders of hemoglobin synthesis and 2) macrocytic anemias which are the result of disturbances in the maturation of erythroid precursors in the bone marrow. In the perioperative period or in the acutely ill patient, more than one of the factors may come into play.

Various factors that may account for acute blood loss in the perioperative period or in the ICU patient include traumatic injury, intraoperative and postoperative surgical losses, or hemorrhage unrelated to the surgical procedure. In the latter case, gastrointestinal hemorrhage represents the most common cause of acute blood loss either from esophageal varicies, carcinomas or stress ulceration. Although the incidence of gastrointestinal bleeding in the perioperative period is generally low, certain patient populations such as burn patients, trauma victims especially those with brain injury, mechanically ventilated patients, and transplant patients are at a higher risk [5–8]. Other associated factors shown to potentially increase the incidence of GI blood loss in the ICU setting include elevated serum creatinine, absence of enteral nutrition and perhaps the choice of pharmacologic agent for GI prophylaxis [9].

Another concern regarding acute blood loss is that it is not always visible. Even intraoperatively, blood may accumulate in the peritoneal or thoracic cavity and be hidden from vision thereby making alterations in vital signs, which is a relatively late indicator of acute blood loss, the first noticeable sign. Bleeding from non-surgical sites is more likely to be hidden thereby mandating that diagnostic tests be repeated at frequent intervals to identify acute blood loss. Various "hidden" sites of bleeding include the thorax and the various intra-abdominal areas including the GI tract, and the retroperitoneum. Perhaps the most common "hidden" cause of blood loss in the ICU and pediatric setting is what is named "iatrogenic" or "nosocomial" anemia caused by repeated blood sampling for laboratory analysis. The latter can be particularly problematic in infants and young children since the amount of blood drawn from central and arterial lines (sample amount plus the "waste" amount as the line is cleared) can be significant. Limiting laboratory analyses to essential testing and returning the "waste" to the patient can help minimize this "hidden" blood loss. Another useful method is utilization whenever feasible of point of care testing (POCT) equipment that requires a very small sample size (generally less than 0.5 mL) [10]. All of these practices are frequently followed in adult Jehovah's Witness patients to limit iatrogenic blood loss and should possibly be expanded to all critically ill patients.

Anemia may also result from decreased production or accelerated destruction of red blood cells. Hemolysis of red blood cells can occur in a variety of conditions related to both immune and non-immune factors. The presence of hemolysis as the cause of anemia can be diagnosed by signs of increased red blood cell turnover including hemoglobinuria, hyperbilirubinemia, and a decreased serum haptoblobin concentration. The latter is the protein that binds free hemoglobin. These findings will co-exist with evidence of increased red blood cell production including increased reticulocyte count, provided that the patient's bone marrow is functioning adequately. As mentioned previously, especially in the perioprative period or the critical care setting, the patient's ability to respond to acute blood loss either from hemolysis or hemorrhage, by augmenting erythropoiesis may be blunted thereby imposing a production problem on top of increased losses. When red cells are destroyed, the hemoglobin molecule is converted to bilirubin, which is then conjugated via the hepatic glucuronyl transferase system to make it water soluble and allow for biliary excretion. Prior to conjugation, the bilirubin is known as unconjugated or indirect while after conjugation, it is known as conjugated or direct bilirubin. In the presence of hemolysis, when the release of bilirubin overwhelms the hepatic glucuronyl transferase system, there is an increase of the amount of free (unconjugated or indirect) bilirubin. This results in the clinical findings of scleral icterus and jaundice. This process can be accelerated when there is an associated hepatic dysfunction. Also, with significant and rapid hemolysis, the concentration of haptoglobin, an alpha-2 globulin that binds to free hemoglobin decreases. Analysis of the serum haptoglobin concentration is readily available in most hospital laboratories. In addition, when the hemoglobin concentration exceeds the haptoglobin binding capacity, the resulting free hemoglobin is filtered in the urine. A fraction of the free hemoglobin may also get oxidized to methemoglobin which is also filtered in the urine. This clinically may appear as hematuria, as the red color of hemoglobin and reddish brown color of methemoglobin are indistinguishable from that of blood. Although urine can be checked for the presence of hemoglobin, a more rapid method is to check the urine for blood which will be positive, while microscopic examination will fail to reveal any red blood cells thereby making the pigment either hemoglobin or myoglobin. The excessive urinary excretion of hemoglobin can cause renal failure, as the hemoglobin pigment crystallizes in the urine causing tubular obstruction. Treatment includes reversal of the inciting process in addition to alkalinization of the urine and maintenance of a diuresis in order to increase the amount of hemoglobin that can exist in solution in the dissolved state and promote the excretion of free hemoglobin.

Various pathologic conditions, both intrinsic and extrinsic to the red blood cell, may result in increased destruction. Disease processes that are intrinsic to the red blood cell include acute infectious processes (malaria), abnormalities of the hemoglobin molecule (hemoglobinopathies such as sickle cell disease or thalassemia), abnormalities of the red blood cell membrane (spherocytosis, paroxysmal nocturnal hemoglobinuria), enzymatic deficiencies (pyruvate kinase deficiency), and immune-mediated hemolytic disorders. The latter are diagnosed by the presence of antibodies directed against the red blood cells either on the surface of the red blood cells themselves (direct Coombs positive hemolytic anemia) or in the serum (indirect Coombs positive hemolytic anemia). Extrinsic causes of hemolysis include trauma to the red blood cells from mechanical devices (intra-aortic balloon pump, extracorporeal circulation, or mechanical heart valves), the rapid infusion of hypotonic fluids, or mechanical problems during the administration of blood products which can occur with the use of excessive pressure on the blood bag, the rapid administration of high volumes through small bore intravenous lines, or when excessive suction is used for intraoperative blood salvage. Increased red blood cell destruction can also be seen in any of a number of pathologic conditions that result in passive congestion of the spleen. This process, known as hypersplenism, results in splenomegaly and the trapping of platelets and red blood cells thereby accelerating their destruction within the spleen.

The third potential mechanism responsible for anemia is decreased production. The hallmark of this condition is anemia with an absent or low reticulocyte count. Decreased production may be the result of an inadequate substrate (deficiency of iron, folate or vitamin B_{12}) for the production of the red blood cells or primary bone marrow failure related to an acute illness or marrow infiltration from a neoplastic process. Although commonly present in the ICU population, substrate deficiency may go unrecognized and therefore untreated as the anemia is attributed to other causes [11]. Absolute iron deficiency may be present in up to one-third of patients admitted to the ICU while nutritional issues (iron, folate or vitamin B_{12} deficiency) responsible for anemia have been found in more than 10% of the ICU population [11, 12]. Guidelines addressing the provision and assessment of nutritional support therapy in critically ill patients have been published [13]. Micronutrients provided in the enteral and parenteral nutrition can reverse or prevent nutritional causes of anemia, protect against oxidative cellular injury, and enhance immune function [14].

Physiologic response to anemia

In the presence of anemia, compensatory mechanisms are called into play to maintain an adequate oxygen delivery to the tissues. These mechanisms can compensate for significant decreases in the hemoglobin concentration. However, eventually a point is reached where the compensatory mechanisms are exhausted and the oxygen consumption of the tissues becomes dependent on oxygen delivery. This is known as the critical hemoglobin.

In the normal state, oxygen transport to the tissues is dependent on processes involving both convection and diffusion. Convection is controlled by the oxygen content of the blood (CaO_2), cardiac output (CO), and the distribution of blood flow (within and between the tissue beds). The significance of the latter can be illustrated by the peripheral vasoconstriction with the resultant decrease of blood flow to the skin and muscles that occurs to maintain blood flow to the vital organs when there is a decrease in cardiac output, alteration in blood volume, or a drop in the hemoglobin concentration.

Diffusion is the primary factor regulating the movement of oxygen from the alveoli to the hemoglobin molecule in the pulmonary capillaries and the delivery of oxygen from the hemoglobin molecule to the tissues at the capillary level. In the peripheral tissues, oxygen delivery is determined by the diffusion gradient (difference between the oxygen tension of the capillary blood and the tissue bed), oxygen conductance of the tissue, and the oxy-hemoglobin affinity (status of the oxy-hemoglobin dissociation curve) [15–17]. As the other factors (diffusion gradients of oxygen from the alveoli to the hemoglobin molecule in the pulmonary capillary system and from the hemoglobin molecule to tissue bed) cannot be readily altered, the primary factor that increases the uptake of oxygen at the alveolar capillary level and augments the unloading of oxygen at the tissue level is a shift of the oxy-hemoglobin dissociation curve.

Several factors can affect the oxy-hemoglobin dissociation curve. These include body temperature, acid-base status, 2,3-diphosphoglycerate (2,3 DPG) levels, and the actual hemoglobin molecule itself [17]. The latter factor rarely comes into play except when a hemoglobinopathy (generally due to a single amino acid substitution in one of the hemoglobin chains) is present whereby there is a permanent shift of the oxy-hemoglobin dissociation curve. Such conditions are exceedingly rare and not amenable to routine therapy. Fetal hemoglobin (with two alpha and two gamma chains) results in altered binding of 2,3-DPG and an inherent leftward shift of the oxy-hemoglobin dissociation curve. This leftward shift or increased affinity of the hemoglobin molecule for oxygen results in improved oxygen uptake at the pulmonary capillary level. This is an advantage in *utero* with the normal low PaO_2 of 30–40 mmHg thereby aiding the oxygen uptake. However, the same increased affinity is a disadvantage at the tissue level as O_2 is not unloaded easily. The physiologic leftward shift of the oxy-hemoglobin dissociation curve associated with fetal hemoglobin is one of the major reasons why isovolemic hemodilution, an alternative strategy to decrease intraoperative autogenic blood transfusion, is not used in neonates and infants. In this technique, whole blood is collected presurgically and replaced with crystalloids or colloids to maintain normovolemia [18]. This technique is not tolerated well until patients are older than 6–9 months, a time when fetal hemoglobin is replaced by adult hemoglobin.

When considering the oxy-hemoglobin dissociation curve, its position relative to the normal state can be expressed as the P_{50} value or the partial pressure of oxygen at which hemoglobin is 50% saturated. In the normal state at a body temperature of 37 °C and with a pH of 7.4, the P_{50} is 26.6 mmHg. This value increases as the affinity of the hemoglobin molecule for oxygen decreases (rightward shift) and decreases when the affinity of the hemoglobin molecule for oxygen increases (leftward shift). Factors that result in a rightward shift of the curve serve to improve the unloading of oxygen at the tissue level and include factors that may occur with exercise such as increased temperature and decreased pH. However, this mechanism does not become operative until the hematocrit reaches 20% [19]. The factor responsible for the shift is an increase in 2,3-DPG in erythrocytes.

Even with effective compensatory mechanism, all organisms will have a critical hemoglobin value, below which the oxygen consumption becomes flow dependent and oxygen delivery to the tissues may fall below the clinical need. Despite the universal presence of a critical hemoglobin concentration in any patient, there is no specific hemoglobin level that can be generally identified as the value below which this occurs. As such, the decision to transfuse any patient should be individualized. Several modifying factors may increase or decrease this critical hemoglobin threshold. In various studies, laboratory animals (dogs and baboons), have tolerated a hemoglobin levels as low as 3–5 gm/dL without major adverse effects [20–22]. However, the importance of modifying features was illustrated by the fact that when dogs with experimentally induced critical coronary stenosis, were subjected to isovolemic hemodilution, electrocardiographic (ECG) evidence of ischemia was noted and myocardial dysfunction occurred even at a higher hemoglobin concentration of

6–7 gm/dL (instead of 3 to 5 gm/dL) [23]. The transfusion of red blood cells corrected both the ECG changes and the myocardial dysfunction [24].

Several mechanisms, both convection and conduction (see above), are activated to maintain tissue oxygen delivery as the hemoglobin concentration decreases. These include increased cardiac output, increased oxygen extraction at the tissue level, and a rightward shift of the oxyhemoglobin dissociation curve. In the awake state, increased cardiac output is due primarily to an increase in both stroke volume and heart rate. In the anesthetized state, stroke volume changes without a significant change in heart rate [25]. This effect is postulated to result from the effects of the anesthetic agents on the autonomic and cardiovascular systems. An increase in heart rate during general anesthesia in response to anemia is more likely to be a sign of hypovolemia or inadequate anesthesia.

In anemia, the factors responsible for the increased stroke volume include decreased systemic vascular resistance and increased venous return due to reduced whole-blood viscosity with improved microcirculatory flow [26, 27]. The increased venous return is demonstrated by an elevation of the left ventricular end-diastolic pressure [28]. The reduced viscosity of the blood noted in anemic states also results in a reduction of flow related resistance thereby decreasing afterload and improving left ventricular ejection [29, 30]. Myocardial contractility also increases, most likely because of activation of cardiac sympathetic fibers [27]. Hence, if intravascular volume is maintained, the cardiac output increase remains stable over a prolonged period of time without adverse hemodynamic consequences [31]. It is interesting to note that although the sympathetic nervous system is activated, it may only play a minor role in the observed hemodynamic changes. The increase in cardiac output with hemodilution may not require an intact autonomic system as laboratory studies in dogs have demonstrated that it occurs in spite of cardiac denervation or in the presence of β-adrenergic blockage [26, 32].

With a decrease in the hemoglobin concentration, there will be a compensatory increase in the plasma component of the blood. This alteration in the relationship between the red cell mass and the plasma volume alters blood viscosity and hence microcirculatory flow. The ratio of shear stress (force required to move a fluid) to shear rate (rate at which a fluid flows) defines viscosity. Fluids with a higher viscosity require a higher shear stress (force) to move. Fluids are considered Newtonian if they maintain a constant viscosity regardless of the velocity of the flow. In such cases, a change in force causes a proportional change in flow rate. Blood is not Newtonian because changes in flow rate produce a change in viscosity and therefore not a linear increase in flow velocity. Viscosity also changes disproportionately to changes in hematocrit in that the change in hematocrit is followed by an exponential increase or decrease in blood viscosity.

As arterial oxygen content and delivery decline, the oxygen extraction ratio increases thereby lowering the mixed venous oxygen saturation. In the resting state, peripheral oxygen extraction does not increase until the hematocrit decreases to less than 20% to 25% [32, 33]. This relationship holds true provided that hypovolemia does not occur. Although a decrease in mixed venous oxygen generally occurs at a hematocrit of 15–20%, more severe degrees of hemodilution may be tolerated in the presence of normal cardiovascular reserve. Van Woerkins and colleagues [27] demonstrated a constant mixed venous partial pressure of O_2 and oxygen saturation in dogs hemodiluted to a mean hematocrit of 9.3 ± 0.3% with an exchange of 50 mL/kg of blood. In this animal model, cardiac output doubled resulting in increased flow to all organs except the liver and adrenals. The greatest increase in flow occurred to the heart and brain. The increased flow rates and cardiac output maintained oxygen delivery down to a hematocrit of 9%. Similar stability with extreme degrees of hemodilution has been demonstrated in other clinical investigations. In a cohort of eight pediatric patients with a mean age of 12 years, Fontana et al. demonstrated no adverse effects with hemodilution to a mean hemoglobin of 3.0 grams/dL [34]. Mixed venous oxygen saturation decreased from 90.8 ± 5.4% to 72.3 ± 7.8% while oxygen extraction increased from 17.3 ± 6.2 to 44.4 ± 5.9%. No adverse effects were noted despite the extreme degree of hemodilution. Hemodilution decreases the absolute amount of hemoglobin available to carry oxygen to the tissues but this is compensated by an increase in cardiac output, usually stroke volume [35]. However, maintenance of euvolemia is mandatory to allow for the increase in stroke volume. Alternatively, if intravascular volume is not maintained, the attenuated or absent compensatory increase in stroke volume cannot compensate the hemodynamic consequences of decreased hemoglobin. In such scenarios, increasing the heart rate is the only mechanism to augment cardiac output.

These compensatory processes allow for the technique of acute normovolemic hemodilution (ANH) which is discussed in greater detail elsewhere in this textbook. Briefly, ANH involves the removal of whole blood from the patient, generally after anesthetic induction, but prior to the start of the surgical procedure and blood loss. The autologous whole blood thus obtained is replaced at a later time. The technique also ensures availability of fresh coagulation factors and active platelets, provided that the blood is maintained at room temperature. As noted above, the presence of fetal hemoglobin up to 6–8 months of age with altered oxygen binding capacity restricts the use of ANH in younger infants. Additionally, children less than 2–4 years of age may not be able to adequately increase their stroke volume to compensate for the decreased hemoglobin concentration. Despite these concerns, the technique has been shown to be beneficial in pediatric cardiac surgery [36, 37].

The compensatory mechanisms to maintain oxygen delivery during hemodilution may not be possible in patients with underlying cardiorespiratory dysfunction. The lowest tolerable hemoglobin concentration at which a decrease in the mixed venous oxygen tension occurs will also be influenced by the use of anesthetic agents and neuromuscular blocking agents. Although these agents decrease peripheral oxygen consumption, they also may blunt the compensatory cardiovascular mechanisms [38, 39].

Although it would be convenient to have a single, specific hemoglobin value to use as a transfusion trigger, several variables play into the decision to transfuse or not. Of significant importance are factors that alter the patient's ability to compensate for the low hemoglobin by increasing cardiac output or factors that place the patients at risk for coronary ischemic when these compensatory cardiovascular responses are activated. Spahn et al. [40] examined left ventricular function following LAD occlusion (decrease by 95% of the vessel's cross-sectional area) and hemodilution in dogs. Only a marginal decrease in function occurred with a hemodilution down to a hematocrit of 24.4 ± 0.1%. The authors concluded that although myocardial function is preserved with moderate hemodilution, the critical level of isovolemic hemodilution in the presence of a critical stenosis of a coronary vessel is between a hematocrit of 15% and 25%. Other factors that might compromise coronary blood flow include factors that alter the myocardial oxygen delivery–demand ratio such as decreased mean arterial pressure and left ventricular hypertrophy. Therefore, the minimal safe hematocrit in patients with compromised cardiac function is defined as the hematocrit at which coronary blood flow can no longer increase sufficiently to meet myocardial demand, which may be a difficult or impossible parameter to measure in the clinical arena.

To reiterate the above points, in spite of several attempts to quantify the critical hemoglobin level, the important points to remember are that it cannot be quantified and that the critical hemoglobin level varies in different patient populations and is influenced by various physiologic states [41–43].

The transfusion threshold

Despite the inability to identify a single number which can be used in any patient as a transfusion trigger, there has been significant work done recently in comparing higher versus lower transfusion triggers in various cohorts of patients. In a 25 center study involving 838 critically ill patients, The Transfusion Requirements in Critical Care (TRICC) Trial randomly assigned patients to a liberal transfusion group (maintenance of the hemoglobin >10 g/dl) or a restrictive transfusion group (maintenance of hemoglobin >7 g/dl) [44]. Patients in the restrictive group received half the volume of transfused blood than the patients in the liberal group. Although the overall 30-day mortality was similar in the two groups (18.7% vs. 23.3%, $p = 0.11$) subset analysis revealed significant differences. The mortality rates were significantly lower with the restrictive transfusion strategy among patients who were less acutely ill (Acute Physiology and Chronic Health Evaluation or APACHE II score $\leq$ 20, 8.7% vs. in 16.1%, $p = 0.03$) and among patients who were less than 55 years of age (5.7% vs. 13.0%, $p = 0.02$). Furthermore, the mortality rate during hospitalization was also significantly lower in the restrictive-strategy group (22.3% vs. 28.1% percent, $p = 0.05$).

Bracey et al. randomized 428 consecutive patients undergoing elective primary coronary artery bypass graft surgery to a postoperative hemoglobin level of 8 gm/dL or the usual institutional guideline of 9 gm/dL [45]. The preoperative and operative clinical characteristics as well as the intraoperative transfusion rate, were similar for both groups. However, between the groups, there was a significant difference in terms of the postoperative transfusion rate of units of red blood cells (0.9 ± 1.5 versus 1.4 ± 1.8 units, $p = 0.005$). Interestingly, there was no difference in clinical outcome including morbidity and mortality rates.

Similarly, decreased blood product use with no difference in clinical outcome has been noted in the pediatric population when comparing restrictive (hemoglobin 7 gm/dL versus liberal (hemoglobin 9.5 gm/dL) transfusion practices [46]. A subgroup analysis of patients in another study also showed no difference in outcome following surgery for congenital heart disease [47]. Remarkably, in another trail, subset analysis of postoperative surgical patients (non-cardiac) revealed a statistically significant decrease in the Pediatric ICU length of stay for the restrictive group (7.7 ± 6.6 versus 11.6 ± 10.2 days, $p = 0.03$) [48].

Finally, a meta-analysis of 10 randomized clinical trials (including the above two studies by Hebert et al. and Bracey et al.) evaluated different transfusion triggers over a 40 year period [49]. The authors suggested that a conservative transfusion trigger reduced the percentage of patients receiving red blood cell transfusions and decreased the total number of red blood cell units transfused. The analysis also suggested that conservative transfusion triggers do not adversely affect mortality, cardiac morbidity, or length of hospital stay when compared to liberal transfusion protocols. Such a strategy might be more prudent especially in countries where there is inadequate testing for blood-borne pathogens. However, a note of caution suggested that the conservative transfusion strategy should be attempted only after a thorough risk–benefit analysis in patients with coexisting cardiovascular disease due to paucity data in this group of patients [49].

Along these same lines, the ASA task force in 2006 on perioperative blood transfusion and adjuvant therapies stated that they strongly agreed red blood cells should usually be administered when the hemoglobin level is less than 6 gm/dl and red blood cells are usually unnecessary when the level is more than 10 g/dl [50]. However, they also stated that these guidelines were systematically developed recommendations that would be expected to assist the practitioner and were not intended as a standard or absolute requirements. Special considerations should also be made for the presence or absence of signs of organ ischemia and rapid blood loss and in complex situations that involve low cardiopulmonary reserve and high oxygen consumption.

Risks of blood transfusion

Over recent years, there has been a shift in the concern regarding blood transfusions away from the transmission of viral agents toward the understanding of the potential effects of allogeneic blood products on underlying immune function and the associated risks of nosocomial infections. In order to come to rational conclusions regarding transfusion triggers, an evaluation of the risk–benefit ratio for allogeneic blood products is necessary [51].

Infectious complications

In the United States, about 4 million patients receive blood products every year to treat anemia, coagulopathy, and thrombocytopenia. Every time a blood product is transfused, there exists the potential for morbidity and even mortality from infectious and non-infections complications related to the use of blood and blood products [52]. For the lay public, much of the concern regarding blood transfusion has centered on the potential for the transmission of infectious diseases, mostly the hepatitis (HBV and HCV) viruses and acquired immunodeficiency syndrome (AIDS) virus. Since 1999, with the implementation of universal donor screening for viral ribonucleic acids through nucleic acid testing, the incidence of HCV and HIV transmission attributed to infected blood products has decreased dramatically [52]. This is a result of the increased sensitivity of the tests which measure antigens of infectious agents rather than antibodies made in response to the infection. This has led to a decrease in the "window period" or the time during which a recently infected donor has not had enough time to produce a detectable antibody response [53]. Current estimates for the risk of receiving a transfusion with infected blood products are in the range of approximately 1 in 500 000 for HBV and 1 in 2 million for HCV. For HIV with nucleic acid testing, the infection window period is about 1 week and the risk of administration of HIV infected blood product is approximately 1 in 2 million [53]. Although advanced and rigorous testing has significantly decreased the risks of the transmission of an infectious agent, it has also added to the cost of blood products.

In the current scenario, of more significance is the possibility of bacterial contamination of blood products. The reported incidence of bacterial contamination of packed RBCs varies from 0.002% and 1%. It is highest for platelets with an incidence estimated at 0.04% up to 10%. Despite these alarming figures, recognized transfusion-related bacteremia is much less frequent with an incidence of only 1 in 100 000 for platelet components and 1 in 5 million for packed RBCs. And the mortality from receiving blood products contaminated with bacteria has been estimated at 1 in 500 000 for platelets and 1 in 8 million for RBCs [53]. The higher risk of bacterial contamination with platelets results from their storage at room temperature.

TRALI

Currently, noninfectious complications, namely transfusion-related acute lung injury (TRALI), transfusion associated circulatory overload (TACO) and hemolytic transfusion reaction are the leading causes of death from transfusion [54]. TRALI is defined as non-cardiogenic pulmonary edema or acute lung injury occurring within 6 hours of transfusion [54, 55]. The etiologic factors involved are thought to be the transfusion of antibodies from the donor which are directed against the host's white blood cells. These antibodies when transfused into a patient with an ongoing inflammatory process and activation of the pulmonary endothelium result in the aggregation of white blood cells in the pulmonary vasculature triggering the release of cytokines and inflammatory mediators thereby provoking acute lung injury. Since a strong association was found between the transfusion of fresh frozen plasma from multiparous women and the incidence of TRALI, several countries including the United States have started the preferential collection of plasma from male donors, and this practice has resulted in a significant reduction in the reported cases of TRALI [56].

TACO

The presenting picture in transfusion-associated circulatory overload is similar to TRALI, but the underlying phenomenon is a cardiogenic circulatory overload resulting in pulmonary edema. This is a preventable situation that can be decreased by slow transfusion rates, use of diuretics, and identification of high risk patients such as those with critical illness, cardiac disease, renal disease and infants [57].

Hemolytic reactions

Hemolytic complications may be immune or non-immune mediated. The classic immune-mediated hemolytic transfusion reaction results from an incompatibility between the administered red cells and the patient. Most are due to the result of the transfusion of incompatible red blood cells related to clerical errors. The incidence is estimated at 1 in 33 000 units with a fatality rate of 1 for every 500 000 units [57, 58]. The signs and symptoms of a hemolytic transfusion reaction are related to activation of the patient's humoral system by the fragmented red blood cells. They vary depending on the amount of incompatible blood that has been transfused. In a conscious patient, the signs and symptoms include chest pain, dyspnea, nausea, vomiting, fever, and chills. In an anesthetized or unconscious patient, the only signs and symptoms may be a change in the color of urine related to hemoglobinuria, coagulopathy, or cardiovascular disturbances. Treatment begins with immediately stopping the transfusion. Serious sequelae of a transfusion reaction include hemoglobinuria with renal failure, activation of the coagulation cascade with disseminated intravascular coagulation (DIC), respiratory failure, and circulatory collapse. Treatment is supportive and includes maintenance of an alkaline diuresis with fluid administration, loop diuretics, and mannitol. Cardiovascular instability is treated with fluid administration and direct-acting adrenergic agents as needed. Respiratory insufficiency related to acute respiratory distress syndrome may require endotracheal intubation and controlled ventilation. DIC and coagulation defects are treated as needed based on the platelet count, prothrombin time, partial thromboplastin time, and fibrinogen level. Documentation of the occurrence of a transfusion reaction is made by obtaining serum for free hemoglobin level and a direct Coomb's test as well as immediate notification and involvement of the blood bank.

Non-immune hemolytic reactions result from external forces that damage the red cells prior to or during their administration. These problems can be prevented by appropriate handling and administration of blood products. Red blood cell lysis can be caused by exposure to hypertonic or hypotonic intravenous fluids, thermal injury during blood transport or storage, and inappropriate methods of warming the blood such as placing the blood in warm water or use of a microwave oven! The signs and symptoms of non-immune transfusion reactions are dependent on the quantity of hemolyzed blood that is administered and in many cases resemble those seen with hemolytic transfusion reactions. Treatment in severe cases is the same as for immune-mediated hemolytic transfusion reactions.

Febrile reactions

Elevation in the core temperature of the recipient is one of the most commonly encountered problems during the administration of blood products. The concern with the development of fever is that it may be the first sign of an immune-mediated hemolytic transfusion reaction. When fever develops, the transfusion should be discontinued and the patient examined for other signs and symptoms of a hemolytic transfusion reaction. Although it is uncommon for fever to be the only sign of a hemolytic transfusion reaction, given the potential morbidity of such events, the transfusion should always be stopped. Other possible causes of fever during transfusion include bacterial contamination of the blood products. Isolated febrile reactions are defined as an increase in core body temperature of greater than 1 °C which cannot be attributed to sepsis or hemolytic reactions, commonly termed a febrile, non-hemolytic transfusion reaction (FNHTR). A FNHTR occurs most commonly in patients who receive numerous transfusions and remains the most common cause of fever during a transfusion. The diagnosis remains one of exclusion by eliminating the possibility of a hemolytic transfusion reaction and bacterial contamination of the transfused blood product. The incidence of FNHTR is related to the patient's history of previous exposure to blood products and the specific component used (1% for packed RBCs versus 20–30% for platelets). FNHTRs are immunologically mediated reactions related to the presence of antibodies in the recipient's plasma to donor's white blood cell antigens. The antibody-antigen reaction leads to the release of endogenous pyrogens from the white blood cells. Pretreating the patient with antihistamines and antipyretics was used routinely in the past, but is no longer recommended. Rather, nowadays, the focus is on the preventive methods that can decrease the amount of causative WBC antigen content in the transfused blood products. The use of leukocyte depletion filters for transfusion has decreased the occurrence of FNHTRs. In many cases, this is performed in the blood bank since the use of these filters during transfusion can significantly slow the rate at which the blood can be transfused.

Metabolic effects

Additional complications of transfusion include the cumulative metabolic effects, the incidence of which increases with the number of units administered. These effects may manifest as hypothermia, metabolic alterations (hypocalcemia, acidosis, hyperkalemia), shift of the oxy-hemoglobin dissociation curve, and coagulation disturbances. With the administration of more than 10–15 mL/kg of any blood product over less than 1 hour, use of a standard blood warming device is recommended to avoid hypothermia. After 2–3 weeks of storage, potassium concentrations of packed red blood cells may reach levels of 20–30 mEq/L. Although there is a limited amount of plasma contained in packed red blood cells, its rapid administration ($\geq$100 mL/min) can limit the time for potassium redistribution and elimination. During rapid administration of blood products, the electrocardiogram should be monitored for signs suggestive of hyperkalemia which include arrhythmias, ST segment and T wave changes. Issues of hyperkalemia are of significant concern especially in neonates and infants and in patients with renal dysfunction or pre-existing hyperkalemia. When transfusion is required in these patients, red blood cells can be washed prior to administration to remove the excess plasma and decrease the potassium concentration of the administered blood product. Alternatively, the blood bank can also frequently provide volume reduced red blood cells where the supernatant (which is rich in potassium) has been removed.

A second metabolic consequence of transfusion is hypocalcemia related to the binding of calcium by the citrate which is used in blood products as an anticoagulant. In practice, especially with slower transfusion rate or low volume replacement, the citrate is metabolized in the liver and hypocalcemia is usually not an issue. However, either hepatic dysfunction leading to inadequate citrate clearance or rapid transfusion can result in citrate overload and precipitate hypocalcemia. Signs and symptoms of hypocalcemia include a prolongation of the QT interval on the ECG, hypotension, and impaired myocardial contractility. The latter effects may be magnified by associated acidosis and hypothermia. In addition to binding calcium, citrate also binds magnesium leading to hypomagnesemia [59]. The latter may impair the normal regulatory responses to hypocalcemia including release of parathormone.

Packed red blood cells also become more acidotic with time as a result of the citrate used as an anticoagulant and the normal metabolic processes of the red blood cells with the production of lactate. With rapid administration, there may be inadequate time for the buffering of the acid load leading to clinically significant acidosis resulting in poor myocardial contractility. Periodic measurement of arterial or venous blood gases and correction of the acidosis with sodium bicarbonate may be needed. The issues of hyperkalemia and acidosis have led some hospital's blood banking committees to institute protocols suggesting the use of relatively fresh blood (less than 7–10 days) in neonates and infants who may be less able to tolerate and compensate the acid and potassium load.

Immunological effects

With the transfusion of allogeneic blood products, immunocompetent T cells are also transfused. Although generally cleared by the host, in certain populations, these T cells may initiate a graft-versus-host response similar to that which occurs with bone marrow transplantation. This may occur more frequently in patients with altered cellular immunity related to congenital defects (DiGeorge syndrome), prematurity, or in patients on chemotherapeutic and immunosuppressive regimens. The irradiation of blood products inactivates the viable lymphocytes and decreases the immunological effects. Irradiation of blood products requires the appropriate equipment which most blood banking facilities have and can be accomplished in a matter of minutes. In general, no significant alteration in the integrity or composition of the blood product occurs; however, there will be an increase in the potassium concentration, which increases even further with time thereby mandating the administration of the irradiated blood product as soon as possible [60].

Several recent investigations also document the potential role of blood product administration on the host's immune system and transfusion-related immunomodulation (TRIM), nosocomial infections and recurrences of malignancy [61–69]. The immunosuppressive effects of transfusion were once thought to be beneficial in the transplant recipient, given the decreased risk of rejection in previously transfused patients [61–63]. However, it is controversial when one also considers the impact of transfusion on nosocomial infections and recurrence of malignancy [64–69]. The increased incidence of infections following the administration of allogeneic blood products has been demonstrated in patients undergoing orthopedic, abdominal and cardiac procedures [64, 65, 67]. These infections have been shown to increase the morbidity and mortality and also the length of ICU stay and hospital costs. Although the potential deleterious role of immunosuppression related to allogeneic blood products is not fully accepted by all experts in the field of transfusion medicine, these data appear to be striking enough that consideration should be given to the potential immunologic impact when evaluating the risk–benefit rationale of transfusion therapy.

Summary

In higher organisms, diffusion is not capable of meeting the oxygen demands of the tissues because of the constraints of time and distance.

Evolution has provided a mechanism whereby oxygen can be delivered to tissues by means of a transfer system that includes an oxygen-binding component (hemoglobin) and a delivery mechanism (cardiovascular system). Although normal hemoglobin levels range from 12 to 14 grams/dL, like many other systems, a redundancy is built in to allow for protection through compensatory mechanisms when homeostasis is altered.

The recent years have seen a move toward limitation of blood products with the goal of providing bloodless surgery. This interest was initially sparked by concerns over the transmission of infectious diseases from the administration of allogeneic blood products. Despite the increased safety of the blood pool with improved screening for the presence of infectious pathogens, a renewed interest in bloodless surgery has been created due to other associated complications of blood product use including TRALI, TACO and hemolytic transfusion reactions. There is also substantial data suggesting the potential immunosuppressive effects of blood products with the potential for increased nosocomial infections and cancer recurrence, especially lymphoma.

As to what is the transfusion level or trigger hemoglobin, each patient must be considered individually based on the associated co-morbid features. In the absence of end-organ dysfunction or disease, clinical data suggest that patients may tolerate a hemoglobin value as low as 5–6 gm/dL without any major problems. And even in the critically ill ICU patients a marginally higher hemoglobin value of 7–8 gm/dL have been shown to be safe. However, associated co-morbid cardiovascular disease may mandate higher hemoglobin values to avoid the risks of coronary ischemia, cardiopulmonary dysfunction and/or compromised coronary perfusion. But even in this population values in excess of 9–10 gm/dL are generally not necessary. With such information in mind, simple maneuvers such as accepting a lower transfusion trigger is a key component in limiting the need for allogeneic blood products.

References

1 Jelkmann W. Erythropoietin: structure, control of production, and function. Physiol Rev. 1992;72:449–89.
2 Ebert BL, Bunn HF. Regulation of the erythropoietin gene. Blood. 1999;94:1864–77.
3 Greenberg AG. Pathophysiology of anemia. Am J Med. 1996;101:7S–11S.
4 Vincent JL, Sakr Y, Creteur J. Anemia in the intensive care unit. Can J Anaesth. 2003;50:S53–9.
5 Pimentel M, Roberts DE, Bernstein CN, et al. Clinically significant gastrointestinal bleeding in critically ill patients in an era of GI prophylaxis. Am J Gastroenterol. 2000;95:2801–6.

6 Devlin JW, Ben Menachem T, Ulep SK, et al. Stress ulcer prophylaxis in medical ICU patients: annual utilization in relation to the incidence of endoscopically proven stress ulceration. Ann Pharmacother. 1998;32:869–74.

7 Czaja AJ, McAlhany JC, Pruitt BA Jr. Acute gastrointestinal disease after thermal injury. An endoscopic evaluation of incidence and natural history. New Engl J Med. 1974;291:925–9.

8 Schiessel R, Starlinger M, Wolf A, et al. Failure of cimetidine to prevent gastroduodenal ulceration and bleeding after renal transplantation. Surgery. 1981;90:456–8.

9 Cook D, Heyland D, Griffith L, et al. Risk factors for clinically important upper gastrointestinal bleeding in patients requiring mechanical ventilation. Crit Care Med. 1999;27:2812–7.

10 Sista R, Hua Z, Thawar P, Sudarsan A. Development of a digital microfluid platform for point of care testing. Lab Chip. 2008;8:2091–104.

11 Streiff RR. Anemia and nutritional deficiency in the acutely ill hospitalized patients. Med Clin North Am. 1993;77:911–89.

12 Rodriguez RM, Corwin HL, Gettinger A, et al. Nutritional deficiencies and blunted erythropoietin response as causes of the anemia of critical illness. J Crit Care. 2001;16:36–41.

13 Martindale M, McClave S, Vincent V, McCarthy M. Guidelines for the provision and assessment of nutrition support therapy in the adult critically ill patient: Society of Critical Care Medicine and American Society for Parentral and Enteral Nutrition: Executive Summary. Crit Care Med. 2009;37:1757–61.

14 Gerlach A, Murphy C. An update on nutrition support in the critically ill. J Pharm Pract. 2011;24:70–7.

15 Groebe K, Thews G. Basic mechanisms of diffusive and diffusion related oxygen transport in biological systems: a review. Adv Exp Med Biol. 1992;317:21–33.

16 Trouwburst A, Van Woerkins ECSM, Tenbrinck R. Hemodilution and oxygen transport. Adv Exp Med Biol. 1992;317:431–40.

17 Marschner JP, Rietbrock N. Oxygen release kinetics in healthy subjects and diabetic patients. I: The role of 2,3-diphosphoglycerate. Int J Clin Pharmacol Ther. 1994;32:533–5.

18 Spahn DR, Casutt M. Eliminating blood transfusions: new aspects and perspectives. Anesthesiology. 2000;93:242–55.

19 Sunder-Plassman L, Kessler M, Jesch F. Acute normovolemic hemodilution: changes in tissue oxygen supply and hemoglobin-oxygen affinity. Bibl Haematol. 1975;41:44–53.

20 Levine E, Rosen A, Sehgal L, et al. Physiologic effects of acute anemia: Implications for a reduced transfusion trigger. Transfusion. 1990;30:11–14.

21 Wilkerson DK, Rosen AL, Sehgal LR, et al. Limits of cardiac compensation in anemia baboons. Surgery. 1988;103:665-670.

22 Geha AS. Coronary and cardiovascular dynamics and oxygen availability during acute normovolemic anemia. Surgery. 1976;80:47–53.

23 Geha AS, Baue AE. Graded coronary stenosis and coronary flow during acute normovolemic hemodilution. World J Surg. 1978;2:645–52.

24 Anderson HT, Kessinger JM, McFarland WJ Jr, et al. The response of hypertrophied heart to acute anemia and coronary stenosis. Surgery. 1978;84:8–15.

25 Ickx BE, Rigolet M, Van der Linden P. Cardiovascular and metabolic response to acute normovolemic anemia. Effects of anesthesia. Anesthesiology. 2000;93:1011–6.

26 Glick G, Plauth WH, Braunwald E. Role of the autonomic nervous system in the circulatory response to acutely induced anemia in unanesthetized dogs. J Clin Invest. 1964;43:2112–24.

27 Van Woerkins J, Trouborst A, Duncker DJ. Catecholamines and regional hemodynamics during isovolemic hemodilution alone and in combination with adenosine-induced controlled hypotension. J Appl Phys. 1992;72:760–9.

28 Guyton AC, Richardson TQ. Effect of hematocrit on venous return. Circ Res. 1961;9:157–65.

29 Crystal GJ, Rooney MW, Salem MR. Regional hemodynamics and oxygen supply during isovolemic hemodilution alone and in combination with adenosine-induced controlled hypotension. Anesth Analg. 1988;67:211–8.

30 Laks H, Pilon RN, Klovekorn WP, et al. Acute normovolemic hemodilution: effects on hemodynamics, oxygen, transport, and lung water in anesthetized man. Surg Forum. 1974;180:103–9.

31 Bowens C, Spahn DR, Frasco PE, et al. Hemodilution induces stable changes in global cardiovascular and regional myocardial function. Anesth Analg. 1993;76:1027–32.

32 Tarnow J, Eberlein HJ, Hess E, et al. Hemodynamic interactions of hemodilution anaesthesia, propranolol pretreatment and hypovolemia. I: Systemic Circulation. Basic Res Cardiol. 1979;74:109–22.

33 Robertie PG, Gravlee GP. Safe limits of isovolemic hemodilution and recommendation for erythrocyte transfusion. Int Anesthesiol Clin. 1990;28:197–203.

34 Fontana JL, Welborn L, Mongan PD, et al. Oxygen consumption and cardiovascular function in children during profound intraoperative normovolemic hemodilution. Anesth Analg. 1995;80:219–25.

35 Verma S, Eisses M, Richards M. Blood conservation strategies in pediatric anesthesia. Anesthesiol Clin. 2009;27:337–51.

36 Friesen RH, Perryman KM, Weigers KR, et al. A trial of fresh autologous whole blood to treat dilutional coagulopathy following cardiopulmonary bypass in infants. Paediatr Anaesth. 2006;16:429–35.

37 Hans P, Collin V, Bonhomme V, et al. Evaluation of acute normovolemic hemodilution for surgical repair of craniosynostosis. J Neurosurg Anesthesiol. 2000;12:33–6.

38 Van der Linden P, De Hert S, Mathieu N, et al. Tolerance to acute hemodilution: Effect of anesthetic depth. Anesthesiology. 2003;99:97–104.

39 Gillies IDS. Anemia and anaesthesia. Br J Anaesth. 1974;46:589–602.

40 Spahn DR, Smith LR, McRae RL, Leone BJ. Effects of acute isovolemic hemodilution and anesthesia on regional function in left ventricular myocardium with compromised coronary blood flow. Acta Anaesthesiol Scand. 1992;36:628–36.

41 Simon TL, Alverson DC, AuBuchon J, et al. Practice parameter for the use of red blood cell transfusions: developed by the Red Blood Cell Administration Practice Guideline Development Task Force of the College of American Pathologists. Arch Pathol Lab Med. 1998;122:130–8.

42 Mallett SV, Peachey TD, Sanehi O, et al. Reducing red blood cell transfusion in elective surgical patients: the role of audit and practice guidelines. Anaesthesia. 2000;55:1013–9.

43 Gibson BE, Todd A, Roberts I, et al. Transfusion guidelines for neonates and older children. Br J Haematol. 2004;124:433–53.

44 Hebert PC, Wells G, Blajchman MA, et al. A multicenter, randomized, controlled clinical trial of transfusion requirements in critical care. N Engl J Med. 1999;340:409–17.

45 Bracey AW, Radovancevic R, Riggs SA, et al. Lowering the hemoglobin threshold for transfusion in coronary artery bypass procedures: Effect on patient outcome. Transfusion. 1999;39:1070–7.

46 Lacroix J, Hébert PC, Hutchison JS, et al. Transfusion strategies for patients in pediatric intensive care units. N Engl J Med. 2007;356:1609–19.

47 Willems A, Harrington K, Lacroix J, et al. Comparison of two red-cell transfusion strategies after pediatric cardiac surgery: a subgroup analysis. Crit Care Med. 2010;38:649–56.

48 Rouette J, Trottier H, Ducruet T, et al. Red blood cell transfusion threshold in postsurgical pediatric intensive care patients: a randomized clinical trial. Ann Surg. 2010;251:421–7.

49 Carson JL, Hill S, Carless P, Hébert P, Henry D. Transfusion triggers: a systematic review of the literature. Transfus Med Rev. 2002;16:187–99.

50 American Society of Anesthesiologists Task Force on Perioperative Blood Transfusion and Adjuvant Therapies. Practice guidelines for perioperative blood transfusion and adjuvant therapies: an updated report by the American Society of Anesthesiologists Task Force on Perioperative Blood Transfusion and Adjuvant Therapies. Anesthesiology. 2006;105:198–208.

51 Squires JE. Risks of transfusion. South Med J. 2011;104:762–9.

52 Zou S, Dorsey KA, Notari EP, Foster GA. Prevalence, incidence, and residual risk of human immunodeficiency virus and hepatitis C virus infections among United States blood donors since the introduction of nucleic acid testing. Transfusion. 2010;50:1495–504.

53 Perkins HA, Busch MP. Transfusion-associated infections: 50 years of relentless challenges and remarkable progress. Transfusion. 2010;50:2080–99.

54 Gilliss BM, Looney MR, Gropper MA. Reducing noninfectious risks of blood transfusion. Anesthesiology. 2011;115:635–49.

55 Lavoie J. Blood transfusion risks and alternative strategies in pediatric patients. Paediatr Anaesth. 2011;21:14–24.

56 Eder AF, Herron RM Jr, Strupp A, Dy B, White J. Effective reduction of transfusion-related acute lung injury risk with male-predominant plasma strategy in the American Red Cross (2006–2008). Transfusion. 2010;50:1732–42.

57 Linden JV, Kaplan HS. Transfusion errors: Cause and effects. Trans Med Rev. 1994;8:169–83.

58 Linden JV, Tourault MA, Schribner CL. Decrease in frequency of transfusion fatalities. Transfusion. 1997;37:243–4.

59 McLellan B, Reid R, Lane P. Massive blood transfusion causing hypomagnesemia. Crit Care Med. 1984;12:146–7.

60 Rivet C, Baxter A, Rock G. Potassium levels in irradiated blood. Transfusion. 1989;29:185–6.

61 Opelz G, Sengar DP, Mickey MR, Terasaki PI. Effect of blood transfusions on subsequent kidney transplants. Transplant Proc. 1973; 5:253–9.

62 Vamvakas EC. Transfusion-associated cancer recurrence and postoperative infection: meta-analysis of randomized, controlled clinical trials. Transfusion. 1996;36:175–86.

63 Opelz G, Vanrenterghem Y, Kirste G, et al. Prospective evaluation of pretransplant blood transfusions in cadaver kidney recipients. Transplantation. 1997;63:964–7.

64 Houbiers JG, van de Velde CJ, Pahlplatz P, et al. Transfusion of red cells is associated with increased incidence of bacterial infection after colorectal surgery: A prospective study. Transfusion. 1997;37:126–34.

65 Ryan T, McCarthy JF, Rady MY, et al. Early bloodstream infection after cardiopulmonary bypass: Frequency rate, risk factors, and implications. Crit Care Med. 1997;25:2009–14.

66 Amato AC, Pescatori M. Effect of perioperative blood transfusion on recurrence of colorectal cancer: meta-analysis stratified on risk factors. Dis Colon Rectum. 1998;41:570–85.

67 Innerhofer P, Walleczek C, Luz G, et al. Transfusion of buffy coat-depleted blood components and risk of postoperative infection in orthopedic patients. Transfusion. 1999;39:625–32.

68 Vamvakas EC, Blajchman MA. Universal WBC reduction: The case for and against. Transfusion. 2001;41:691–712.

69 Vamvakas EC, Blajchman MA. Transfusion-related immunomodulation (TRIM): An update. Blood Rev. 2007;21:327–48.

CHAPTER 5

Blood transfusion in surgery

Sharad Sharma[1], Lance W Griffin[2], and Nicolas Jabbour[3]

[1]Department of Transplant Surgery, UTMB, Galveston, TX, USA
[2]University of Texas Medical Branch, Galveston, TX, USA
[3]Service de Chirurgie et Transplantation Abdominale, Cliniques Universitaires
Saint-Luc, Bruxelles, Belgium

Introduction

This chapter will serve as an overall guide to understanding the availability, cost, and usage of blood products in the surgical discipline. This
discussion will include techniques used during operative procedures,
such as cell saver and acute normovolemic hemodilution, which play
a role in minimizing the need for blood products. We will also address
post-operative issues regarding careful use of blood testing and an understanding of the relationship between oxygen consumption and delivery.
In addition, artificial blood products and their potential applications
in the future will be considered. The potential benefits of avoidance of
unnecessary blood transfusion in surgical patients will be explained with
the express goal of improving patient outcomes in the future.

The cost-effectiveness of blood products: a surgical perspective

Traditional notions about blood transfusions, including arbitrary cutoff
values of hemoglobin and theories supporting multiple unit transfusions,
have been challenged in recent years in light of a better understanding
of blood products in surgical and medical practice [1]. While the use of
blood products can be lifesaving, it comes at a price. Blood is a precious,
fast-depleting commodity with a sizable price tag and significant adverse
effects associated with it, like any other intervention in medicine.

The wide-ranging impact of transfusion-free surgery cannot be fully
realized before considering the status of blood donation and transfusion in

Transfusion-Free Medicine and Surgery, Second Edition. Edited by Nicolas Jabbour.
© 2014 John Wiley & Sons, Ltd. Published 2014 by John Wiley & Sons, Ltd.

the United States. Reports from the National Blood Data Resource Center reveal that in 2008 approximately fifteen million units of blood were used in the treatment of five million eight hundred thousand patients, most of whom were older than 65 [2]. As the current population of the United States ages, these blood requirements will only continue to rise. If this trend is not met by supply, and that is not likely given the increasing exclusionary criteria placed on collected blood along with declining donation rates, shortages are predicted to occur by the year 2030. This shortage of blood products will likely have a deleterious effect on the public's well-being, especially during unforeseen events such as trauma, acts of terrorism, and war. Often, the survival of a trauma patient is related directly to the adequate availability of blood products.

The cost of the practice of blood transfusion includes more than just acquisition, banking, work-up, and dispensation of blood. Additional indirect expenditures arise surrounding the administration of blood products, which encompass, for example, the work-up and treatment of side effects of blood transfusion. Fever, the most common side effect of homologous blood transfusion, occurs at a rate of 1% to 2% and, in many instances, requires extensive radiographic and microbiologic evaluations. Taking into account all of these factors, the burden blood transfusion bears to society can amount to several billion dollars a year. Surgery influences this value significantly since greater than half of all transfused blood is administered to surgical patients.

Financial concerns aside, transfusion-associated health risks are an important consideration as well. Screening has significantly reduced the rate of viral transmission but the risk has not been eliminated [3]. Further, there has been little improvement in the risk of bacterial sepsis. The risk of clinically apparent sepsis following blood transfusion exceeds the risk of HIV, HBV, and HCV transmission [4]. Transmission of prion-associated diseases, such as Creutzfeldt–Jakob disease, and of parasitic infections, such as Leishmaniasis or Chagas' disease, has been documented in small but significant numbers. ABO incompatibility occurs at a rate of one in 33 000 and acute anaphylaxis at one in 20 000 to 50 000 [3]. Transfusion-related acute lung injury (TRALI) is another rare, poorly understood, but potentially fatal, complication of blood transfusion.

Additionally, the immunomodulatory effects of allogenic blood can have adverse consequences. A number of studies have indicated that homologous blood transfusions may increase the risk of post-operative bacterial infection [3, 5, 6]. In a meta-analysis of prospective trials comparing transfused versus non-transfused patients, Hill et al. showed that transfused patients, especially trauma victims, were 3.45 times more likely to develop a post-operative bacterial infection [7]. In a prospective study of transfusion in intensive care units, Shorr et al. showed by multivariate analyses that packed red cell transfusion independently increases the risk of ventilator-associated pneumonia [8]. Several studies also have documented a strong association between blood transfusion and cancer recurrence, although a causal relation has not been established. In a meta-analysis, Vamvakas reported a 3.6 times increase in risk of cancer recurrence with blood transfusion in head and neck cancers, 2.4 times in gastric cancers, and 1.6 times in prostate cancers [9]. Similarly, while examining colorectal cancers, Amato et al. reported a 1.68 times increase in odds of recurrence with blood transfusion, irrespective of all patient or disease-specific factors [10]. The risk of recurrence was directly related to the number of units transfused, with transfusion of greater than three units resulting in double the risk associated with transfusion of one or two units. Following transfusion of at least two units of allogenic blood, the serum of patients begins to show a significant increase in vascular endothelial growth factor and a concomitant drop in endostatin, thereby rendering it favorable for angiogenesis – a potential mechanism that mediates cancer recurrence. This angiogenic potential of the serum has been documented *in vitro* by a significant increase in endothelial cell proliferation and whole assay angiogenesis [11].

Blood product transfusions are similar to organ transplantation and must be treated with as much care, attention and consideration, and must be used only when absolutely indicated. The goal of utilizing blood products should be limited to improving tissue oxygenation and facilitating coagulation.

Pre-operative optimization of the surgical patient

Pre-operative optimization is not a novel surgical practice. A number of patient variables have been studied in association with surgical outcome. Much focus has been placed on the link between a patient's nutritional status and the morbidity and mortality from surgical procedures. Interestingly, the need for transfusion during surgery also has been linked to a patient's nutritional status. Stephenson et al. categorized 99 patients with end-stage liver disease requiring liver transplantation into mild, moderate, and severe malnutrition based on subjective global assessment of nutritional status [12]. After correcting for several patient variables such as age, sex, platelet count, serum creatinine, and hemoglobin levels, those with severe malnutrition were found to require significantly more packed red blood cell transfusion than those in the mild and moderate categories.

Traditionally, less emphasis has been placed on a patient's hematological status prior to surgery. Patients who are anemic prior to surgery are clearly more likely to receive transfusions than those who are not. In fact, in a multivariate analysis conducted in the study described above, the only other factor predictive of intra-operative transfusion was pre-operative hemoglobin levels [12]. The surgical community is not in the habit of enhancing hematologic values prior to surgery, a fact partially due to the perception of safety and universal availability of blood products. Anemia and coagulopathy should be addressed decisively pre-operatively to improve the patient's hemoglobin levels prior to surgery and to minimize operative blood loss. Clotting disorders as a result of vitamin K deficiency, for example, secondary to biliary obstruction, long-term parenteral nutrition, etc., should be alleviated via supplementation. When coagulopathy due to liver disease prevents response to this intervention, components of the clotting pathway may need to be replenished directly.

Anemia, with a wide array of causative factors such as chronic disease, bone marrow suppression, malnutrition, iron deficiency, hemolysis etc., can be a particular challenge to manage. One of the preferred approaches to managing pre-operative anemia is directly enhancing the patient's red cell mass, which, in many ways, can be considered equivalent to autologous donation without the use of blood banking. We view the patient's bone marrow as an untapped well of blood products and reason that before asking of the general public, the patient can and should serve as a source of this precious product. By carefully and adequately stimulating the bone marrow, patients can produce an average of one unit of blood per week, resulting in more than five units of blood within four to six weeks [13].

To stimulate the bone marrow, it is important to understand the cause of anemia and also provide the bone marrow with the elements necessary for synthesis. Recombinant human erythropoietin (rHuEPO) has gained widespread popularity to enhance the possibility of autologous donation in a number of orthopedic surgical procedures as well as for Jehovah's Witness patients [14–18]. Subcutaneous administration of rHuEPO (with a half-life of 19 to 22 hours) has been preferred to the intravenous route (with half-life of 4 to 5 hours) due to its increased ability to maintain effective stimulatory levels in the blood, cost-effectiveness, and greater convenience of application [19]. In addition, a dosing interval of 72 hours has been reported to result in greater reticulocyte responses than an interval of 24 hours, with a maximum absolute dose of 900 IU/kg/week [20]. Bone marrow stimulation with rHuEPO can be employed in most patients even in the presence of malnutrition, liver disease, or portal hypertension.

However, in response to inflammation either from chronic or acute infections or neoplasm, the stimulatory effect of rHuEPO may be blunted. Kalantar-Zadeh et al. examined erythropoietic responsiveness in a cohort of patients with anemia secondary to end-stage renal disease, a condition normally treated with rHuEPO [21]. During a 13-week period, patients were given, on average, 217 U/kg of rHuEPO along with iron supplementation. Patients with higher Malnutrition Inflammation Scores (MIS) and increased inflammatory markers, such as IL-6, were found to have greater resistance to treatment. Ozguroglu et al. studied the effect of endogenous erythropoietin in 40 anemic cancer patients and in 20 otherwise healthy patients with iron deficiency anemia [22]. They found a diminished response in the cancer patients at all observed hemoglobin levels. In addition, because the anemic cancer patients were found to have higher measured levels of erythropoietin than 34 cancer patients without anemia, the study attributed the findings to a blunted response to erythropoietin. Although the precise pathophysiology of this clinical effect has not been fully elucidated, it is believed that inflammatory cytokines, such as IL-1 and TNFα, directly inhibit erythropoiesis and induce iron sequestration by the reticuloendothelial system, promoting the synthesis of ferritin at the expense of red cell formation [23].

In addition to stimulation, supplemental minerals and vitamins are required for efficient erythropoiesis. Several studies have evaluated the effects of iron supplementation. Erythropoietin has been shown to hasten the depletion of iron stores by phlebotomy in iron-replete adults [24]. Physiologically normal amounts of mobilizable iron are frequently insufficient to meet the needs of the expanded pool of transferrin receptors on red cell precursors, resulting in relative iron deficiency and limiting rHuEPO-driven erythropoiesis [24]. Iron requirements (in milligrams) can be estimated by multiplying the factor of 150 by the amount of desired elevation in hemoglobin (in g/dl). Pre-treatment iron stores can be evaluated by measuring serum iron, total iron binding capacity, transferrin saturation, and ferritin levels. A functional iron deficiency occurs when transferrin saturation falls below 20%, the serum ferritin declines to less than 100 µg/L, or the proportion of hypochromic RBCs rises above 10%. Daily 200 mg doses of oral elemental iron, or 900 mg of iron sulfate, can be given during the first four to six weeks of treatment. The enteral route of supplementation, however, may not meet the requirements of a highly promoted erythropoiesis and may be poorly tolerated by patients. As a result, additional intravenous iron dextran or iron saccharate at a dose of 200 mg per week for three to four weeks may help meet the accelerated needs. Administration of parenteral iron, however, is associated with rare but potentially serious complications including life-threatening anaphylactoid reactions and possibly acute iron toxicity, a risk that may be even smaller with the use of the saccharate form [25].

Attempts must be made pre-operatively to minimize sources of blood loss. For example, in patients with massive esophageal varices or severe portal hypertension, minimizing pre-operative blood loss may be just as important as the correction of anemia. A discriminatory use of a transjugular intrahepatic portosystemic shunt (TIPS) may be indicated in such select cases.

Intra-operative approach to blood conservation

There are some cardinal principles that need to be adhered to intra-operatively to minimize blood loss and preclude the need for transfusions. These include sound surgical judgment, accurate surgical technique, application of acute normovolemic hemodilution (ANH) and blood salvage techniques, optimizing the coagulation system, etc.

A. Surgical judgment

Peri-operative decision making and judgment are as important as the surgical technique and are crucial to successful outcomes. Good decision making involves flexibility and the acknowledgment that operative procedures should not proceed under unfavorable circumstances. At the time of writing, with the routine application of highly innovative technology to the practice of medicine, less focus is directed toward clinical management and thought processes involved in overall patient care. Clearly, there is no substitute for good surgical judgment, and astute clinical management continues to play a pivotal role in patient outcome [26].

B. Surgical technique

As long as a patient's hemoglobin is sufficient to provide tissues with adequate oxygen, the only indication for blood transfusion is to replace operative blood loss. Transfusion is not a therapeutic goal in itself. Of all the indications for intra-operative blood product utilization, most are related directly to the amount of blood lost. Surgeons, therefore, are the only health care providers that can effectively decrease the use of blood products. To provide a safe, transfusion-free surgical practice, therefore, surgical techniques should be driven by a zero tolerance for blood loss. Precise technique and meticulous hemostasis must be the cornerstones of any surgical procedure. The patient's coagulation system should not be relied upon, and simple physical packing, even of minor bleeding, should not be considered sufficient. We recommend resorting to more dependable measures such as argon beam electrocautery, suture ligation, etc.

In many cases, patients with psychosocial reasons for wishing to avoid blood product delivery require innovative thinking and extra attention on the conservation of blood loss to avoid such transfusion. We believe that application of these principles across nature or type of procedure should be feasible and should result in diminished blood product utilization following any surgical procedure.

C. Intra-operative cell salvage (ICS)

ICS serves as an effective tool in blood conservation by allowing the retrieval and reuse of blood lost in the operative field. Several studies have documented the intact structure and function of red cells recycled in this fashion. Electron microscopy has revealed only minor alterations in red cell morphology with ICS [27]. The red cells maintain near normal survival and 2,3 diphosphoglycerate concentration as well [28, 29]. ICS is regarded as a reliable method of auto-transfusion and is embraced even by Jehovah's Witness patients if administered via a contained system continuous with the patient at all times. ICS has been successfully employed to reduce the need for allogenic blood in a wide variety of surgical procedures including gynecologic, cardiac, orthopedic, and liver transplant surgery [30–33]. McGill et al., in a randomized controlled trial, documented that when undertaken with ICS, patients undergoing coronary artery bypass were 0.47 times less likely to require blood products [34].

However, the use of ICS brings with it a new set of important considerations prior to its integration into any program. Probably the most controversial issue surrounding ICS is cost. The cell-saver device, associated components and disposables, and the services of a perfusionist add up to a significant financial undertaking. Several studies have evaluated the ICS economic burden in comparison to blood transfusions [35, 36]. Shuhaiber et al. evaluated the impact of introducing ICS into a community hospital for use in abdominal aortic aneurysm repairs [37]. The authors retrospectively looked at 93 elective and 25 emergent aortic aneurysm repairs. Thirty-three percent of elective repairs and 84% of emergent repairs exclusively received allogenic blood, while the rest received some combination of allogenic and autologous blood. The use of ICS did not statistically significantly reduce the need for allogenic blood or impact the length of hospital stay or post-operative hemoglobin levels. However, the incorporation of ICS doubled the expenditure associated with blood product utilization. In a study of orthotopic liver transplants, Kemper et al. compared the cost of intra-operative blood salvage based on the duration of the surgery with the absolute cost of transfusing equivalent amounts of allogenic packed red cells [38]. On average, autologous ICS cost $1048/patient, while an equivalent amount of allogenic blood was calculated at $429/patient. Their case-by-case analysis revealed that in only three patients (4.8%) who received between 16.4 and 46.6 units of recycled cells did the use of ICS result in cost savings. In stark contrast, other studies that have looked at all surgical patients in a general hospital setting or exclusively abdominal trauma victims have reported significant financial savings with the use of ICS [39, 40]. A retrospective review of patients who underwent elective abdominal aortic aneurysm repair examined the cost effectiveness of a standby cell-saver for all patients [41]. Factoring in the expenses associated with acquisition, laboratory services, administration, and overhead, the authors computed a cost of $169 for a unit of autologous blood that compared favorably with $155 for a unit of allogenic blood. From this data, the authors concluded that operations involving at least 1000 mL blood loss with cell salvage of at least 750 mL would benefit from ICS.

Szpisjak et al. examined the economic factors involved in the incorporation of an intra-operative auto-transfusion service using four differing economic models [42]. The fully outsourced model evaluated the cost when the entire service was outsourced; in the partially outsourced model, the equipment and disposables were provided by the hospital while the technician was contracted; the new employee model involved hiring a full-time technician exclusively for the ICS service; and, finally, in the cross-trained model, the equipment and disposables were provided by the hospital and the technician was an employee who was cross-trained in the operation of ICS. Their analysis assumed a maximum of one case per day using ICS and a fixed cost of ICS per use. The authors found that the fully outsourced model was the most economical for caseloads below 55 cases annually, beyond which the cross-trained model was predicted to generate the lowest cost. In reality, the cost analysis of ICS is complex and depends on a variety of factors including the type of cell salvage device, the nature of surgical procedures, amount of blood loss, annual caseload, etc. More important, studies of cost are an index of the direct financial burden. What cannot be included in these analyses is the price of allogenic blood transfusion, far more important than the mere cost of it. For all the reasons we have discussed earlier, ICS will certainly ease the burden on the need for blood products and, we believe, may even lead to an eventual financial benefit.

Another important consideration with the use of ICS is that only red blood cells are salvaged. The blood that is recycled is depleted of clotting factors and platelets. Large volume ICS may, therefore, lead to a coagulopathy if clotting factors are not appropriately replenished. If heparin is used in the ICS circuit to prevent clotting, the returned blood cells must be washed carefully of any residual heparin. Some of the other complications associated with the use of ICS include air embolism, infection, and DIC [29]. To minimize these risks, ICS is contraindicated in patients with intra-abdominal infections and in cases with potential for contamination with gastric or amniotic fluid. Certain local clotting agents, such as gelatin sponges, powders, or collagen hemostatic material should also be avoided in conjunction with ICS.

Caution also should be exercised with the use of ICS in patients with malignancy. Animal studies have suggested that tumor cells are capable of maintaining viability even after filtration and centrifugation in ICS, and there is hence at least a theoretical potential for systemic dissemination of malignant cells [43]. In a study of 408 patients who underwent radical retropubic prostatectomy for cancer, Davis et al. monitored PSA levels post-operatively as a surrogate for cancer recurrence [44]. They found no difference in recurrence rates between patients that received ICS, autologous blood, or no transfusion at all. Furthermore, there is evidence that the application of specific techniques may even further reduce the likelihood of malignant cell transmission. Hansen et al. investigated the effect of irradiating salvaged blood that contains neoplastic cells *in vitro* [45]. Tumor cells obtained from a number of cell lines and solid tumors, such as breast, colon, pancreatic, and prostate cancers, were added to washed red cells. At a radiation dose of 50 Gy, they documented complete eradication of the proliferative capacity and DNA metabolism of all neoplastic cells, even when the mixtures contained 10^7 to 10^{10} tumor cells prior to irradiation. The erythrocytes remained unaffected, maintaining their 2,3-DPG and ATP levels, as well as their rheologic properties and structural integrity. Leukocyte depletion filters (LDF) also have been studied *in vitro* to limit re-infusion of cancer cells. Edelman et al. ran suspensions containing 10^6 cells from renal cell, prostate, and transitional cell carcinoma cell lines through a standard ICS, a standard blood filter, and an LDF [46]. The LDF, but not the other two, was effective at completely eliminating tumor cells from the suspension. Both irradiation and LDF come at an additional expense, but they may be justifiable when the use of ICS may be lifesaving in say a Jehovah's Witness patient, to avoid the alternative of potentially life-threatening anemia.

In sum, while the technology of ICS is rapidly evolving, significant controversy surrounds the utility of ICS, and several precautionary measures need to be undertaken for its successful use. We believe a judicious expansion of the application of intra-operative cell salvage will significantly assist in the maturation of a transfusion-free program.

D. Acute normovolemic hemodilution (ANH)

A promising complement to ICS is acute normovolemic hemodilution. It is normally considered if the potential for blood loss exceeds 20% of the patient's blood volume [47]. ANH involves collection of blood and its replacement with a colloid or crystalloid infusion just prior to incision, followed by re-infusion of the collected blood at the conclusion of the surgery. By inducing a moderate isovolemic anemia during surgery, the blood lost is diluted and by withdrawing and later re-infusing whole blood, ANH spares not only the red cell mass but platelets and clotting factors as well. Experience with ANH has revealed that normovolemic anemia is well-tolerated in most patients [48]. As the hematocrit falls (usually to the low twenties), cardiac output rises while the central venous pressure is maintained at its initial level throughout surgery. In addition to the increased cardiac output, the main compensatory responses seen include an increased oxygen extraction at the tissue along with a right-ward shift of the oxyhemoglobin dissociation curve (see Chapter 6). Under anesthesia, these responses can occur without significant elevations in heart rate. Several studies have corroborated these findings in cardio-vascular parameters. Weiskopf et al. studied 32 healthy volunteers in whom ANH was instituted to hemoglobin levels of 5 g/dL [49]. Oxygen consumption, plasma lactate concentration, and electrocardiographic changes were monitored. Even after 2.4 hours of isovolemic anemia, there was no evidence of inadequate oxygenation, no change was observed in right or left side filling pressures, nor was a significant alteration seen in lactate levels. The ECG findings were mostly normal, except for ST elevations in two patients, which resolved without sequelae. A mild increase in oxygen consumption was detected, but the compensatory responses were mainly due to an increased heart rate (75%) and cardiac output (25%). In a meta-analysis of the effect of normovolemic anemia following surgery in Jehovah's Witness patients, the risk of post-operative mortality was found to be significantly higher in patients with underlying cardiovascular disease [50]. Consequently, ANH is not recommended in patients with myocardial disease or in infants and neonates.

ANH offers a few advantages over pre-operative autologous donation (PAD). There are added benefits of greater convenience and reduced expense. Blood collection as part of ANH is performed only once, on the day of surgery in the operating room, whereas PAD can involve multiple clinic visits depending on the quantity of blood desired. This additional administrative cost when coupled with the extra expenditure associated with discarded or unused blood units diminishes the appeal of PAD [51]. PAD does not guarantee against clerical errors or mishandling leading to a host of other complications. Furthermore, the quality of blood used in PAD often can be compromised in manners that are unlikely to occur within ANH. For example, stored blood can develop abnormal 2,3-DPG levels and other biochemical alterations that can reduce the oxygen-carrying capacity. Finally, ANH has gained acceptance among Jehovah's Witnesses because collected blood can be kept within an extracorporeal circuit that is in continuity with the patient [52].

E. Anesthesia management

Vital to the management and maintenance of a patient's hematologic system is clear communication with the anesthesiologist. The role of anesthesiologists in blood management is critical, especially given their involvement in ICS and ANH. The explicit goals of anesthesia during transfusion-free surgery should include the maintenance of normovolemic status and the potential need for hyperoxic ventilation and controlled hypotensive anesthesia. For example, a low CVP may markedly reduce blood loss during parenchymal transection for liver resection. In a similar fashion, blood loss during spinal surgery can be curtailed significantly by relative hypotensive anesthesia. Avoidance of hypothermia can help avoid temperature-related coagulopathy.

F. Coagulation management

Meticulous surgical technique aside, an understanding and an optimization of the coagulation system during surgery are essential to minimize blood loss. This approach must go beyond the standard coagulation tests, such as PT, PTT, and platelet count, which reflect the quantity of clotting factors but convey little in regard to the quality of clot formation. While these basic measurements suffice in most patients, in select instances, more sophisticated monitoring may be required. For example, fibrinolysis can be a major cause of coagulopathy unresponsive to conventional treatment in patients with end-stage liver disease. However, the diagnosis of fibrinolysis cannot be made by the usual coagulation tests, mandating the need for a thomboelastogram.

The correction of coagulopathy implied the infusion of blood products such as FFP, cryoprecipitate, and platelets. Significant inroads have been made into the understanding of and ability to manipulate several other factors that play a major role in enhancing coagulation. The use of epsilon aminocaproic acid to limit fibrinolysis may be of significant benefit.

In a randomized, prospective study, the use of both epsilon aminocaproic acid and tranexamic acid significantly reduced blood loss, transfusion requirements, and sternal closure times in children undergoing corrective surgery for cyanotic heart disease [53]. A multicenter, randomized study examined the effectiveness of aprotinin in orthotopic liver transplantation [54]. Porte el al. divided 137 patients with similar clinical characteristics, pre-operative laboratory parameters, and surgical variables into three groups based on pre-operative administration of high dose aprotinin, regular dose aprotinin, or placebo. Both high dose aprotinin, which served to inhibit kallekrein, and regular dose aprotinin, at a plasmin inhibiting level, were administered at a loading dose of 2×10^6 kallekrein inhibiting units (KIU) followed by an infusion of 1×10^6 KIU/hr and 0.5×10^6 KIU/hr, respectively, until two hours after graft reperfusion. Aprotinin administration resulted in significant reduction in blood loss by 60% in the high dose group and 44% in the regular dose group ($p = 0.03$), with a concomitant fall in the need for homologous and autologous blood ($p = 0.02$) and blood products ($p = 0.01$). All of these benefits were observed in the absence of any pro-thrombotic complication.

Recombinant activated factor VII (rFVIIa) was initially introduced as an alternative therapy for hemophiliacs with inhibitors for human factors. Extracted from transfected hamster kidney cells, rFVIIa is characterized by an amino acid sequence and biological activity that are identical to activated human factor VII. rFVIIa binds to exposed tissue factor at sites of injury only, thereby promoting the formation of a localized clot, without increasing the risk of systemic thrombosis. Its initial role in the management of hemophilia has been expanded (an off-label use outside of the FDA-approved indication) to include liver disease, drug-induced coagulopathy, platelet disorders such as Glanzmann thrombasthenia, pregnancy-related clotting disorders, DIC, etc. rFVIIa has shown significant promise for the control of bleeding in several surgical procedures such as liver transplantation, trauma, vascular surgery, prostatectomy, etc. [55–58]. Egan et al. retrospectively reviewed the records of six children who underwent cardiac surgery that was complicated by persistent bleeding unresponsive to conventional therapy consisting of aprotinin, FFP, and cryoprecipitate [59]. Two intravenous doses of rFVIIa given two hours apart significantly curtailed the bleeding. The authors, hence, support the use of rFVIIa as a safe tool for hemostasis that may serve to limit the need for repeat thoracotomy in this population.

Given that most clotting factors are synthesized by the liver, and FVIIa, with a half-life of less than two hours, is depleted most rapidly in liver failure, rFVIIa is thought to hold significant promise in liver transplantation.

In a Cochran Central Database review, rFVIIa, in addition to aprotinin and thromboelastography, was felt to potentially reduce blood loss and transfusion requirements [60]. However, one should bear in mind the potential for creation of pro-thrombotic state and side effects likely induced by such state in an inherently fragile patient population.

Post-operative care

Appropriate post-operative management of the hematologic system begins with prevention and early recognition of blood loss. Any sudden drop in hematocrit or ongoing blood loss from drains should warrant consideration of active bleeding and be dealt with promptly. Further work-up, including laboratory testing, should not delay institution of appropriate interventions. Phlebotomy represents a major and under-appreciated source of blood loss, especially in the intensive care setting. Restricting investigations to the absolute essential, avoidance of blood draw from large bore or high-flow lines, and minimizing the quantity of blood drawn by using pediatric collection tubes can significantly limit iatrogenic post-operative anemia. MacIsaac et al. investigated the effects of a blood-conserving device on anemia in a randomized trial of 160 patients [61]. After matching for age, sex, and severity of illness, the use of the venous arterial management protection plus (VAMP Plus) system reduced the amount of blood used for lab testing by 53% when compared with routine blood draws from standard arterial lines.

There is an increasing body of evidence that moderate degrees of anemia are well-tolerated by a majority of patients in the post-operative recovery phase. Hebert et al. conducted a randomized trial examining the relationship between transfusion strategies and patient outcomes [62]. Among 838 patients with hemoglobin levels less than 9 g/dL within 72 hours of admission to an intensive care unit, approximately half were managed using a liberal strategy of transfusing blood for hemoglobin values below 10 g/dL, while the rest were assigned to a more restrictive strategy of transfusion for levels below 7 g/dL. The overall in-hospital mortality was significantly lower in the restrictive group, as was 30-day mortality among patients under 55 years of age or those less acutely ill. The overall 30-day mortality was similar between both groups. Patients with cardiac disease, however, represent a unique population for whom additional consideration is warranted. In an investigation of the effect of anemia on surgical morbidity and mortality in patients with cardiovascular disease, the cases of 1958 Jehovah's Witnesses who declined transfusions were reviewed by Carson et al. [50]. They found that mortality increased from 1.3% in patients with hemoglobin levels exceeding 12 g/dL to 33.3% in those with hemoglobin levels less than 6 g/dL.

The adverse effects of blood transfusion are particularly more pronounced in the post-operative period. In a prospective, multi-center study of 4,892 ICU patients, Corwin et al. [63]. reported that 44% received at least one unit of packed red cells. Only 19% of the 213 participating hospitals followed established guidelines governing transfusion, and low hemoglobin value (at a mean of 8.6 g/dL) was cited 90% of the time as the reason for the transfusion. Blood transfusion was associated with a significantly increased incidence of acute respiratory distress syndrome, pneumonia, and infection. In addition, after correcting for baseline hemoglobin levels and severity of illness, transfusion had a strong correlation with prolonged hospitalization and increased mortality.

Studies that have evaluated the role of rHuEPO in the post-operative period have produced mixed results, largely related to the heterogeneity of the patients studied and the high degree of variability among drug administration protocols [64]. In two, large, randomized, prospective studies, Corwin et al. showed that the use of rHuEPO resulted in significantly higher hemoglobin levels and reduced blood transfusion requirements [65, 66]. No improvement was observed, though, in the duration of hospitalization or mortality. Gabriel et al. observed that in patients with multiple organ dysfunction, despite increased cytokine levels, rHuEPO resulted in increased reticulocyte counts, though it did not translate into a reduction in transfusion requirement [67]. Still et al. also observed no change in transfusion requirements despite rHuEPO administration [68].

Additional goals that complement reducing blood loss and improving hemoglobin levels in the post-operative period include augmenting oxygen delivery and reducing oxygen consumption. Oxygen delivery can be improved by increasing the inhaled oxygen content (via supplemental oxygen, mechanical ventilation, or hyperbaric oxygen), maintaining adequate intra-vascular volume and optimizing cardiac performance. Appropriate cardiac and respiratory support, control of fevers and shivering, and bed rest with sedation or complete paralysis in selected instances, can help minimize oxygen consumption.

Trends in transfusion-free surgery

Ongoing investigation into the understanding and application of oxygen-carrying blood substitutes is bound to further reduce our dependence on allogenic blood products. Blood substitutes that can serve the function of tissue oxygenation may have significant utility, while at the same time eliminate the risk of transmission of infections, allow longer shelf-times, and lead to a predictable supply and availability with universal compatibility. The use of blood substitutes also may allow for greater intra-operative normovolemic hemodilution. In recent years, aggressive investigations as to the understanding and application of oxygen-carrying blood substitutes has led to the development of a number of investigational products that have been proposed as potential alternatives to our current transfusion supplies. Most notably, hemoglobin-based oxygen carriers have progressed to a number of clinical trials for evaluation as true substitutes. While a number of these products have been demonstrated to successfully transport oxygen, they are fraught with negative cardiovascular effects and have failed to gain regulatory approval [69].

In addition to these oxygen carrying blood substitutes, synthetic coagulation factors also play an important role in the future of blood product utilization. The clinical success observed with rFVIIa has triggered a multitude of studies evaluating recombinant proteins that shift the procoagulant/anticoagulant balance toward a more pro-coagulant state at the site of blood loss. Newer agents currently in laboratory trials have the potential to decrease blood loss even in the absence of an obvious underlying hemostatic defect or in the setting of coagulopathies resulting from dilution and consumption as in trauma and surgery [70]. The availability of these transfusion-sparing hemostatic agents will further facilitate the practice of transfusion-free medicine.

Conclusion

Blood transfusion in surgery has long been understood to carry a fair amount of clinical risk despite its obvious benefits for improved oxygen delivery. For these reasons, the improved blood loss conservation and novel methods for avoidance of potentially unnecessary transfusion is of paramount importance for further advancement in the total care of the surgical patient. As novel techniques and products continue to emerge and be proven for such a goal, the clinical communities' dependence upon blood products will continue to decrease and patient outcomes will improve.

References

1 Varghese R, Myers ML. Blood conservation in cardiac surgery: let's get restrictive. Semin Thorac Cardiovasc Surg. 2010 Summer;22(2):121–6.
2 Report of the US Department of Health and Human Services. The 2009 national blood collection and utilization survey report. Washington, DC: US Department of Health and Human Services, Office of the Assistant Secretary for Health; 2011.

3 Carson JL, Altman DG, Duff A, Noveck H, Weinstein MP, Sonnenberg FA, et al. Risk of bacterial infection associated with allogeneic blood transfusion among patients undergoing hip fracture repair. Transfusion. 1999;39:694–700.

4 Wagner SJ. Transfusion-transmitted bacterial infection: risks, sources and interventions. Vox Sang. 2004;86:157–63.

5 Duffy G, Neal KR. Differences in post-operative infection rates between patients receiving autologous and allogeneic blood transfusion: a meta-analysis of published randomized and nonrandomized studies. Transfus Med. 1996;6:325–8.

6 Vamvakas EC. Possible mechanisms of allogeneic blood transfusion-associated postoperative infection. Transfus Med Rev. 2002;16:144–60.

7 Hill GE, Frawley WH, Griffith KE, Forestner JE, Minei JP. Allogeneic blood transfusion increases the risk of postoperative bacterial infection: a meta-analysis. J Trauma. 2003;54:908–14.

8 Shorr AF, Duh MS, Kelly KM, Kollef MH; CRIT Study Group. Red blood cell transfusion and ventilator-associated pneumonia: A potential link? Crit Care Med. 2004;32:666–74.

9 Vamvakas EC. Perioperative blood transfusion and cancer recurrence: meta-analysis for explanation. Transfusion. 1995;35:760–8.

10 Amato AC, Pescatori M. Effect of perioperative blood transfusions on recurrence of colorectal cancer: meta-analysis stratified on risk factors. Dis Colon Rectum. 1998;41:570–85.

11 Patel HB, Nasir FA, Nash GF, Scully MF, Kakkar AK. Enhanced angiogenesis following allogeneic blood transfusion. Clin Lab Haematol. 2004;26:129–35.

12 Stephenson GR, Moretti EW, El-Moalem H, Clavien PA, Tuttle-Newhall JE. Malnutrition in liver transplant patients: preoperative subjective global assessment is predictive of outcome after liver transplantation. Transplantation. 2001;72: 666–70.

13 Goodnough LT, Monk TG, Andriole GL. Erythropoietin Therapy. N Engl J Med. 1997;336:933–8.

14 Sans T, Bofil C, Joven J, Cliville X, Simo JM, Llobet X, et al. Effectiveness of very low doses of subcutaneous recombinant human erythropoietin in facilitating autologous blood donation before orthopedic surgery. Transfusion. 1996;36:822–6.

15 Price TH, Goodnough LT, Vogler WR, Sacher RA, Hellman RM, Johnston MF, et al. Improving the efficacy of preoperative autologous blood donation in patients with low hematocrit: a randomized, double-blind, controlled trial of recombinant human erythropoietin. Am J Med. 1996;101:22S–27S.

16 Sarac TP, Clifford C, Waters J, Clair DG, Ouriel K. Preoperative erythropoietin and blood conservation management for thoracoabdominal aneurysm repair in a Jehovah's Witness. J Vasc Surg. 2003;37:453–5.

17 Nelson CL, Stewart JG. Primary and revision total hip replacement in patients who are Jehovah's Witnesses. Clin Orthop. 1999;(369):251–61.

18 Bennett DR, Shulman IA. Practical issues when confronting the patient who refuses blood transfusion therapy. Am J Clin Pathol. 1997;107:S23–7.

19 Ng T, Marx G, Littlewood T, Macdougall I. Recombinant erythropoietin in clinical practice. Postgrad Med J. 2003;79:367–76.

20 Cazzola M, Mercuriali F, Brugnara C. Use of recombinant human erythropoietin outside the setting of uremia. Blood. 1997;89:4248–67.

21 Kalantar-Zadeh K, McAllister CJ, Lehn RS, Lee GH, Nissenson AR, Kopple JD. Effect of malnutrition-inflammation complex syndrome on EPO hyporesponsiveness in maintenance hemodialysis patients. Am J Kidney Dis. 2003;42:761–73.

22 Ozguroglu M, Arun B, Demir G, Demirelli F, Mandel NM, Buyukunal E, et al. Serum erythropoietin level in anemic cancer patients. Med Oncol. 2000;17:29–34.

23 Weiss G. Pathogenesis and treatment of anaemia of chronic disease. Blood Rev. 2002;16:87–96.

24 Brugnara C, Chambers LA, Malynn E, Goldberg MA, Kruskall MS. Red blood cell regeneration induced by subcutaneous recombinant erythropoietin: iron-deficient erythropoiesis in iron-replete subjects. Blood. 1993;81:956–64.

25 Goodnough LT, Skikne B, Brugnara C. Erythropoietin, iron, and erythropoiesis. Blood. 2000;96:823–33.

26 Jabbour N, Gagandeep S, Mateo R, Sher L, Henderson R, Selby R, et al. Live donor liver transplantation: staging hepatectomy in a Jehovah's Witness recipient. J Hepatobiliary Pancreat Surg. 2004;11:211–4.

27 Paravicini D, Wasylewski AH, Rassat J, Thys J. Red blood cell survival and morphology during and after intraoperative autotransfusion. Acta Anaesthesiol Belg. 1984;35:43–9.

28 Ray JM, Flynn JC, Bierman AH. Erythrocyte survival following intraoperative autotransfusion in spinal surgery: an in vivo comparative study and 5-year update. Spine. 1986;11:879–82.

29 Williamson KR, Taswell HF. Intraoperative blood salvage: a review. Transfusion. 1991;31:662–75.

30 Yamada T, Yamashita Y, Terai Y, Ueki M. Intraoperative blood salvage in abdominal uterine myomectomy. Int J Gynaecol Obstet. 1997;56:141–5.

31 Rosengart TK, Helm RE, DeBois WJ, Garcia N, Krieger KH, Isom OW. Open heart operations without transfusion using a multimodality blood conservation strategy in 50 Jehovah's Witness patients: implications for a "bloodless" surgical technique. J Am Coll Surg. 1997;184:618–29.

32 Huo MH, Paly WL, Keggi KJ. Effect of preoperative autologous blood donation and intraoperative and postoperative blood recovery on homologous blood transfusion requirement in cementless total hip replacement operation. J Am Coll Surg. 1995;180:561–7.

33 Williamson KR, Taswell HF, Rettke SR, Krom RA. Intraoperative autologous transfusion: its role in orthotopic liver transplantation. Mayo Clin Proc. 1989;64:340–5.

34 McGill N, O'Shaughnessy D, Pickering R, Herbertson M, Gill R. Mechanical methods of reducing blood transfusion in cardiac surgery: randomised controlled trial. BMJ. 2002;324:1299–306.

35 Guerra JJ, Cuckler JM. Cost effectiveness of intraoperative autotransfusion in total hip arthroplasty surgery. Clin Orthop. 1995;315:212–22.

36 Simpson MB, Georgopoulos G, Eilert RE. Intraoperative blood salvage in children and young adults undergoing spinal surgery with predeposited autologous blood: efficacy and cost effectiveness. J Pediatr Orthop. 1993;13:777–80.

37 Shuhaiber JH, Whitehead SM. The impact of introducing an autologous intraoperative transfusion device to a community hospital. Ann Vasc Surg. 2003;17:424–9.

38 Kemper RR, Menitove JE, Hanto DW. Cost analysis of intraoperative blood salvage during orthotopic liver transplantation. Liver Transpl Surg. 1997;3:513–7.

39 Keeling MM, Gray LA Jr, Brink MA, Hillerich VK, Bland KI. Intraoperative auto-transfusion. Experience in 725 consecutive cases. Ann Surg. 1983;197:536–41.

40 Smith LA, Barker DE, Burns RP. Autotransfusion utilization in abdominal trauma. Am Surg. 1997;63:47–9.

41 Goodnough LT, Monk TG, Sicard G, Satterfield SA, Allen B, Anderson CB, Thompson RW, Flye W, Martin K. Intraoperative salvage in patients undergoing elective abdominal aortic aneurysm repair: an analysis of cost and benefit. J Vasc Surg. 1996;24:213–8.

42 Szpisjak DF, Potter PS, Capehart BP. Economic analysis of an intraoperative cell salvage service. Anesth Analg. 2004;98:201–5.

43 Homann B, Zenner HP, Schauber J, Ackermann R. Tumor cells carried through autotransfusion. Are these cells still malignant? Acta Anaesthesiol Belg. 1984;35:51–9.

44 Davis M, Sofer M, Gomez-Marin O, Bruck D, Soloway MS. The use of cell salvage during radical retropubic prostatectomy: does it influence cancer recurrence? BJU Int. 2003;91:474–6.

45 Hansen E, Knuechel R, Altmeppen J, Taeger K. Blood irradiation for intraoperative autotransfusion in cancer surgery: demonstration of efficient elimination of contaminating tumor cells. Transfusion. 1999;39:608–15.

46 Edelman MJ, Potter P, Mahaffey KG, Frink R, Leidich RB. The potential for reintroduction of tumor cells during intraoperative blood salvage: reduction of risk with use of the RC-400 leukocyte depletion filter. Urology. 1996;47:179–81.

47 Napier JA, Bruce M, Chapman J, Duguid JK, Kelsey PR, Knowles SM, et al. Guidelines for autologous transfusion. II. Perioperative haemodilution and cell salvage. British Committee for Standards in Haematology Blood Transfusion Task Force. Autologous Transfusion Working Party. Br J Anaesth. 1997;78:768–71.

48 Oriani G, Pavesi M, Oriani A, Bollina I. Acute normovolemic hemodilution. Transfus Apher Sci. 2011 Dec;45(3):269–74. Epub 2011 Oct 22.

49 Weiskopf RB, Viele MK, Feiner J, Kelley S, Lieberman J, Noorani M, et al. Human cardiovascular and metabolic response to acute, severe isovolemic anemia. JAMA. 1998;279:217–21.

50 Carson JL, Duff A, Poses RM, Berlin JA, Spence RK, Trout R, et al. Effect of anemia and cardiovascular disease on surgical morbidity and mortality. Lancet. 1996;348: 1055–60.

51 Etchason J, Petz L, Keeler E, Calhoun L, Kleinman S, Snider C, et al. The cost effectiveness of preoperative autologous blood donations. N Engl J Med. 1995;332: 719–24.

52 Hughes DB, Ullery BW, Barie PS. The contemporary approach to the care of Jehovah's witnesses. J Trauma. 2008 Jul;65(1):237–47.

53 Chauhan S, Das SN, Bisoi A, Kale S, Kiran U. Comparison of epsilon aminocaproic acid and tranexamic acid in pediatric cardiac surgery. J Cardiothorac Vasc Anesth. 2004;18:141–3.

54 Porte RJ, Molenaar IQ, Begliomini B, Groenland TH, Januszkiewicz A, Lindgren L, et al. Aprotinin and transfusion requirements in orthotopic liver transplantation: a multicentre randomised double-blind study. Lancet. 2000;355:1303–9.

55 Midathada MV, Mehta P, Waner M, Fink LM. Recombinant factor VIIa in the treatment of bleeding. Am J Clin Pathol. 2004;121:124–37.

56 Kenet G, Walden R, Eldad A, Martinowitz U. Treatment of traumatic bleeding with recombinant factor VIIa. Lancet. 1999;354:1879.

57 Stratmann G, Russell IA, Merrick SH. Use of recombinant factor VIIa as a rescue treatment for intractable bleeding following repeat aortic arch repair. Ann Thorac Surg. 2003;76:2094–7.

58 Friederich PW, Henny CP, Messelink EJ, Geerdink MG, Keller T, Kurth KH, et al. Effect of recombinant activated factor VII on perioperative blood loss in patients undergoing retropubic prostatectomy: a double-blind placebo-controlled randomised trial. Lancet. 2003;361:201–5.

59 Egan JR, Lammi A, Schell DN, Gillis J, Nunn GR. Recombinant activated factor VII in paediatric cardiac surgery. Intensive Care Med. 2004;30:682–5.

60 Gurusamy KS, Pissanou T, Pikhart H, Vaughan J, Burroughs AK, Davidson BR. Methods to decrease blood loss and transfusion requirements for liver transplantation. Cochrane Database Syst Rev. 2011 Dec 7;12:CD009052.

61 MacIsaac CM, Presneill JJ, Boyce CA, Byron KL, Cade JF. The influence of a blood conserving device on anaemia in intensive care patients. Anaesth Intensive Care. 2003;31:653–7.

62 Hebert PC, Wells G, Blajchman MA, Marshall J, Martin C, Pagliarello G, et al. A multicenter, randomized, controlled clinical trial of transfusion requirements in critical care. Transfusion Requirements in Critical Care Investigators, Canadian Critical Care Trials Group. N Engl J Med. 1999;340:409–17.

63 Corwin HL, Gettinger A, Pearl RG, Fink MP, Levy MM, Abraham E, et al. The CRIT Study: Anemia and blood transfusion in the critically ill--current clinical practice in the United States. Crit Care Med. 2004;32:39–52.

64 Pajoumand M, Erstad BL, Camamo JM, Use of Epoetin Alfa in Critically Ill Patients, Ann Pharmacother. 2004;38:641–8.

65 Corwin HL, Gettinger A, Pearl RG, Fink MP, Levy MM, Shapiro MJ, et al; EPO Critical Care Trials Group. Efficacy of recombinant human erythropoietin in critically ill patients: a randomized controlled trial. JAMA. 2002;288:2827–35.

66 Corwin HL, Gettinger A, Rodriguez RM, Pearl RG, Gubler KD, Enny C, et al. Efficacy of recombinant human erythropoietin in the critically ill patient: a randomized, double-blind, placebo-controlled trial. Crit Care Med. 1999;27:2346–50.

67 Gabriel A, Kozek S, Chiari A, Fitzgerald R, Grabner C, Geissler K, et al. High-dose recombinant human erythropoietin stimulates reticulocyte production in patients with multiple organ dysfunction syndrome. J Trauma. 1998;44:361–7.

68 Still JM Jr, Belcher K, Law EJ, Thompson W, Jordan M, Lewis M, et al. A double-blinded prospective evaluation of recombinant human erythropoietin in acutely burned patients. J Trauma. 1995;38:233–6.

69 Chen JY, Scerbo M, Kramer G. A review of blood substitutes: examining the history, clinical trial results, and ethics of hemoglobin-based oxygen carriers. Clinics (Sao Paulo). 2009;64(8):803–13.

70 Chiu J, Ketchum LH, Reid TJ. Transfusion-sparing hemostatic agents. Curr Opin Hematol. 2002;9:544–50.

CHAPTER 6

Current view of coagulation system

Yoogoo Kang and Elia Elia

Department of Anesthesiology, Thomas Jefferson University,
Jefferson Medical College, Philadelphia, PA, USA

The coagulation system serves several vital functions to provide normal physiology. It maintains fluidity of blood stream to deliver oxygen and nutrients to tissues, repairs interruption in vascular integrity, and participates in inflammatory process to control or limit the harmful effects of injury or pathologic process. In surgical settings, major emphasis has been placed on clot formation to avoid excessive blood loss, and control of excessive clot formation to avoid thrombosis. In this chapter, basic principles and clinical hemostasis including monitoring and management are described.

Normal hemostasis

In order for blood to freely flow through the vasculature, it must stay in the liquid state. Yet, it should be able to transform into gelatinous glue to seal any breaches in the vascular integrity to prevent exsanguinations. If this property were compromised, even minor injuries or surgical procedures would be life threatening. An intricately balanced system, therefore, exists to achieve these two seemingly mutually exclusive end points.

Hemostasis refers to the process by which liquid blood is transformed first into a solid state, followed by a liquid state, and is achieved by a delicate balance of forces promoting bleeding (anticoagulants and prolysins) or clotting (procoagulants and antilysins) (Figure 6.1). It is divided into five distinctive, interactive phases:

1 *vascular phase*, in which intense vasoconstriction reduces blood flow to the injured site to minimize bleeding;

2 *platelet phase*, or primary hemostasis, in which platelets amass at the site of injury and form a mechanical seal or "platelet plug";

Transfusion-Free Medicine and Surgery, Second Edition. Edited by Nicolas Jabbour.
© 2014 John Wiley & Sons, Ltd. Published 2014 by John Wiley & Sons, Ltd.

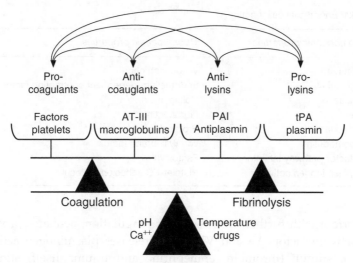

Figure 6.1 Hemostatic balances between clot formation and fibrinolysis.

3 *fibrin formation* phase or secondary hemostasis, in which a dense interwoven meshwork of fibrin invests and reinforces the plug;
4 insoluble *fibrin formation, which follows the soluble fibrin* network formation; and
5 *fibrinolysis,* which involves clot resorption and recanalization.

These five equally important steps take place simultaneously and interdependently in a concert of vascular endothelium, platelets and coagulation proteins.

Vascular phase

Trauma results in intense vasoconstriction of the injured vessel within a few seconds. The response is primarily myogenic but may be enhanced by neural elements and humoral mediators, such as thromboxane A_2, serotonin, norepinephrine produced by activated platelets. Vasoconstriction may last up to 30 min. In addition, tissue edema and bleeding into the tissue increase extravascular pressure to minimize extravasation.

The next important vascular phase involves vascular endothelial cells to initiate and modulate clot formation. Endothelial cells lining blood vessels play an important role in maintaining perfusion, permeability and blood fluidity, and have dual function (Table 6.1). Endothelial cells are nonthrombogenic because their surface is negatively charged to repel negatively charged platelets. They produce an inhibitor of platelet aggregation (prostaglandin I_2), thrombomodulin, and heparan sulfate, which activates antithrombin [1–3]. Thrombomodulin binds to thrombin

Table 6.1 Endothelial cell function.

Nonthrombogenic properties	Thrombogenic properties
Vasodilatation	Vasoconstriction
Prostaglandin I_2	Endothelium-dependent contracting factor (EDCF)
Nitric oxide	Collagen
ADPase	Fibronectin
Heparin sulfates	Proteoglycans
Thrombomodulin	von Willebrand factor
Tissue factor pathway inhibitor	Factor VIII
Tissue plasminogen activator	Platelet-EC adhesion molecule

to interfere with further progression of coagulation, activates protein C to inactivate factors Va and VIIIa, and releases plasminogen activator. Further, stimuli (thrombin, epinephrine and trauma itself) stimulate endothelial synthesis of PGI_2 to inhibit platelet aggregation as a negative feedback mechanism [4]. Endothelial cells are also thrombogenic and metabolically active: they produce collagen, fibronectin, proteoglycans, and von Willebrand factor (vWF), and release vWF, Factor VIII and prostanoids. Endothelium is a barrier between the blood and vessel wall, and its permeability is maintained by the junctional adaptations. Large molecules pass across the endothelium into the vessel wall through patent intercellular junctions (endocytosis), and via transendothelial pores. Its fenestration is affected by serotonin and norepinephrine released by platelets.

Therefore, impaired endothelial function results in a variety of hemostatic defects. For example, insufficient quantity of protein C interferes with the feedback inhibition of coagulation mediated by the thrombin-thrombomodulin complex, resulting in systemic thrombosis [5]. Thrombotic condition also develops when the release of tissue plasminogen activator is insufficient [6]. On the other hand, an increase in endothelial fenestration leads to petechiae or idiopathic thrombocytopenic purpura (ITP) [7].

Platelet phase

Platelets are disc-shaped anucleated cellular elements, measuring 2–3 μm in diameter. Their production from bone marrow megakaryocytes is regulated by thrombopoietin [8], and the average adult has 150–400 billion platelets per liter of blood. Platelets have a life span of 7–10 days, and aging cells are removed from circulation by the reticuloendothelial system. Platelets are the cornerstone of hemostasis and participate in multiple phases of coagulation [9]. Their cytoplasm is rich in mitochondria and various granules, and their cell surface receptors allow interaction with and adhesion to diverse elements of the subendothelial matrix. They adhere to the injured vessel wall and entice other platelets, leucocytes and erythrocytes into the enlarging platelet aggregate. This primary hemostasis begins within a few seconds following injury, and platelets provide a phospholipid surface on which various enzyme complexes are assembled. Additionally, platelets release growth factors that assist in wound healing and tissue repair.

Platelets normally circulate in a quiescent, "non-sticky" state. They do not adhere to the negatively charged vascular endothelium and do not stick to one another, since these aggregates are rapidly eliminated by the reticuloendothelial system. Vascular injury, however, removes the endothelial barrier and allows platelets to come in direct contact with highly thrombogenic subendothelium to cause adhesion (Figure 6.2). In venous blood, adhesion is achieved by the attachment of platelet GP Ia/IIa receptors to subendothelial collagen matrix. In arterial circulation, however, the interaction between a constitutively active adhesive protein complex (GP Ib/V/IX) present on the platelet surface and vWF of the subendothelial matrix slows down platelets before adhesion.

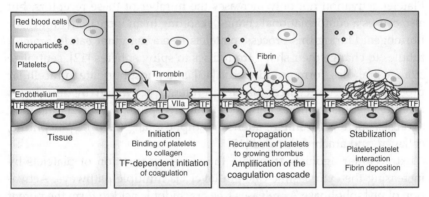

Figure 6.2 Interactions between platelets and subendothelium. In a healthy individual, TF expressed by vascular smooth muscle cells, pericytes, and adventitial fibroblasts in the vessel wall is physically separated from its ligand FVII/FVIIa by the endothelium. Vessel injury leads to the rapid binding of platelets to the subendothelium and activation of the coagulation cascade by TF. Propagation of the thrombus involves recruitment of additional platelets and amplification of the coagulation cascade by the intrinsic pathway, and possibly by TF-positive MPs and TF stored in platelets. Finally, fibrin deposition stabilizes the clot. De novo synthesis of TF by platelets may also play a role in stabilization of the clot. Modified with permission from Mackman N, Tilley RE, Key NS. Arterioscler Thromb Vasc Biol. 2007;27:1687–93.

Adhesion is a fairly slow process, and platelet plug formation is greatly amplified by platelet activation. Platelet activation is induced by binding of ligands (i.e., vWF and collagen) to platelet surface receptors, platelet adhesion per se, and agonists released during platelet degranulation (e.g., ADP, 5-HT, epinephrine, thromboxane A_2) or produced by the coagulation cascade. Platelets undergo morphological as well as functional changes on activation. Activated platelets extend cytoplasmic processes from their cell bodies, lose their surface undulation and appear smooth. They spread, flatten and increase their surface area by as much as 400% to cover an endothelial defect and also to assemble procoagulant "factories." During the activation process, phosphotidyl serine from the inner cell membrane migrates to the outer layer to increase the amount of negatively charged phospholipid from virtually 0% to 12% [10]. Simultaneously, the binding of ligands to cell membrane receptors signals platelets to express and activate GP IIb/IIIa receptors, thus converting them from low to high affinity receptors. This process is referred to as inside-out signaling and enhances the ability of platelets to aggregate via fibrinogen bridges [11].

As platelet adhesion to the subendothelium progresses, they recruit additional platelets to form a mass of aggregated platelets. Platelet aggregation is an important step in hemostasis. A resting platelet has 40,000–80,000 GPIIb/IIIa receptors with a low affinity for fibrinogen. Platelet activation not only increases the number of these receptors, but also causes a conformational change, resulting in an increased affinity for fibrinogen. During this process, platelets lose a marginal band of microtubules to change their shape from discs to spiny spheres [12], centralize storage granules, form pseudopodia [13], and phosphorylate intracellular proteins [14]. Aggregated platelets undergo activation by forming a receptor–agonist complex between surface receptors of platelets and their agonists, such as thrombin, adenosine diphosphate (ADP), epinephrine, collagen, and arachidonic acid [15].

Extracellular agonists stimulate the secretory function of platelets by increasing the cytoplasmic calcium level via multiple pathways. Activation of phospholipase A_2 releases free arachidonic acid to form the potent platelet aggregator thromboxane A_2 and this in turn transports calcium from intracellular stores to cytoplasm [16, 17]. Phospholipase A_2, in addition, promotes synthesis of PGD_2, an inhibitor of platelet activation, to modulate platelet activities. ADP, platelet activating factor (PAF), and activation of phospholipase C and protein kinase C also raise cytoplasmic calcium concentration to potentiate platelet aggregation [18].

Activation of platelets results in the release of intracellular granules, exposure of platelet receptors for plasma proteins, and structural change in the platelet surface membrane. Several types of granules containing a variety of chemicals are present in platelets. Dense bodies contain serotonin, adenosine triphosphate (ATP), ADP, pyrophosphate, and calcium. Alpha-granules store adhesive proteins, such as fibrinogen, vWF, factor V, high-molecular-weight kininogen, fibronectin, α_1-antitrypsin, β-thromboglobulin, platelet factor 4, and platelet-derived growth factor. Lysosomes include acid hydrolases that are released during the inflammatory process [12].

Receptors for specific plasma proteins are found in the platelet membrane. Receptors for fibrinogen (glycoprotein IIb-IIIa complex) are essential in platelet aggregation and are activated by any agonists inducing platelet aggregation [19]. Therefore, lack of glycoproteins seen in patients with Glanzmann's thrombasthenia leads to significant bleeding [20]. A glycoprotein receptor for vWF (Ib) is known to be present, and interactions between glycoprotein receptors and fibronectin and thrombospondin also participate in platelet aggregation [21]. Additionally, platelets develop receptors for specific plasma coagulation factors during the course of activation. Activated factor V (Va) secreted by the platelet or circulating in the plasma serves as a binding site for factor Xa.

Cyclic 3',5'-adenosine monophosphate (cyclic AMP) is one of the most important regulatory substance that modulates activation of platelets [22]. Cyclic AMP, with the support of PGD_2 in platelets, reduces cytoplasmic free calcium to regulate platelet activation by stimulating a calcium/magnesium ATPase-dependent pump [23]. Other regulatory substances include an ADP-destroying ectoenzyme (ADPase) on the endothelial cell surface and thrombomodulin, a thrombin inhibitor.

Understanding of platelet activation and its regulation process led to the development of new classes of antiplatelet drugs: GPIIb/IIIa receptor antagonists (abciximab and eptifibatide) and ADP receptor antagonists (clopidogrel and ticlopidine).

Coagulation phase

Clotting factors involved in the coagulation cascade are listed in Table 6.2. The liver synthesizes most coagulation protein factors, and the majority are serine proteases. Factor VIII is produced partially in the liver and partially by megakaryocytes and endothelial cells. Factors II, VII, IX and X are vitamin K-dependent factors and contain γ-glutamyl carboxyl acid (GIa) residues at the N-terminal end of the molecule [24], which require vitamin K for their hepatic synthesis. The carboxyl groups of the GIa residue bind to calcium to serve as a bridge for protein binding to the phospholipid surface. Factors VII, IX and X are structurally similar with two epidermal

Table 6.2 Clotting factors.

Factors	Name
I	Fibrinogen
II	Prothrombin
III	Tissue thromboplastin (or tissue factor)
IV	Calcium
V	Proaccelerin
VII	Proconnectin
VIII	Antihemophilic factor
IX	Christmas factor
X	Stuart Power factor
XI	Plasma thromboplastin antecedent
XII	Hageman factor
XIII	Fibrin stabilizing factor

growth factor-like domains. Prothrombin, instead, has a kringle domain, (so named because it resembles a Scandinavian pastry). Coumadin, a vitamin K antagonist, inhibits activation of factors II, VII, IX, and X and, consequently, interferes with coagulation. Factors V and VIII are not proteases, but large molecular weight cofactors for the proteases. They have a structural similarity to ceruloplasmin and are referred to as labile factors owing to their short half-life. They are present in plasma in inactive forms and need to be activated by minor proteolytic cleavage.

For the surface activation or intrinsic system, factor XII (Hageman factor) binds to negatively charged surfaces such as kaolin, dextran sulfate, and sulfatides, and binding to these surfaces activates factor XII to XIIa by exposing its catalytic site [25, 26]. Two of the major substrates of factor XIIa are prekallikrein and factor XI, both of which exist in a noncovalent molecular complex with HMWK [27]. Factor XIa activates factor IX in the presence of calcium (Figure 6.3). Factor IX is one of the vitamin K-dependent proteins, and is synthesized as prozymogens and converted to serine proteases by a limited number of proteolytic cleavages. Factor IXa, in turn, activates factor X in the presence of calcium, phospholipids and a large protein cofactor, factor VIII. Factor VIII is found in the form of a noncovalent complex with vWF [28], and accelerates the conversion of factor X to Xa. The absence of factor VIII and IX results in hemophilia A and hemophilia B, respectively.

In addition to the intrinsic system developed within the vascular system, the extrinsic system also converts factor X to Xa with tissue factor (thromboplastin) being a cofactor. Tissue thromboplastin is a lipoprotein with a

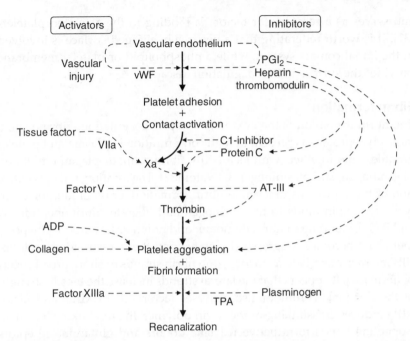

Figure 6.3 Overview of hemostasis. The process of hemostasis is illustrated by the series of cellular and coagulation factor events shown by the solid vertical arrows in the center. Activators and other procoagulants influence hemostasis as noted by the dotted arrows at left. Inhibitors of hemostasis and processes acting to degrade coagulant proteins or inhibit platelet aggregation are shown as dashed arrows at right. With permission from Cohnan RW, Marder VJ. Salzman EW, Hirsh J. Overview of hemostasis. In: Colman RW, Hirsh J, Marder VJ, Salzman EW, eds. *Hemostasis and Thrombosis*. Philadelphia: Lippincott; 1987, p. 4.

single polypeptide chain bound noncovalently to phospholipid [29]. Its cofactor activity is similar to HMWK in the contact phase, to factor VIII in the intrinsic system, and to factor V in the final common pathway. Factor VII is an important next protein in the extrinsic system [30]. The coagulant activity of factor VII is potentiated by factor XIIa or factor IXa and requires tissue thromboplastin, suggesting the intrinsic and extrinsic pathway interacts at several levels of the cascade.

Factor Xa formed by either the extrinsic or the intrinsic pathway converts prothrombin to thrombin. Factor Xa removes the N-terminal GIa portion from prothrombin, resulting in separation of the two-chain thrombin molecule from the phospholipid surface. The interaction of factor Xa, factor V, phospholipid, and calcium (prothrombinase complex) leads to an explosive activation of prothrombin on the platelet membrane. The factor V in the prothrombinase complex is secreted from α-granules and serves as a receptor for factor Xa binding to the activated platelets [31]. It is worth reiterating that a negatively charged surface is involved in the initial contact system, while a phospholipid or platelet membrane provides the surface in the coagulation cascade.

Fibrin formation

The fibrin formation is the next major step in coagulation. Fibrinogen, a large glycoprotein, is present in high concentration in plasma and platelet granules, and interacts with factor XIII, fibronectin, α_2-plasmin inhibitor, plasminogen, and plasminogen activator [32]. The location and concentration of these proteins determine fibrin formation, cross linking or fibrin lysis. Thrombin binds to the fibrinogen and liberates fibrinopeptides A and B [33], resulting in fibrin monomer and polymer formation. The polymer chain becomes progressively longer, and the two-stranded protofibrills interact laterally to form long, thin fibrin strands or short, broad sheets of fibrin [34]. It appears that the lateral strands increase the tensile strength of the clot [35]. Thrombin also activates factor XIII to XIIIa, and factor XIIIa induces crosslinking of the fibrin polymer. In crosslinking, covalent isopeptide bonds form between lysine donors and glutamine receptors [36], with two γ-chains cross-linked rapidly to form γ-γ dimers; α-chains are cross-linked more slowly, each with two other such chains, to form a polymer network [37]. The cross-linked fibrin fiber contains approximately 100 protofibrills linked and branched together in a random fashion and is plasmin-resistant.

The fibrin mesh binds the platelets together and attaches itself to the vessel wall by binding to platelet receptor glycoproteins and by interactions with thrombospondin, fibronectin, and fibrinogen released from platelet granules [38]. These proteins serve as bridges between plasma proteins and the platelet interior, between platelets and the vessel wall, and between plasma fibrin fibers and the subendothelial matrix. Platelets play another important role: Their glycoprotein IIb/IIIa joins plasma fibrinogen (or α-granule fibrinogen) to intracellular actin to induce clot retraction and vasoconstriction [39]. A high local thrombin concentration (approximately 150 nM) inside a thrombus results in activation of thrombin activatable fibrinolysis inhibitor (TAFI) [40, 41], and activated TAFI cleaves lysine residues from the fibrin surface, thereby preventing the binding of tPA and plasminogen [42, 43].

Fibrinolysis

Fibrinolysis is the process of removing unwanted clot. Fibrinogen is broken down by plasmin into fibrin degradation products (FDPs), which are then removed from circulation by the reticuloendothelial system. The production of plasmin from its inactive precursor, plasminogen, is a closely regulated process that is accomplished by one of two activators: tissue plasminogen activator (tPA) and urokinase (uPA) [44]. Tissue plasminogen activator is present in plasma in a large quantity and plays a major role in removing intravascular clot. uPA is produced by tissue macrophages and is present only in small concentrations in plasma and may play a role in removing fibrin from tissue. Thrombin is a potent stimulus for release of tPA by endothelial cells [45]. tPA has a short plasma half life (4 min) as it is rapidly inactivated by plasminogen activator inhibitor type 1 (PAI-1) and subsequently eliminated by hepatic clearance. PAI-1 is a serine protease inhibitor synthesized in the liver and endothelium, and its expression is increased in inflammatory states [46]. PAI-1 rapidly binds to and neutralizes tPA in plasma and uPA, but not streptokinase. However, binding to fibrinogen not only protects TPA from inactivation, but also increases its affinity for plasminogen. It activates plasminogen to plasmin, which then degrades the fibrin. Bound plasmin is protected from α_2-antiplasmin, while free plasmin in the plasma is quickly inactivated [47]. Thrombin modulates fibrinolytic activation by activating Factor XIIIa and TAFI.

Although this coagulation cascade, developed in 1964, has been well accepted [48], it has been modified to a cell-based model which describes the complex networking of various elements of coagulation (Figure 6.4) [49]. In this model, tissue factor expressed by vascular smooth muscle cells, pericytes, and adventitial fibroblasts in the vessel wall is physically separated from its ligand factor VII/VIIa by the endothelium. Vessel injury leads to the rapid binding of platelets to the subendothelium and activation of the coagulation cascade by tissue factor. Propagation of the thrombus involves recruitment of additional platelets and amplification of the coagulation cascade by the intrinsic pathway, and possibly by tissue factor-positive microparticles and tissue factor stored in platelets. Finally, fibrin deposition stabilizes the clot. De novo synthesis of TF by platelets may also play a role in stabilization of the clot.

Recently, blood has been found to contain microparticles (MPs) derived from a variety of cell types, including platelets, monocytes, and endothelial cells [50]. In addition, tumor cells release MPs into the circulation. MPs are formed from membrane blebs that are released from the cell surface by proteolytic cleavage of the cytoskeleton. All MPs are procoagulants because they provide membrane surfaces for the assembly of components of the coagulation protease cascade. Importantly, procoagulant activity is increased by the presence of anionic phospholipids, particularly

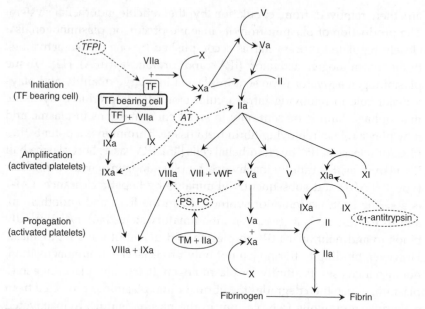

Figure 6.4 Cell-based model of hemostasis comprising initiation, amplification, and propagation. Solid arrows indicate activation and dotted arrows indicate inhibition. TF, tissue factor; TFPI, tissue factor pathway inhibitor; AT, antithrombin; PS, protein S; PC, protein C; TM, thrombomodulin Modified with permission from Vine AK. Recent advances in haemostasis and thrombosis. Retina. 2009;29:1–7.

phosphatidylserine (PS), and the procoagulant protein tissue factor (TF), which is the major cellular activator of the clotting cascade.

Regulation of hemostasis

Excessive activation of coagulation can cause thrombosis and tissue ischemia. Inadequate clot formation, on the other hand, can precipitate organ injury either directly from hemorrhage into tissue or indirectly as a consequence of hemorrhagic shock. Coagulation, therefore, needs to be closely regulated to ensure that neither extreme is attained. This balance is achieved by regulating procoagulant, anticoagulant and prolysins and antilysins.

The propensity to form intravascular clot has been summarized into Virchow's triad of endothelial injury, hypercoagulability, and blood stasis. Flow of blood discourages coagulation by diluting and washing away any activated coagulation factors. Intact endothelium also discourages clot formation by preventing blood from coming into contact with the subendothelium and produces heparin, a cofactor for antithrombin (AT). Endothelial cells also produce nitric oxide and prostacyclin to inhibit platelet activation and to discourage vascular stasis by vasodilation. Endothelial cells express a membrane protein, thrombomodulin, which binds and changes the nature of thrombin from a procoagulant to an anticoagulant protease. After binding with thrombomodulin, thrombin loses its affinity for fibrinogen but activates protein C. The activated protein C forms a complex with protein S to inhibit VIIIa and Va. The importance of Protein S and C as anticoagulants is exemplified by factor V Leiden abnormality. In this condition, production of genetically altered factor V resistant to inhibition by protein C leads to the most common prothrombotic condition in Caucasians.

Coagulation is regulated by the positive and negative feedback mechanisms. The process of positive feedback is repeated in many stage of coagulation. For example, kallikrein cleaves factor XII to accelerate contact activation and cleaves HMWK to liberate the nonapeptide bradykinin. The activated HMWK allows more prekallikrein (and factor XI) to interact with the activating surfaces [27]. An example of negative feedback is found in the conversion of factor XIIa to factor XIIf by kallikrein to turn off surface-bound coagulation. Factor XIa also cleaves the light chain of HMWK to limit its cofactor activity [51].

Plasma proteolytic inhibitors also participate in controlling the extent and speed of coagulation and fibrinolysis. Cl inhibitor is the major inhibitor of the intrinsic system, which inhibits factor XIIa and kallikrein [52]. α_1-antitrypsin inhibits factor Xia [53] and neutrophil elastase, and its deficiency results in emphysema due to the unopposed effects of elastase in the lung.

Antithrombin is the major inhibitor of factors IXa, Xa and thrombin by forming inactive antithrombin-serine protease complexes. The inhibition is potentiated by heparin by its binding to a lysine group in antithrombin [54]. It is known that approximately 40–50% reduction in antithrombin may lead to thrombotic conditions. α_2-macroglobulin is a secondary inhibitor for many plasma coagulants and fibrinolytic enzymes, including kallikrein, thrombin, and plasmin. α_2-macroglobulin-enzyme complexes possess some enzymatic activity and may be utilized for inhibition of certain enzymes protected from other inhibitors.

Abnormal hemostasis

Disorders of hemostasis may be encountered in the perioperative period, and they may arise from an abnormality in any phase of coagulation.

Spontaneous bleeding in the absence of trauma, however, is unusual and indicative of major defect in the hemostatic system. Medical bleeding is a term that refers to excessive spontaneous or traumatic hemorrhage in the presence of some aberration of hemostasis. Bleeding is usually controlled once the underlying hemostatic defect is corrected. While postoperative bleeding may be exacerbated by preexisting hemostatic defects, its primary cause is usually surgical.

Congenital hemostatic disorders
Von Willebrand disease (vWD)
This autosomal dominant disorder is the most common congenital hemostatic disorder with a prevalence of 1% and is the result of quantitative or qualitative defects in von Willebrand factor (vWF) [55]. Since vWF mediates platelet adhesion to the subendothelial matrix, platelet dysfunction is the common finding. Additionally, vWF is a carrier for factor VIII and prevents its rapid enzymatic degradation. Patients with vWD, therefore, have a variable factor VIII deficiency that contributes to bleeding [56, 57]. Laboratory tests reveal a prolonged bleeding time and activated partial thromboplastin time (aPTT). Diagnosis is made by ristocetin-induced platelet agglutination and by quantitation of vWF antigen. Bleeding in patients with a mild form of vWD can be controlled with desmopressin (DDAVP), which stimulates the release of endogenous vWF from endothelial cells. The drug is ineffective in subtypes of the disease producing either normal quantities of functionally abnormal vWF or no vWF at all. Treatment of the latter forms requires administration of factor VIII/vWF concentrates in the form of either cryoprecipitate (CRYO) or commercially available alternatives that have been heat-treated to destroy human immunodeficiency virus (HIV).

Hemophilia A and B
Hemophilia A is an X-linked recessive disorder resulting in a deficiency of coagulation factor VIII. It occurs in 1 in 10,000 live male births. Phenotypic expression varies with the degree of factor activity. Children with severe disease (factor VIII < 1%) present with cephalhematoma at birth or neonatal bleeding after circumcision. Children with the moderate form of the disease (factor VIII, 1–5%) often present with bleeding episodes into soft tissues and joints following mild trauma. Patients with mild disease (factor VIII > 5%) may be seen in adolescence with hemarthrosis and arthropathies involving weight-bearing joints or with serious bleeding following major trauma or surgery [58, 59]. aPTT is usually prolonged, and specific factor assays are required to distinguish it from hemophilia B.

Hemophilia B occurs less frequently (1 in 100 000 live births) and is due to factor IX deficiency. Treatment of acute bleeding episodes hinges on restoration of plasma factor levels. Rarer conditions that might be encountered are found elsewhere [52].

Hemophilia C
Unlike the X-linked hemophilias, hemophilia C, is an autosomal disorder and caused by factor XI deficiency [60]. Its incidence is approximately 1:1,000,000, and severe hemophilia C is more common in Ashkenazi Jewish descendants, with an incidence of 1:450 [61]. The association between abnormal hemostasis and mild factor XI deficiency is controversial, ranging from poor correlation between factor XI levels and bleeding [62], to minimal bleeding in minor surgery such as tooth extraction, tonsillectomy, nasal surgery, and urologic surgery [63]. In patients with moderate to severe hemophilia C, fresh frozen plasma (FFP) or factor XI concentrate are effective, and activated prothrombin complex concentrates and recombinant factor VIIa have been used successfully for major surgery in patients with factor XI inhibitors [64].

There are other types of rare congenital hemostatic disorders [65]. Congenital afibrinogenemia/hypofibrinogenemia is treated by FFP, CRYO, and fibrinogen concentrate, hypoprothrombinemia by FFP and prothrombin complex, Factor V deficiency by FFP, and Factor VII deficiency by recombinant activated factor VII.

Acquired hemostatic disorders
Acquired disorders are more frequently encountered than their hereditary counterparts.

Vitamin K deficiency
Vitamin K is a fat-soluble vitamin that acts as a cofactor for γ-carboxylation of certain glutamic acid residues in prothrombin and factors VII, IX, and X. Vitamin K deficiency can arise from inadequate dietary intake or defective intestinal absorption [66]. Prolonged administration of broad-spectrum antibiotics may cause vitamin K deficiency, as vitamin K-producing gut flora is destroyed. Early in its course, vitamin K deficiency presents with a prolonged prothrombin time (PT) and a normal aPTT owing to deficiency of factor VII with the shortest half-life [67]. When other vitamin K-dependent factors become depleted, aPTT is also prolonged. Parenteral vitamin K ameliorates the condition within 12–24 h. For a more rapid correction, fresh frozen plasma (FFP) is required.

Liver disease

The etiology of coagulation disorders in patients with chronic liver disease is multifactorial, and it affects all phases of coagulation [68, 69]. Thrombocytopenia may result from reduced production and splenic sequestration and destruction of platelets. Synthesis of coagulation factors is also impaired by chronic liver disease, since the liver produces all coagulation factors except VIII and vWF. Liver disease may also impair the absorption and storage of vitamin K, resulting in vitamin K deficiency. The diseased reticuloendothelial component of the liver impairs the clearance of activated coagulation factors resulting in hypercoagulation and possibly consumptive coagulopathy. In addition, impaired clearance of tPA, together with excessive activation of coagulation, triggers fibrinolysis.

Massive transfusion

Massive transfusion (greater than 10 units of packed red blood cells in 24 hours) to correct hemorrhage can precipitate coagulopathy and exacerbate bleeding. This has been referred to as the 'bloody vicious cycle' [70]. The cause of coagulopathy following massive transfusion is multifactorial. Dilutional coagulopathy is the primary cause of coagulopathy in patients with acute bleeding, since a large quantity of coagulation factors and platelets can be lost. In uncomplicated major bleeding, dilutional coagulopathy is self-limiting once platelets and coagulation factors are replenished. The dilutional coagulopathy, however, can be compounded by complications of massive transfusion and impaired tissue perfusion. Metabolic acidosis is a common occurrence from acids in the transfused blood and tissue lactic acidosis, and impairs coagulation by inhibiting the enzymatic reactions involved in the coagulation cascade. Massive transfusion together with inadequate hepatic perfusion leads to ionic hypocalcemia or citrate intoxication to impair coagulation [71]. Hypothermia can be another factor that may interfere with coagulation. Hypovolemia and inadequate tissue perfusion are the primary causes of hypothermia seen during massive transfusion [72], and exposure to cold environment and the use of cold resuscitating solutions are contributory factors. Hypothermia produces a number of detrimental effects on coagulation. It increases splenic and hepatic platelet sequestration [73], alters platelet morphology [74], and inhibits platelet function [75]. The coagulation cascade, an enzymatic process, is also inhibited [76, 77]. Decreasing the body temperature to 35 °C, 33 °C and 31 °C prolongs PT equivalent to that achieved by reducing factor IX activity to 39%, 16% and 2.5% of normal value, respectively [78]. It should be noted, however, that impaired coagulation in hypothermia may be protective, because 'normal' coagulation in slow circulation at the capillary level may precipitate thrombosis. The role of hypothermia-induced vasoconstriction on clinical bleeding is unknown.

Drugs

Many patients are placed on inhibitors of coagulation to treat or prevent thrombotic events, such as stroke, coronary thrombosis, and deep venous thrombosis, and these drugs affect hemostasis in a predictable way.

Disseminated intravascular coagulation (DIC)

DIC has been extensively reviewed in the past [79, 80]. Briefly, DIC is characterized by an excessive, uncontrolled activation of coagulation triggered by various stimuli, followed by secondary fibrinolysis. Bleeding is a consequence of depletion of coagulation factors and platelets, and fibrinolysis. Laboratory diagnosis is made by prolonged PT and aPTT, hypofibrinogenemia, thrombocytopenia, and the presence of a large quantity of fibrin(ogen) degradation products and D-dimer. DIC is managed by the treatment of underlying pathology and replacement therapy. Administration of FFP replaces coagulation inhibitors (i.e., antithrombin) in addition to coagulation factors, and platelet infusion restores platelet function. The use of coagulation inhibitors (i.e., heparin) is still controversial.

Heparin induced thrombocytopenia

Heparin-induced thrombocytopenia (HIT) is an IgG-mediated hypersensitivity reaction to heparin [81, 82]. It is characterized by a decrease in platelet count and a propensity for venous or arterial thrombosis. Heparin binds to platelets via PF4 and elicits IgG antibody production. These antibodies activate platelets by binding to platelet FCγIIa receptors by their Fe tails. HIT antibodies also facilitate thrombin generation by mediating tissue factor expression by endothelial cells and macrophages. While this condition is primarily prothrombotic, concurrent bleeding may occur in the face of severe thrombocytopenia.

Cardiopulmonary bypass

Cardiopulmonary bypass (CPB) is associated with a qualitative and quantitative platelet dysfunction characterized by an increase in bleeding time and a decrease in platelet aggregation and granular contents [83]. This defect is caused by the excessive activation of platelets by CPB and removal of aggregated platelets by the reticuloendothelial system [84]. The degree of platelet dysfunction is related to the duration of CPB, and bleeding time and platelet function returns to normal after about 1 h of uncomplicated CPB.

Circulating anticoagulants

Circulating anticoagulants are immunoglobulins formed against any enzymes of the coagulation cascade, and the most common ones are antibodies against factor VIII. The lupus anticoagulant is an antibody against phospholipids, which was initially described in patients with systemic lupus erythematosus. Whilst excessive bleeding has been described in patients with lupus anticoagulant [85], this is primarily a prothrombotic condition.

Evaluation of hemostasis

History and physical examination

History and physical examination are helpful in identifying patients with underlying coagulation disorders and assessing the risk of bleeding in the intra- and postoperative period. An inquiry should be made into bleeding tendencies following minor or major trauma, dental procedure, or various types of surgery. A family history of bleeding may indicate an inherited coagulation disorder. Medication history is useful in identifying drugs or nutritional supplements that can affect coagulation. Coexisting medical conditions that may affect coagulation (e.g., congestive heart failure, renal dysfunction and cirrhosis) should be investigated. Certain malignancies may also be associated with bleeding dyscrasia. For example, 15% of patients with acute myelocytic leukemia develop DIC.

A physical examination might reveal evidence of underlying medical conditions. The presence of petechia and ecchymosis may suggest primary hemostatic defect. Stigmata of chronic liver disease (ascites, hepatosplenomegaly and jaundice) should alert the clinician of the possibility of hemostatic dysfunction.

Coagulation tests

Laboratory tests are conducted to confirm preliminary suspicions and to identify the site of the coagulation disorder, either at the coagulation proteins or at platelets.

Prothrombin time

In this test, tissue thromboplastin containing tissue factor and phospholipid are added to the citrated blood specimen, and the specimen is then recalcified. PT is the time to form the initial clot and is the expression of the extrinsic pathway. Since various sources of thromboplastin are used, a great variation is observed in its results. The International Normalized Ratio (INR) was introduced in an effort to overcome this shortcoming. It standardizes the measurement both with respect to values for normal patients and standard human thromboplastin sensitivity established by the World Health Organization. INRs obtained from different laboratories with different sources of thromboplastin are, therefore, comparable. PT monitors activities of factors V, VII, X, prothrombin and thrombin, and is prolonged in defects of the extrinsic and common pathways. It is abnormal in vitamin K deficiency and is considered to be the most sensitive hepatic synthetic function test. It is also used to monitor the anticoagulant effects of coumadin.

Activated partial thromboplastin time
aPTT evaluates the intrinsic and common pathways. Phospholipid, calcium and a contact activator (i.e., kaolin or silica) are added to the citrated specimen, and clotting is activated via the intrinsic pathway. This is a reliable test with less than 10% variability and used to monitor heparin activity. Abnormal prolongation may be seen in the presence of circulating antibodies or when insufficient quantity of blood is mixed into the anticoagulant.

Thrombin time and reptilase time
Thrombin is added to the citrated blood specimen, and the time to clot formation is noted. The thrombin time (TT) is prolonged in hypofibrinogenemia, dysfibrinogenemia and in the presence of thrombin inhibitors, such as heparin and FDPs. The Reptilase Time (RT) is a modification of the thrombin time. Reptilase, like thrombin, cleaves fibrinogen. Unlike thrombin, the cleavage fragments formed can spontaneously polymerize even in the presence of FDPs. Additionally, reptilase is not inhibited by AT and is unaffected by heparin. An abnormal TT in the presence of a normal RT suggests the presence of a thrombin inhibitor.

Bleeding time and platelet count
For bleeding time, a blood pressure cuff is applied to the upper arm and inflated to 40 mmHg in order to achieve a standardized venous pressure. One or two incisions are made on the forearm (9 mm long and 1 mm deep). A filter paper is used to blot the incision every 30 s until bleeding ceases. The bleeding time is a sensitive indicator of platelet dysfunction as long as platelet count is greater than $100,000/mm^3$. Therefore, simultaneous determination of platelet count is important in interpretation of bleeding time.

Bleeding time is prolonged in patients on aspirin and with von Willebrand disease and Glanzmann's thrombasthenia. It has a number of drawbacks. It is prolonged in the absence of platelet dysfunction in patients with anemia, severe hypofibrinogenemia, and vascular defects. It is labor intensive, and results may vary depending on location, technical expertise, and age and sex of the patient.

Specialized platelet function tests

Platelet aggregometry measures platelet aggregation induced by ADP, thrombin or collagen. Aggregation cytometry utilizes monoclonal antibodies to determine platelet surface receptor density. A detailed discussion of these tests is beyond the scope of this chapter.

Platelet function analyzer

The platelet function analyzer (PFA) evaluates primary hemostasis by measuring the time required for whole blood to occlude an aperture in the membrane of the test cartridge, which is coated with platelet agonist. It requires only 500 µL of blood, and is conducted at 37 °C. The test can be conducted at the patient's bedside and is simple, quick, reliable, and reproducible [86].

Activated clotting time

Blood is added to a test tube containing an activator, such as kaolin or diatomaceous earth. The blood in the test tube is placed in a well where it is gently rotated to mix its contents and warmed to 37 °C. The time to clot formation is the activated clotting time (ACT), and it monitors clot formation by the intrinsic pathway. Unlike aPTT, which is unreliable after a large dose of heparin, ACT is reliable even after a large dose of heparin given during CPB. ACT has the greatest utility in this setting and can be used as a bedside monitor for coagulation.

Ecarin clotting time

Direct thrombin inhibitors (DTIs) such as hirudin, lepirudin, argatroban and bivalirudin are frequently used in patients with HIT or thrombosis. At low DTI concentrations, TT, aPTT, and ACT provide reasonable correlations with DTI concentration. The correlation, however, is poor when a high concentration is required during CPB, and ecarin clotting time is a better monitoring test [87]. The test employs the venom of the saw-scaled viper (*Echis carinatus*). The metalloprotease in the venom converts normal prothrombin to meizothrombin, which is still capable of converting fibrinogen to fibrin in a dose-dependent manner [88]. Thromboelastography using ecarin-treated blood to initiate coagulation has also been reported to provide a better correlation with bivalirudin levels than with ACT [89].

Anti-Xa activity assay

Anti-factor Xa activity assay is used to monitor the effects of low-molecular -weight heparins, indirect factor Xa inhibitors and, occasionally, unfractionated heparin. Patient plasma is mixed with a reagent containing a known amount of factor Xa and excess antithrombin. A chromogenic substrate of factor Xa is added, and a color change reaction indicates the proportion to the factor Xa not bound by anti-factor Xa activity in the patient's serum.

Preoperative screening tests

Determination of PT, aPTT, platelet count and bleeding time is commonly employed for screening surgical patients who may develop excessive bleeding. They are, however, very poor screening tools for the general population and do not per se predict the risk of bleeding. For example, Eisenberg et al. reviewed 750 patients who required general surgical or gynecological procedures [90]. Abnormal PT and/or aPTT results were obtained in 2.7% of 480 patients with no clinical history and signs of bleeding – an incidence similar to that occurring by chance (2.28%) – and none of the patients with prolonged PT developed bleeding complications. A similar observation was made by Velanovich in 520 patients undergoing elective surgical procedures, in which neither PT nor aPTT had independent or associated value in predicting surgical bleeding [91]. The lack of correlation between screening tests and the degree of bleeding in surgical patients is also found in bleeding time [92]. In a retrospective analysis on 1800 patients undergoing various surgical procedures, the bleeding time was prolonged in 110 (6%) patients. Of these, 66 ingested drugs that affect platelet function, 6 had uremia, 11 had platelet count less than $100,000/mm^3$, and 27 with unknown etiology. Seven patients experienced postoperative bleeding: three patients experienced minor bleeding and four had bleeding unrelated with platelet dysfunction.

Thromboelastography

Thromboelastography (TEG) is a method of assessing whole blood coagulation, and technical aspects of the test have been extensively reviewed [93, 94]. Briefly, a small quantity of blood (0.36 ml) is placed into a cuvette, and a central piston (*pin*) suspended by a torsion wire is lowered into the blood specimen (Figure 6.5). A rim of blood about 1 mm in width is created between the cuvette and the piston. The cuvette rotates with a 4.5° angle

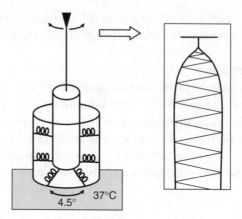

Figure 6.5 Schematic diagram of thromboelastography.

in either direction at every 4.5 seconds, with a midcycle oscillatory pause of 1 s. Most commonly, TEG recording begins at 4 minutes from blood sampling. Before clot formation, the pin is stationary. As a clot begins to form, increasing elastic force of fibrin strands couples the pin and the cuvette and oscillatory movement of the cuvette is transmitted to the pin. The torque experienced by the pin is plotted graphically on paper, or digitally on a computer screen (Hemoscope, Skokie, Illinois). The reaction or gelation time (R) is the latency period between the initiation of the test (when the specimen was placed in the cup) and measurable fibrin formation (amplitude of 2 mm) (Figure 6.6). The clot formation time (K) begins from the initiation of clot formation to the point where amplitude becomes 20 mm. R and K are prolonged in patients with coagulation factor deficiency, thrombocytopenia and in the presence of anticoagulants

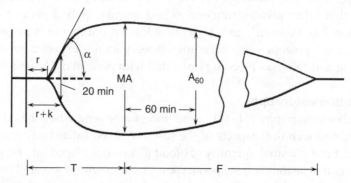

Figure 6.6 Typical thromboelastographic variables measured (*Source*: Kang et al. [102] with permission).

(e.g., heparin). The alpha angle (α) measures the rate of clot formation and is affected by coagulation protein deficiencies and/or platelet dysfunction. Maximum amplitude (MA) is affected by platelet function and fibrinogen concentration. TEG parameters have been compared with conventional coagulation tests [95]. R and K times correlate with aPTT, and amplitude (A, mm) with the clot strength or shear elastic modulus, G [G (dynes cm^{-2}) = (5,000A)/(100 − A)]. A positive relation between maximum amplitude and platelets and fibrinogen has been demonstrated [96, 97].

TEGs of various clinical conditions are shown in Figure 6.7 [98]. Deficiency of coagulation factors (e.g., hemophilia), hypocalcemia, hypothermia, and heparin effect are seen as a prolonged reaction time and slow clot formation rate. Thrombocytopenia is seen as small maximum amplitude and prolonged reaction time and slow clot formation rate, because platelet function is essential to the progression of the coagulation cascade. In patients with fibrinolysis, prolonged reaction time, slow clot formation rate and small maximum amplitude are accompanied by a gradual decrease in amplitude to zero, because the net amount of fibrin is reduced in the presence of active digestion of fibrins. Excessive activation of coagulation is seen as very short reaction time and rapid clot formation rate. Once DIC develops, all TEG variables deteriorate and a straight line is formed.

TEG has several advantages over standard methods of coagulation monitoring. It is portable and the test can be performed at the patient's bedside. Results can be obtained fairly quickly: the onset of clot formation within a few minutes and platelet function within 45 minutes. While

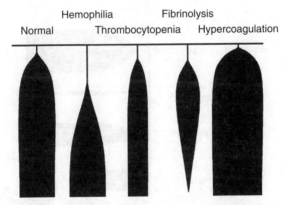

Figure 6.7 Thromboelastographic patterns of normal and disease states. (*Source*: Kang et al. [98] with permission).

conventional coagulation tests end observation once fibrin begins to form, TEG assesses dynamic changes of the complete coagulation process, from coagulation to fibrinolysis. Further, it is possible to make definitive differential diagnosis of coagulopathy by comparing multiple channels of TEG. For example, a comparison between TEG of untreated blood (0.36 mL) and that of blood treated with FFP (0.03 mL of FFP in 0.33 mL of whole blood) elucidates the presence of coagulation factor deficiency and beneficial effects of FFP administration. A similar comparison can be made by comparing TEGs of blood treated with other blood products (platelets and CRYO) and pharmacologic agents (e-aminocaproic acid (EACA), protamine sulfate, aprotinin, DDAVP, etc.) [99–101].

Differential diagnosis of pathologic coagulation during liver transplantation is shown in Figure 6.8. Coagulation deteriorated rapidly on reperfusion of the grafted liver by prolonged clot formation rate, small amplitude, and rapid decrease in amplitude. A blood specimen treated with EACA improved coagulation by a shortened reaction time, increased amplitude and disappearance of fibrinolysis, suggesting active fibrinolysis. The same blood specimen treated with protamine sulfate normalized the reaction time and increased amplitude with persistent fibrinolysis, indicating the heparin effect. This patient received EACA (250 mg) and protamine sulfate (25 mg) to normalize coagulation.

TEG has been proved valuable in intraoperative management of coagulation during liver transplantation, in which the etiology of bleeding is multifactorial and changes in coagulation are rapid and dramatic [102]. Its clinical effectiveness also has been shown in cardiac surgery and other major surgical procedures [103]. Most importantly, it is a valuable educational tool in understanding the global coagulation process.

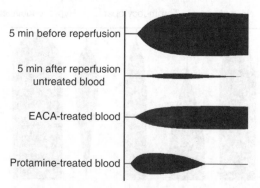

Figure 6.8 Differential diagnosis of fibrinolysis and heparin effect after reperfusion of the graft liver during orthotopic liver transplantation. (*Source*: Kang et al. [98] with permission).

Rotational thromboelastometry (ROTEM®)

ROTEM was introduced to the clinical arena recently. The principle of ROTEM is essentially similar to that of TEG, and both techniques measures shear viscoelasticity of the blood clotting process. The major difference is found in its design. In TEG, viscoelasticity is measured by the electromechanical force between the rotating cuvette with blood specimen and the fixed torsion wire, while ROTEM uses optomechanical mode between the fixed cuvette and rotating pin. Graphic results of ROTEM and TEG are similar, although ROTEM uses a different set of nomenclature. Differential diagnosis of coagulopathy can be made using both TEG and ROTEM by testing blood treated with various activators or inhibitors (heparinase, aprotinin and platelet inhibitor).

Management of intraoperative coagulation

Clinical coagulation

Although major advances have been made in understanding coagulation in the past three decades, clinicians are often puzzled by the complexity of coagulation and lack of relationship between laboratory values and clinical presentation. This may stem from over simplification of coagulation, analytic interpretation of coagulation instead of appreciation of global coagulation, and, possibly, insufficient education of clinical coagulation. It is worthwhile to review coagulation in the perspective of clinicians.

Coagulation is a part of systemic inflammatory response. As described in the contact activation of coagulation, vascular injury leads to activation of Hageman factor, which activates kallikrein, bradykinin, fibrinolysis, and the complement system. For example, tissue injury caused by various stimuli (laceration, thermal injury, ischemia, rejection, acidosis, etc.) activates inflammation and coagulation simultaneously to repair damaged tissue. Therefore, coagulation management should be directed to the treatment of underlying pathology.

Coagulation has five distinctive, equally important, interacting phases. However, major emphasis has been placed on the intrinsic and extrinsic system. The extent of vascular injury by the surgical team, local vasoconstriction and platelet aggregation may play a more important role in determining surgical blood loss, although its clinical significance has not been elucidated.

Hemostasis is a net balance between the clot formation and fibrinolysis with the positive and negative feedback, and is influenced by activities and interactions of procoagulants, anticoagulants, lysins, antilysins, physiologic variables, drugs and other chemical substances (Figure 6.1).

Commonly used coagulation tests (PT, aPTT and platelet count) represent only a fraction of the coagulation balance and do not provide clinicians with necessary clinical information.

Another puzzling issue is that the surgical field appears to be 'wet' particularly at the end of major surgical procedure, although the coagulation profile at this time may be relatively normal. It is speculated that this is a delayed bleeding phenomenon, possibly caused by the loss of incomplete clot formed in the presence of dilutional coagulopathy or by ongoing fibrinolysis after excessive activation of coagulation.

Coagulation management

Intraoperative hemorrhage can be life-threatening, and rapid and decisive intervention is essential. Surgical hemostasis is the most important part of coagulation management in most cases. The goal of medical management of coagulation is to maintain normal blood coagulability by frequent monitoring and specific therapy using minimal amounts of blood components or pharmacologic agents while avoiding thrombosis. The first step of coagulation management is maintaining optimal physiologic state (normovolemia, normothermia and normal electrolyte balance and acid-base state), since impaired tissue perfusion caused by the altered physiologic state triggers inflammatory response and coagulation. This is followed by replacement therapy and pharmacologic therapy.

Most clinicians agree that normal blood coagulability does not necessarily require a normal quantity or activity of coagulation elements, and the reverse is also true. The hypothetical relationship between blood coagulability and coagulation profiles is shown in Figure 6.9 [104]. Normal blood coagulability is expected in patients with normal coagulation profiles and is well maintained until levels of coagulation factors gradually decrease below the critical level. This is indirectly observed in hemophiliac patients in whom normal hemostasis is maintained unless factor VIII level reaches below 30% of normal value, and platelet function is relatively normal until platelet counts fall below 50,000/mm^3 [105, 106]. Blood coagulability, however, is impaired rapidly and becomes a clinical concern once coagulation factor levels decrease below this critical level. If this relationship exists, normal blood coagulability can be achieved by maintaining coagulation profiles above the critical level (shaded area), while administering a minimal quantity of blood products. This concept can be extended to patients undergoing surgical procedure with major bleeding (Figure 6.10).

Intraoperatively, coagulability and coagulation profiles deteriorate by dilution and/or pathologic coagulation, and can be corrected by

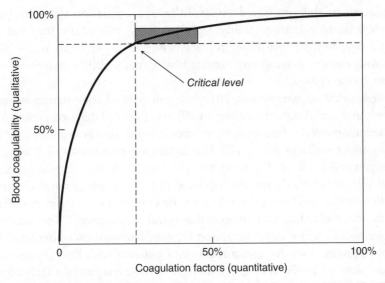

Figure 6.9 Hypothetical relationship between blood coagulability and coagulation profiles. (*Source*: Kang et al. [104] with permission.)

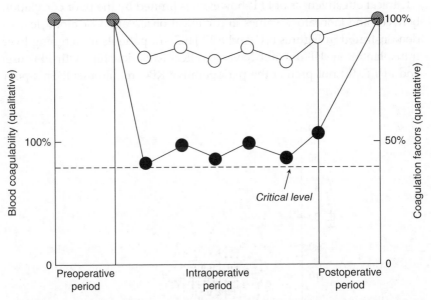

Figure 6.10 Blood coagulability and coagulation profiles during liver transplantation. Solid circles represent a hypothetical patient without coagulation monitoring and therapy, and open circles represent a patient with monitoring of coagulability and treatment. (*Source*: Kang [104] with permission.)

replacement therapy based on quantity of coagulation elements (open circles) or blood coagulability (solid circles). It is likely that patients with quantitative test-based replacement therapy receive more blood products while maintaining similar blood coagulability compared with their counterparts.

Monitoring of coagulation is an integral part of coagulation management, and serial determinations of PT, aPTT and platelet count are commonly employed. The conventional recommendation is to administer FFP to a patient with a prolonged PT. FFP contains approximately 400mg of fibrinogen and 1 unit of clotting factors per 1 ml of solution. Labile factors (V and VIII) are easily destroyed in thawed FFP unless refrigerated. Common indications of FFP are: (1) reversal of the effects of coumadin in patients with active bleeding or anticipated surgical procedures; (2) documented or suspected factor deficiency; and (3) supplementation of depleted factors following massive transfusion or in patients with liver disease. The usual dose of 15–20 ml/Kg is expected to raise coagulation factor levels by 2–3%. CRYO is rich in fibrinogen, factors VIII and vWF. It is indicated in vWD, hemophilia A, and the fibrinolytic state in which fibrinogen, factor V and VIII are selectively destroyed by plasmin.

Clinical effectiveness of FFP, however, is limited by the poor correlation between the laboratory values and clinical observation or blood loss as demonstrated in Figures 6.11 and 6.12 [107]. In patients undergoing liver transplantation, PT did not have significant relationship with FFP use, and aPTT did not predict the perioperative RBC requirement. This poor

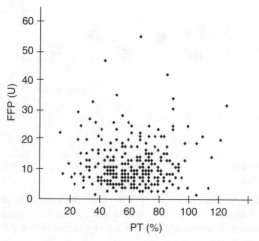

Figure 6.11 The relationship between FFP requirement and prothrombin time during liver transplantation. (*Source*: Gerlach et al. [107] with permission.)

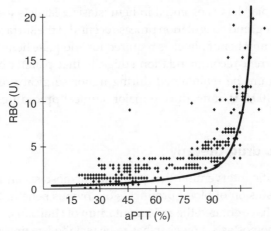

Figure 6.12 The relationship between RBC requirement and aPTT during liver transplantation. (*Source*: Gerlach et al. [107] with permission.)

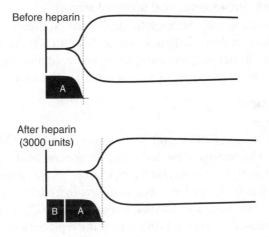

Figure 6.13 The clinical significance of moderately prolonged clot formation.

correlation may be explained by a comparison of TEG before and after heparin administration (Figure 6.13). Normal TEG pattern is observed before heparin administration. Bleeding, however, is expected to occur until clot is formed in the injured vessel, and the area under the curve (A) represents blood loss. Heparin administration typically prolongs the reaction time and shifts the TEG to the right. The area under the curve or bleeding becomes larger and includes (B). Therefore bleeding is greater with heparin administration, but the increase in the area under the curve (B) may not be large enough to cause clinically significant bleeding.

The role of platelets is essential in hemostasis: platelets form the initial hemostatic plug, and coagulation process occurs on the surface of platelets. Although the number of platelets required for adequate hemostasis is controversial, current recommendation suggests that platelet count greater than $50,000/mm^3$ be maintained during minor surgical procedures and greater than $100,000/mm^3$ during major surgical procedures and neurosurgery [108].

Hemostatic drug therapy

Any therapeutic intervention that promotes hemostasis and reduces the need for transfusion of blood product is of obvious benefit. Drugs of different classes have entered the armamentarium of clinicians. The benefit of augmenting hemostasis, however, has to be weighed against the potential for thrombotic sequelae that may arise.

Prolysins (tPA, urokinase, and streptokinase)

Acute interventions with fibrinolytic drugs can be lifesaving in patients with pulmonary emboli, ischemic stroke (e.g., middle cerebral arterial occlusion), and in patients suffering acute myocardial infraction without immediate access to percutaneous coronary interventions [109–111].

Antifibrinolytics
Lysine analogs

The lysine analogs, EACA and tranexamic acid (AMCA), accelerate activation of plasminogen by inducing conformational change in the molecule, but inhibit fibrinolysis by blocking the lysine-binding site of plasmin. Antifibrinolytics have been shown to reduce blood loss and transfusion requirements in cardiac surgery [112, 113], liver transplantation [114], prostate surgery [115], and joint replacement surgery [116, 117]. For cardiac surgery, either drug is given IV following the induction of anesthesia as a bolus followed by an infusion. The dose for EACA is 150 mg/kg bolus followed by 15 mg/kg/hr, and for AMCA it is 10 mg/kg followed by 1 mg/kg/hr. It is noteworthy that a recent study showed that a small, single dose of EACA (<500 mg) is effective in treating fibrinolysis during liver transplantation [118]. Since fibrinolysis is a natural protective mechanism against thrombosis; indiscriminate use of antifibrinolytics may lead to thrombosis.

Aprotinin

Aprotinin is a polypeptide serine protease inhibitor that reversibly binds to, and inactivates a number of serine proteases including trypsin, chymotrypsin, plasmin, kallikrein, Hageman factor, and most coagulation factors. As a result, it is expected to inhibit both coagulation and fibrinolysis [101]. It also prevents platelet activation during CPB and has been shown to preserve platelet GPIb receptors. Aprotinin is used in cardiac surgery to reduce blood loss and transfusion requirements, possibly by inhibiting excessive activation of coagulation and fibrinolysis. It is indicated when excessive blood loss is anticipated (i.e., redo cardiac surgery or patients on antiplatelet agents) or when blood transfusion is refused. Aprotinin is commonly given as 2 million KIU (kallikrein inactivation units) bolus followed by an infusion of 0.5 KIU/h. Aprotinin has been shown to reduce blood loss and transfusion requirements during liver transplantation [119]. However, recent literatures question the clinical effectiveness of aprotinin, and its use has been reduced in many centers. Although the incidence of thromboembolic complication was not different from patients who received placebo, fatal pulmonary embolism following administration of the drug has been reported [120], and the drug is withdrawn from clinical use to avoid thrombotic complications. Other possible side-effects are anaphylaxis and renal injury.

Procoagulants
Eltrombopag (Promacta)
This drug is a thrombopoietin receptor agonist indicated for the treatment of thrombocytopenia in patients with chronic immune (idiopathic) thrombocytopenic purpura who have had an insufficient response to corticosteroids, immunoglobulins, or splenectomy. Its use should be limited to those with ITP whose degree of thrombocytopenia and clinical condition increase the risk for bleeding.

Desmopressin (DDAVP)
DDAVP (1-deamino 8-d-arginine vasopressin) is a synthetic analog of the naturally occurring posterior pituitary hormone, vasopressin (ADH, anti-diuretic hormone). It stimulates endothelial cells to release both factor VIII and subtypes of vWF, and their level can increase up to four-fold, peaking 30–60 minutes after an IV dose [121]. DDAVP improves hemostasis in patients with hemophilia A and vWD [122, 123], and improves bleeding time in patients with uremia [124], congenital platelet defects [125], end-stage liver disease [100, 126], and possibly those undergoing cardiac surgery [127]. The dose of DDAVP is 0.3 µg/kg IV or subcutaneously; or 300 µg (150 µg in children) intranasally. It may be repeated 12–24 h after the initial dose. Tachyphylaxis may develop after the fourth dose.

Recombinant factor VIIa (rVIIa)

As described previously, factor VIIa-TF complex activates factor X to a small amount of Xa, and subsequently small amounts of thrombin are generated. This small quantity of thrombin activates factors V, VIII, and IX and platelets to set the stage for platelet surface-mediated burst of thrombin generation. Factor VIIa has low affinity for platelet surfaces and does not attach to these surfaces in physiologic concentrations. However, in high concentrations, it does bind to the surface of activated platelets and directly activates factor X, resulting in platelet surface thrombin generation without factors VIIIa and IXa. Therefore, a high dose rVIIa restores platelet surface thrombin generation and promotes clot formation in hemophilia A and B. In the USA, rVIIa is approved for use in patients with congenital FVII deficiency and in a subset of hemophilia patients in whom the presence of inhibitors substantially reduces the efficacy of conventional therapy with factor concentrates. In 2008, approximately 20,000 patients received rVIIa with 97% of cases being off-label use. The drug appears to reduce blood loss, but thromboembolic events and acute respiratory distress syndrome may be observed in up to 20% of patients [128]. Similar observations were made in cardiac surgical patients: blood transfusion requirement is reduced, but thromboembolic risk increased [129, 130].

Anticoagulants
Antiplatelet agents

In the arterial circulation, platelet activation is the triggering event for thrombosis, a process which cannot be adequately suppressed with heparin and warfarin. Thus, antiplatelet therapy is the primary strategy for the prevention or treatment of arterial thrombosis. The main drugs for this purpose are aspirin and clopidogrel (Plavix®). Other parenteral antiplatelet drugs, including GP IIb/IIIa inhibitors, may be administered during percutaneous coronary artery interventions. Pharmacology and clinical use of antiplatelet drugs are currently being investigated and reviewed [131].

Aspirin (acetylsalicylic acid) irreversibly acetylates and inactivates the enzyme cyclooxygenase, which is necessary for the conversion of platelet arachidonic acid to thromboxane A2, a powerful platelet-aggregating agent. Other nonsteroidal anti-inflammatory drugs (NSAIDs), such as ibuprofen, act as reversible inhibitors of cyclooxygenase, and cyclooxygenase-2 inhibitors are not antiplatelet drugs.

Ticlopidine and clopidogrel impair platelet function by interfering with ADP-induced aggregation and are to be used as a substitute for aspirin in patients who could not take it or where aspirin failed [132]. Clopidogrel has emerged as an extremely valuable and safe antiplatelet drug. In a clinical trial in patients at risk of ischemic events, clopidogrel was superior to aspirin and less toxic. The onset of action is moderately delayed (2–3 h) following an initial loading dose of 300 mg, and it persists for the life of the platelet. The usual daily dose of clopidogrel is 75 mg orally, and it is used in combination with aspirin in unstable angina, in percutaneous cardiac intervention procedures, and postprocedure follow-up.

GP IIb-IIIa Inhibitors are potent antiplatelet agents. A monoclonal antibody (abciximab) inhibits fibrinogen receptors on the platelet surface (GP IIb/IIIa) and is widely used in high-risk coronary artery disease. Abciximab, forming an irreversible complex with receptors, inhibits platelet function for the life of the individual platelet. The inhibiting effect of abciximab appears at first to be transient due to its short half-life and binding sites other than platelets, and additional dosing is required to inhibit appearance of 'new' GP IIb/IIIa molecules from within platelets. Abciximab may cause transient severe thrombocytopenia in the first 2–4 h after administration, and platelet count monitoring is required. Two other GP IIb/IIIa inhibitors (tirofiban and eptifibatidec) are low-molecular-weight competitive inhibitors and are available only for IV use in high-risk coronary artery disease. Effects of these two drugs are reversible and transient.

Phosphodiesterase Inhibitors are another group of antiplatelet agents. Sustained-release dipyridamole is an old member of antiplatelet agents. Its effectiveness is relatively weak, and is used as an adjuvant to warfarin for prophylaxis against embolization from mechanical heart valves [133]. Recently, reformulated dipyridamole with low-dose aspirin (25 mg) has been introduced for prevention of stroke in patients with transient ischemic attacks or in the secondary prevention of stroke [134]. Cilostazol is a relatively weak antiplatelet agent and is used in peripheral vascular disease [135].

Antithrombotics

After the clinical diagnosis of thrombophilia manifests as arterial and venous thrombosis, prophylactic and therapeutic antithrombotic therapies are usually necessary to prevent the reoccurrence of thrombosis, and to reduce morbidity and mortality from a vascular occlusion in major organs. Since the beginning of the twentieth century, warfarin derivatives, and unfractionated heparin have been used for these purposes [136]. Over the past several years, new drugs with more predictable pharmacokinetics have been introduced, including low molecular weight heparin

Table 6.3 Antithrombotic drugs.

Drug	Mechanism of Action	Indication	Route	Half Life	Elimination	Monitoring
Heparin	Inhibit thrombin/fXa	PCI, CPB, Thrombosis	IV, SQ	1–2.5 h	Hepatic	aPTT/ACT
LMWH	Inhibit fXa> thrombin	DVT/ PE Prophylaxis	SQ	3–5 h	Renal	Anti-Xa
Warfarin	Reduce Vitamin K	Stroke/DVT Prophylaxis	oral	36–42 h	Hepatic	Pt/INR
Fondaparinux	Inhibit fXa	DVT/ PE Prophylaxis	SQ	17 h	Renal	AntiXa
Rivaroxaban	Inhibit fXa	DVT/ PE Prophylaxis	Oral	5–10 h	Renal	AntiXa
Apixaban	Inhibit fXa	DVT/ PE Prophylaxis	Oral	5–18 h	Renal	AntiXa
Argatroban	Inhibit thrombin	HIT/HITT, PCI	IV	40–50 min	Hepatic	aPTT/ ACT
Lepirudin	Inhibit thrombin	HIT/HITT	IV	1.3 h	Renal	aPTT/ACT
Bivalirudin	Inhibit thrombin	PCI, CPB,	IV	25 min	Plasma/ Renal	aPTT/ACT
APC	EPCR Modulation of fVa/fVIIIa	Severe Sepsis	IV	13 min	Plasma/ Renal	
sTM	Protein C activation	DIC, DVT prophylaxis	IV	3–4 h	Renal (>50%)	aPTT

PCI, percutaneous coronary intervention; CPB, cardiopulmonary bypass, DVT, deep vein thrombosis; PE, pulmonary embolism; APC, activated protein C; endothelial protein C receptor; sTM, soluble thrombomodulin.

(LMWH) and a synthetic pentasaccharide (fondaparinux) [137]. The list of antithrombotic drugs is listed in Table 6.3 [138].

References

1 Vasiiev JM, Gelfand IM. Mechanism of non-adhesiveness of endothelial and epithelial surfaces. Nature. 1978;274:710–11.
2 Mustard JF, Kinlough-Rathbone RL, Packham MA. The vessel wall in thrombosis. In Colman RW, Hirsh J, Marder V. Salzman EW, eds. Thrombosis and Hemostasis: Basic Principles and Clinical Practice. Philadelphia: JB Lippincott; 1982, pp. 703–15.
3 Mason RG, Mohammad SF, Chuang HY, Richardson PD. The adhesion of platelets to subendothelium, collagen and artificial surfaces. Semin Thromb Hemost. 1976;3: 98–116.
4 MacIntyre DE, Pearson JD, Gordon JL. Localization and stimulation of prostacyclin production in vascular cells. Nature. 1978: 271;549–51.

5 Marder VJ. Molecular bad actors and thrombosis. N Engl J Med. 1984;310: 588–9.

6 Stead NW, Kinney 1, Lewis JG Campbell EE, Shifman MA, Rosenberg RD, Pizzo SV. Venous thrombosis in a family with defective release of vascular plasminogen activator and elevated plasma factor VIII/von Willebrand's factor. Am J Med. 1983;74:33–9.

7 Kitchens CS. The anatomical basis of purpura. Prog Hemost Thromb. 1980;5:211–44.

8 Kaushansky K. Thrombopoietin: the primary regulator of platelet production. Blood. 1995;86:419–31.

9 Shattil SI, Bennett IS. Platelets and their membranes in hemostasis: physiology and pathophysiology. Ann Intern Med. 1981;94:108–18.

10 Marcus AJ, Weksler BB, Jaffe EA. Enzymatic conversion of prostaglandin endoperoxide H2 and arachidonic acid to prostacyclin by cultured human endothelial cells. J Biol Chem. 1978;253:7138–41.

11 Shattil SJ, Hoxie JA, Cunningham MJ, Vrass LF. Changes in the platelet membrane glycoprotein IIb-IIIa complex during platelet activation. J Biol Chem. 1985;78:340–8.

12 Holmsen H, Weiss HJ. Secretable storage pools in platelets. Ann Rev Med. 1979;30:119–34.

13 White JG. Current concepts of platelet structure. Am J Clin Pathol. 1979;71:363–78.

14 Lyons RM, Stanford N, Majerus PW. Thrombin-induced protein phosphorylation in human platelets. J Clin Invest. 1975;56:924–36.

15 Pickett WC, Jesse RL, Cohen P. Initiation of phospholipase A2 activity in human platelets by the calcium ionophore A23187. Biochim Biophys Acta. 1977;486:209–13.

16 Hamberg M, Svensson I, Samuelsson B. Prostaglandin endoperoxides: A new concept concerning the mode of action and release of prostaglandins. Proc Natl Acad Sci. 1974;71:3824–8.

17 Hamberg M, Svensson J, Samuelsson B. Thromboxanes: A new group of biologically active compounds derived from prostaglandin endoperoxides. Proc Natl Acad Sci. 1975;72:2994–8.

18 Gerrard JM, White JG. Prostaglandins and thromboxanes: "middlemen" modulating platelet function in hemostasis and thrombosis. Prog Hemost Thromb. 1978;4:87–125.

19 Phillips DR. An evaluation of membrane glycoproteins in platelet adhesion and aggregation. Prog Hemost Thromb. 1980;5:81–109.

20 Nurden AT, Caen JP. The different glycoprotein abnormalities in thrombasthenic and Bernard-Soulier platelets. Semin Hematol. 1979;16:234–50.

21 Packham MA, Mustard JF. Platelet adhesion. Prog Hemost Thromb. 1984; 7:211–88.

22 Haslam RJ, Davidson MM, Fox JE, Lynham JA. Cyclic nucleotides in platelet function. Thromb Haemost. 1978;40:232–40.

23 Kaser-Glanzmann R, Jakabova M, George JN, Luscher EF. Stimulation of calcium uptake in platelet membrane vesicles by adenosine 3′,5′-cyclic monophosphate and protein kinase. Biochim Biophys Acta. 1977;466:429–40.

24 Bucher D, Nebelin E, Thomsen J, Steflo J. Identification of gamma–carboxyglutamic add residues in bovine factors IX and X, and in a new vitamin K-dependent protein. FEBS Letter. 1976;68:293–6.

25 Mandle RJ Jr, Kaplan AP. Hageman factor substrates. Human plasma prekallikrein: Mechanism of activation of Hageman factor and participation in Hageman factor – dependent 11-fibrinolysis. J Biol Chem. 1977;252:6097–7001.

26 Ratnoff OD, Colopy JE. A familial hemorrhagic trait associated with deficiency of clot-promoting fraction of plasma. J Clin Invest. 1955;34:602–13.

27 Mandle RJ Jr, Colman RW, Kaplan AP. Identification of prekallikrein and high molecular weight kininogen as a complex in human plasma. Proc Natl Acad Sci USA. 1976;73:4179–83.

28 Cooper HA, Griggs TR, Wagner RH: Factor VIII recombination after dissociation by CaC12. Proc Natl Acad Sci USA. 1973;70:2326–9.

29 Bjorklid E, Storm E, Prydz H. The protein component of human brain thromboplastin. Biochem Biophys Res Commun. 1973;55:969–76.

30 Radcliffe R, Nemerson Y. Activation and control of factor VII by activated factor X and thrombin: Isolation and characterization of a single chain form of factor VII. J Biol Chem. 1974;250:388–95.

31 Miletich JP, Jackson CM, Majerus PW. Properties of the Factor X binding site on human platelets. J Biol Chem. 1978;253:6908–16.

32 Doolittle RF, Goldbaum DM, Doolittle LR. Designation of sequences involved in the "coiled-coil" interdomainal connector in fibrinogen: constructions of an atomic scale model. J Mol Biol. 1978;120:311–25.

33 Blomback B, Blomback M. The molecular structure of fibrinogen. Ann NY Acad Sci. 1972;202:77–97.

34 Ferry JD. The conversion of fibrinogen to fibrin: events and recollections from 1942 to 1982. Ann N Y Acad Sci. 1983;27;408:1–10.

35 Hermans J, McDonagh J. Fibrin: Structure and interactions. Semin Thromb Hemost. 1982;8:11–24.

36 Folk JE, Finlayson JS. The epsilon-(γ-glutamyl) lysine crosslink and the catalytic role of transglutaminase. Adv Protein Chem. 1977;31:1–133.

37 McKee PA, Mattock P. Hill RL. Subunit structure of human fibrinogen, soluble fibrin, and cross-linked insoluble fibrin. Proc Natl Acad Sci USA. 1970;66: 738–44.

38 Kaplan KL, Broekman MJ, Chernoff A, Lesznik GR, Drillings M. Platelet alpha-granule proteins: studies on release and subcellular localization. Blood. 1979;53:604–18.

39 Nachmias V, Sullender J, Asch A. Shape and cytoplasmic filaments in control and lidocaine-treated human platelets. Blood. 1977;50:39–53.

40 Broze GJ Jr, Higuchi DA. Coagulation-dependent inhibition of fibrinolysis: role of carboxypeptidase-U and the premature lysis of clots from hemophilic plasma. Blood. 1996;88:3815–23.

41 Mosnier LO, Bouma BN. Regulation of fibrinolysis by thrombin activatable fibrinolysis inhibitor, an unstable carboxypeptidase B that unites the pathways of coagulation and fibrinolysis. Arterioscler Thromb Vasc Biol. 2006;26:2445–53.

42 Felez J, Chanquia CJ, Fabregas P, Plow EF, Miles LA. Competition between plasminogen and tissue plasminogen activator for cellular binding sites. Blood. 1993;82:2433–41.

43 Nesheim M, Wang W, Boffa M, Nagashima M, Morser J, Bajzar L. Thrombin, thrombomodulin and TAFI in the molecular link between coagulation and fibrinolysis. Thromb Haemost. 1997;78:386–91.

44 Lijnen HR, Collen D. Interaction of plasminogen activators and inhibitors with plasminogen and fibrin. Semin Thromb Hemost. 1982;8:2–10.

45 Alkjaersig N, Fletcher AP, Sherry S. The mechanism of clot dissolution by plasmin. J Clin Invest. 1959;38:1086–95.

46 Juhan-Vague I, Alessi MC, Mavri A, Morange PE. Plasminogen activator inhibitor-1, inflammation, obesity, insulin resistance and vascular risk. J Thromb Haemost. 2003;1:1575–9.

47 Sakata Y, Aoki N. Cross-linking of alpha2-plasmin inhibitor to fibrin by fibrin-stabilizing factor. J Clin Invest. 1980;65:290–7.

48 Davie EW. A brief historical review of the waterfall/cascade of blood coagulation. J Biol Chem. 2003;278:50819–32.

49 Hoffman M, Monroe DM 3rd. A cell-based model of hemostasis. Thromb Haemost. 2001;85:958–65.

50 Owens P III, Mackman N. Microparticles in Hemostasis and Thrombosis. Circ Res. 2011;108:1284–97.

51 Scott CF, Silver LD, Purdon DA, Colman RW. Cleavage of human high molecular weight kininogen by factor XI, in vitro: Effect on structure and function. J Biol Chem. 1985;260:10856–863.

52 Schapira M, Scott CF, Colman RW. Protection of human plasma kallikrein from inactivation by Cl inhibitor and other protease inhibitors: The role of high molecular weight kininogen. Biochemistry. 1981;20:2738–43.

53 Scott CF, Schapira M, James HL, Cohen AB, Colman RW. Inactivation of factor XIa by plasma protease inhibitors: predominant role of alpha 1-protease inhibitor and protective effect of high molecular weight kininogen. J Clin Invest. 1982;69:844–52.

54 Rosenberg RD, Damus PS. The purification and mechanism of action of human antithrombin-heparin cofactor. J Biol Chem. 1973;248:6490–505.

55 Murray EW, Lillicrap D. Von Willebrand disease: pathogenesis, classification and management. Transfusion Med Rev. 1996;10:93–110.

56 Wagner DD. Cell biology of von Willebrand factor. Ann Rev Cell Biol. 1990;6:217–46.

57 Bloom AL. von Willebrand factor: clinical features of inherited and acquired disorders. Mayo Glin Proc. 1991;66:743–51.

58 Brinkhous KM, Graham JH. Hemophilia and the hemophilioid states. Blood. 1954;9:254–7.

59 Levine PH. Clinical manifestations and therapy of hemophilia A and B. In: Colman RW, Hirsh J, Marder V. Salzman EW, eds. Thrombosis and Hemostasis: Basic Principles and Clinical Practice. Philadelphia: JB Lippincott; 1987, pp. 97–111.

60 Rosnethal R, Dreskin O, Rosenthal N. Plasma thromboplastin antecedent (PTA) deficiency: Clinical, coagulation, therapeutic and hereditary aspects of a new hemophilia-like disease. Blood. 1955;10:120–31.

61 Shpilberg O, Peretz H, Zivelin A, Yatuv R, Chetrit A, Kulka T, Stern C, Weiss E, Sligsohn U. One of the two common mutations causing factor XI deficiency in Ashkenazi Jews (type II) is also prevalent in Iraqi Jews, who represent the ancient gene pool of Jews. Blood. 1995;85:429–32.

62 Brenner B, Laor A, Lupo H, Zivelin A, Lanir N, Seligsohn U. Bleeding predictors in factor-XI-deficient patients. Blood Coagul Fibrinol. 1997;8:511–5.

63 Asakai R, Chung DW, Davie EW, Seligsohn U. Factor XI deficiency in Ashkenazi Jews in Israel. N Engl J Med. 1991;325:153–8.

64 Hedner U. Mechanism of action of recombinant activated factor VII: An update. Semin Hematol. 2006;43(Suppl 1):S105–7.

65 Triplett DA. Coagulation and bleeding disorders: review and update. Clin Chem. 2000;46:1260–9.

66 Olson RE. Vitamin K. In: Colman RW, Hirsh J, Marder V. Salzman EW eds. Thrombosis and Hemostasis: Basic Principles and Clinical Practice. Philadelphia: JB Lippincott; 1987, pp. 846–60.

67 Green G, Poller L, Thompson SM, Dymock 1W. Factor VII as a marker of hepatocellular synthetic function. J Clin Pathol. 1976;29:971–5.

68 Violi F, Ferro D, Quintarelli C, Saliola M, Corrado C, Balsano F. Clotting abnormalities in chronic liver disease. Dig Dis. 1991;10:162–72.

69 Mammen EF. Coagulation defects in liver disease. Med Clin N Am. 1994;78: 545–54.

70 Cosgriff N, Moore EE, Sauaia A, Kenny-Moynihan M, Burch JM, Galloway B. Predicting life-threatening coagulopathy in the massively transfused trauma patient: hypothermia and acidosis revisited. J Trauma. 1997;42:857–61.

71 Marquez J, Martin D, Virji MA, Kang YG, Warty VS, Shaw B Jr, Sassano JJ, Waterman P, Winter PM, Pinsky MR. Cardiovascular depression secondary to ionic hypocalcemia during hepatic transplantation in humans. Anesthesiology. 1986;65:457–61.

72 Bergenstein JM, Slakey DP, Wallace JR, Gottlieb M. Traumatic hypothermia is related to hypotension, not resuscitation. Ann Emerg Med. 1996;27:39–42.

73 Hessel, II, EA, Schmer G, Dillard DH. Platelets kinetics during deep hypothermia. J Surg Res. 1980;28:23–34.

74 White T, Krivit W. An ultrastructural basis for the shape changes induced in platelets by chilling blood. Blood. 1967;30:635–75.

75 Valeri CR, Feingold H, Cassidy G, Ragno G, Khuri S, Altschule MD. Hypothermia-induced reversible platelet dysfunction. Ann Surg. 1987;205: 175–81.

76 Rohrer MJ, Natale AM. Effect of hypothermia on the coagulation cascade. Crit Care Med. 1992;20:1402–5.

77 Kurrek MM, Reed RL. Effect of hypothermia on enzymatic activity of thrombin and plasmin. Surg forum. 1987;38:221–3.

78 Johnston TD, Chen Y, Reed RI. Relative sensitivity of the clotting cascade to hypothermia. Surg Forum. 1989;40:199–201.

79 Sick RL. Disseminated intravascular coagulation and related syndromes: a clinical review. Sem Thromb Hemost. 1989;14:299–338.

80 Marder VJ, Martin SE, Frances CW, Colman RW. Consumptive thrombohemorrhagic disorders. In: Colman RW, Hirsh J, Marder V. Salzman EW, eds. Thrombosis and Hemostasis: Basic Principles and Clinical Practice. Philadelphia: JB Lippincott; 1987, pp. 975–1015.

81 Warkentin TE. An overview of the heparin-induced thrombocytopenia syndrome. Semin Thromb Hemost. 2004;30:273–83.

82 Comunale ME, Van Cott EM. Heparin-induced thrombocytopenia. Int Anesthesiol Clin. 2004;42:27–43.

83 George JN, Shattil SJ. The clinical importance of acquired abnormalities of platelet function. N Engl J Med. 1991;324;27–39.

84 Weerasinghe A, Taylor KM. The platelet in cardiopulmonary bypass. Ann Thor Surg. 1998;66:2145–52.

85 Manoharan A, Gottlieb P. Bleeding in patients with lupus anticoagulant. Lancet. 1984;2:171.

86 Mammen EF, Comp PC, Gosselin R, Greenberg C, Hoots WK, Kessler CM, Larkin EC, Liles D, Nugent DJ. PFA-100 system: a new method of assessment of platelet dysfunction. Semin Thromb Hemost. 1998;24:195–202.

87 Casserly IP, Kereiakes DJ, Gray WA, Gibson PH, Lauer MA, Reginelli JP, Moliterno DJ. Point-of-care ecarin clotting time versus activated clotting time in correlation with bivalirudin concentration. Thromb Res. 2004;113: 115–21.

88 Murphy GS, Marymont JH: Alternative anticoagulation management strategies for the patient with heparin-induced thrombocytopenia undergoing cardiac surgery. J Cardiothorac Vasc Anesth. 2007;21:113–26.

89 Carroll RC, Chavez JJ, Simmons JW, Snider CC, Wortham DC, Bresee SJ, Cohen E. Measurement of patients' bivalirudin plasma levels by a thrombelastograph ecarin clotting time assay: a comparison to a standard activated clotting time. Anesth Analg. 2006;102:1316–19.

90 Eisenberg JM, Clarke JR, Sussman SA. Prothrombin and partial thromboplastin times as preoperative screening tests. Arch Surg. 1982;117:48–51.

91 Velanovich V. The value of routine preoperative laboratory testing in predicting postoperative complications: A multivariate analysis. Surgery 1991;109: 236–43.

92 Barber A, Green D, Galuzzo T, Ts'ao CH. The bleeding time as a preoperative screening test. Am J Med. 1985;78:761–4.

93 Kang Y. Thromboelastography in liver transplantation. Semin Thromb Hemost. 1995;21 (Suppl 4):34–44.

94 Mallett SV, Cox DJA. Thromboelastography. BJA. 1992;69:307–13.

95 Zuckerman L, Cohen E, Vagher JP, Woodward E, Caprini JA. Comparison of thromboelastography with common coagulation test. Thromb Haemostas. 1981;46:752–6.

96 Gottumukkala VN, Sharma SK, Philip J. Assessing platelet and fibrinogen contribution to clot strength using modified thromboelastography in pregnant women. Anesth Analg. 1999;89:1453–5.

97 Khurana S, Mattson JC, Westley S, O'Neill WW, Timmis GC, Safian RD. Monitoring platelet Glycoprotein IIb/IIIa-fibrin interaction with tissue-factor activated thromboelastography. J Lab Clin Med. 1997;130:401–11.

98 Kang YG. Monitoring and treatment of coagulation. In: Winter PM, Kang YG, eds. Hepatic Transplantation, Anesthetic and Perioperative Management. Philadelphia: Praeger Publisher; 1986, pp. 151–73.

99 Kang YG, Lewis JH, Navalgund A, Russell MW, Bontempo FA, Niren LS, Starzl TE. Epsilon-aminocaproic acid for treatment of fibrinolysis during liver transplantation. Anesthesiology. 1987;66:766–73.

100 Kang Y, Scott V, DeWolf A, Roskoph J, Aggarwal S. In vitro effects of DDAVP during liver transplantation. Transplant Proc. 1993;25:1821–2.

101 Kang Y, DeWolf A, Aggarwal S, Campbell E, Martin LK. In vitro study on the effects of aprotinin on coagulation during orthotopic liver transplantation. Transplant Proc. 1991;23:1934–5.

102 Kang YG, Martin DJ, Marquez J, Lewis JH, Bontempo FA, Shaw BW Jr., Starzl TE, Winter PM. Intraoperative changes in blood coagulation and thrombelastographic monitoring in liver transplantation. Anesth Analg. 1985;64:888–96.

103 Shore-Lesserson L, Manspeizer HE, DePerio M, Francis S, Vela-Cantos F, Ergin MA. Thromboelastography-guided transfusion algorithm reduces transfusions in complex cardiac surgery. Anesth Analg. 1999;88:312–9.

104 Kang Y. Transfusion based on clinical coagulation monitoring does reduce hemorrhage during liver transplantation. Liver Transpl Surg. 1997;3:655–9.

105 Post M, Telfer MC. Surgery in hemophilic patients. J Bone Joint Surg Am. 1975;57:1136–45.

106 Miller RD, Robbins TO, Tong MJ, Barton SL. Coagulation defects associated with massive blood transfusions. Ann Surg. 1971;174:794–801.

107 Gerlach H, Slama KJ, Bechstein WO, Lohmann R, Hintz G, Abraham K, Neuhaus P, Falke K. Retrospective statistical analysis of coagulation parameters after 250 liver transplantations. Semin Thromb Hemost. 1993;19:223–32.

108 Consensus conference: Platelet transfusion therapy. JAMA. 1987;257:1777–80.

109 Hefer DVF, Munir A, Khouli H. Low-dose tenecteplase during cardiopulmonary resuscitation due to massive pulmonary embolism: a case report and review of previously reported cases. Blood Coagul Fibrinolysis. 2007;18: 691–4.

110 Albers GW, Amarenco P, Easton JD, Sacco RL, Teal P. Antithrombotic and thrombolytic therapy for ischemic stroke: the Seventh ACCP Conference on Antithrombotic and Thrombolytic Therapy. Chest. 2004;126:483S–512S.

111 Singh KP, Harrington RA. Primary percutaneous coronary intervention in acute myocardial infarction. Med Clin North Am. 2007;91:639–55.

112 Vander Salm TJ, Kaur S, Lancey RA, Okike ON, Pezzella AT, Stahl RF, Leone L, Li JM, Valeri CR, Michelson AD. Reduction of bleeding after heart operations through the prophylactic use of epsilon-amino caproic acid. J Thorac Cardiovasc Surg. 1996;112:1098–107.

113 Katasaros D, Petricevic M, Snow NJ, Woodhall DD, Van Bergen R. Tranexamic acid reduces postbypass blood use: a double blinded, prospective, randomized study in 210 patients. Ann Thorac Surg. 1996;61:1131–5.

114 Boylan JF, Klinck JR, Sandler AN, Arellano R, Greig PD, Nierenberg H, Roger SL, Glynn MF. Tranexamic acid reduces blood loss, transfusion requirements, and coagulation factor use in primary orthotopic liver transplantation. Anesthesiology. 1996;85:1043–8.

115 Stefanini M, English HA, Taylor AE. Safe and effective, prolonged administration of epsilon aminocaproic acid in the bleeding urinary tract. J Urol. 1990;143:559–61.

116 Benoni G, Fredin H. Fibrinolytic inhibition with tranexamic acid reduces blood loss and blood transfusion after knee arthroplasty: a prospective randomized, double-blind study in 86 patients. J Bone Joint Surg Br. 1996;78:434–40.

117 Hiippala ST, Strid LJ, Wennerstrand MI, Arvela JV, Niemela HM, Mantyla SK, Kuisma RP, Ylinen JE. Tranexamic acid radically decreases blood loss and transfusion associated with total knee arthroplasty. Anesth Analg. 1997;84:839–44.

118 Kang Y. Clinical use of synthetic antifibrinolytic agents during liver transplantation. Semin Thromb Hemost. 1993;19:258–61.

119 Porte RJ, Molenaar IQ, Begliomini B, Groenland TH, Januszkiewicz A, Lindgren L, Palareti G, Hermans J, Terpstra OT. Aprotinin and transfusion requirements in orthotopic liver transplantation: a multicentre randomized double-blind study. Lancet. 2000;355:1303–9.

120 Baubillier E, Cherqui D, Dominique C, Khalil M, Bonnet F, Fagniez PL, Duvaldestin P. A fatal thrombotic complication during liver transplantation after aprotinin administration. Transplantation. 1994;57:1664–6.

121 Lethagen S, Harris AS, Sjorin E, Nilsson IM. Intranasal and intravenous administration of desmopressin: effect on F VIII/vWF, pharmacokinetics and reproducibility. Thromb Haemost. 1987;58:1033–6.

122 Mannucci PM, Ruggeri ZM, Pareti FI, Capitanio A. 1-Deamino-8-D-arginine vasopressin: a new pharmacological approach to the management of hemophilia and von Willebrand's diseases. Lancet. 1977;1:869–72.

123 Kobrinsky NL, Israels ED, Gerrard JM, Cheang MS, Watson CM, Bishop AJ, Schroeder ML. Shortening of bleeding time by 1-deamino-8-D-arginine vasopressin in various bleeding disorders. Lancet. 1984;1:1145–8.

124 Steiner RW, Coggins C, Carvalho AC. Bleeding time in uremia: a useful test to assess clinical bleeding. Am J Hematol. 1979;7:107–17.

125 Rao AK, Ghosh S, Sun L, Yang X, Disa J, Pickens P, Polansky M. Mechanism of platelet dysfunction and response to DDAVP in patients with congenital platelet function defects: a double-blind placebo-controlled trial. Thromb Hemost. 1995;74:1071–8.

126 Mannucci PM, Vicente V, Vianello L, Cattaneo M, Alberca I, Coccato MP, Faioni E, Mari D. Controlled trial of desmopressin in liver cirrhosis and other conditions associated with a prolonged bleeding time. Blood. 1986;67:1148–53.

127 Salzman EW, Weinstein MJ, Weintraub RM, Ware JA, Thurer RL, Robertson L, Donovan A, Gaffney T, Bertele V, Troll J. Treatment with desmopressin acetate to reduce blood loss after cardiac surgery: a double-blind randomized trial. N Engl J Med. 1986;314:1402–6.

128 Aaron C, Logan AC, Yank V, Stafford RS. Off-Label Use of Recombinant Factor VIIa in U.S. Hospitals: Analysis of Hospital Records. Ann Intern Med. 2011;154:516–22.

129 Yank V. Tuohy CV, Logan AC, Bravata D, Staudenmayer K, Eisenhut R, Sundaram V, McMahon D, Olkin I, McDonald KM, Owens DK, Stafford RS. Systematic Review: Benefits and Harms of In-Hospital Use of Recombinant Factor VIIa for Off-Label Indications. Ann Intern Med. 2011;154:529–40.

130 Diprose P, Herbertson MJ, O'Shaughnessy D, Gill RS. Activated recombinant factor VII after cardiopulmonary bypass reduces allogeneic transfusion in complex non-coronary cardiac surgery: randomized double-blind placebo controlled pilot study. Br J Anaesth. 2005;95:596–602.

131 Angiolillo DJ, Capranzano P. Pharmacology of emerging novel platelet inhibitors. Am Heart J. 2008;156:S10–S15.

132 Becker RC, Meade TW, Berger PB, Ezekowitz M, O'Connor CM, Vorchheimer DA, Guyatt GH, Mark DB, Harrington RA. The primary and secondary prevention of coronary artery disease: American College of Chest Physicians Evidence-Based Clinical Practice Guidelines (8th Edition). Chest. 2008;133:776S–814S.

133 Altman R, Rouvier J, Gurfinkel E, D'Ortencio O, Manzanel R, de La Fuente L, Favaloro RG. Comparison of two levels of anticoagulant therapy in patients with substitute heart valves. J Thorc Cardiovasc Surg. 1991;101:427–31.

134 Aw D, Sharma JC. Antiplatelets in secondary stroke prevention: should clopidogrel be the first choice? Postgrad Med J. 2012;88:34–7.

135 Sobel M, Verhaeghe R. Antithrombotic therapy for peripheral artery occlusive disease: American College of Chest Physicians Evidence-Based Clinical Practice Guidelines (8th Edition). Chest. 2008;133:815S–43S.

136 Bates SM, Weitz JI. New anticoagulants: beyond heparin, low-molecular-weight heparin and warfarin. Br J Pharmacol. 2005;144:1017–28.

137 Kearon C, Kahn SR, Agnelli G, Goldhaber S, Raskob GE, Comerota AJ. American College of Chest Physicians. Antithrombotic therapy for venous thromboembolic disease: ACCP Evidence-Based Clinical Practice Guidelines (8th Edition). Chest. 2008;133:454S–545S.

138 Hall R, Mazer CD. Antiplatelet drugs: a review of their pharmacology and management in the perioperative period. Anesth Analg. 2011;112:292–318.

CHAPTER 7

Topical hemostatic agents

Fabrizio Di Benedetto and Giuseppe Tarantino

Hepato-pancreato-biliary Surgery and Liver Transplantation Unit,
University of Modena and Reggio Emilia Modena, Italy

Introduction

Management of hemostasis in the operating theatre has always been an issue of fundamental importance in any surgical procedure. This goal is reached through many key components that start, first of all, with good and accurate surgical techniques and anesthetic support. Good hemostasis provides several advantages to patients, to the surgical team and, in terms of cost-effectiveness, to the health care facilities. The amount of blood loss may greatly vary between different surgical procedures and depends on both surgical and non-surgical factors Even if in most cases surgical hemostasis is able to stop bleeding, it may be necessary to make use of pro-hemostatic agents, especially in non-surgical bleedings, or in difficult to access bleedings.

Generally, it is well established that perioperative bleeding and the need for blood transfusions is related to increased morbidity, mortality and costs [1, 2]. In combination with the continued concern for the risk of transmitting transfusion-mediated infections, this has renewed the interest in strategies to reduce perioperative blood loss.

Several different topical agents can be used to achieve or maintain hemostasis in surgical patients. The mechanism of action in the vast majority of these agents is based on local activation of the endogenous coagulation system, local vasoconstriction, and a combination of local clotting activation and mechanical compression. These compounds can be viewed as an extension of the more conventional surgical techniques to obtain or stimulate local hemostasis.

History of hemostatics

Historically, to stop a bleed has always been a specific task of the surgeon, both in healing war wounds and in spontaneous hemorrhages. Until

Transfusion-Free Medicine and Surgery, Second Edition. Edited by Nicolas Jabbour.
© 2014 John Wiley & Sons, Ltd. Published 2014 by John Wiley & Sons, Ltd.

the 17th century, surgeons achieved hemostasis mainly using local heat, directly with cauteries or by hot oil. This kind of hemostasis was the only known practice until 1600 when Ambroise Parè (1509–1590), a French surgeon, introduced vascular ligation as the preferable method to provide bleeding control; since then, hemostasis has been achieved largely by mechanical means (ligatures, stitches and clips).

Topical hemostasis, hemostasis by ligatures and heat application can be found in all the history of surgery. Direct heat application and the consequent protein coagulation always remained in force until the improvement of the different forms of electro-coagulation, which are the electrical scalpel (1924), the bipolar forceps (1940s) and recently the radio frequency and ultrasonic scalpel (2000s).

Research and large-scale application of proper hemostatics leading to what we know today, originated mainly from war experience. Most of the topical agents were originally developed to improve wound healing in soldiers with severe burn injuries during WWI, WWII, the Vietnam War, and more recently the Afghan and Iraqi wars.

As regards topical agents the first to be used was cyanoacrylate, synthesized for the first time by Harry Coover (Eastmann Kodak) during WWII to make more precise gun sights; however, the project was never finished. The idea was then taken back to Europe by Bernd Braun who used it as a tissue adhesive in 1964 with the name of "Histocoll®", well-known as "Hystoacryl®" (Braun) by 1968. The first experimental studies on albumin and glutaraldehyde-based glue as hemostatic agents were run by N. Braunwald in 1965 and their first clinical use is thanks to D. Guilmet in 1979. First largely used in liver and kidney surgery, these products were then used in cardiovascular surgery. These semi-synthetic products contained toxic agents such as resorcinol and formaldehyde, causing severe inflammatory reactions. In 2001 the Food and Drug Administration (FDA) approved the usage of Bioglue® (Cryolife Inc.), albumin and glutaraldehyde based and formaldehyde free. Polyethylene glycol-based synthetic sealants are the most recent products. Their use in clinical trials in thoracic surgery started in 1997, and thereafter they were used in neurosurgery.

The biology of hemostasis

It is important for the surgeon to understand the mechanisms of hemostasis and thrombosis; this is fundamental for a patient undergoing any surgical procedure. Hemostasis can be defined as a tightly regulated process that maintains the blood flow through the vasculature simultane- ously as a thrombotic response to tissue damage occurs [3]. Hemostasis is reached and maintained through a complex interaction and perfect balance of the vessel wall, platelets, and the coagulation system [4, 5]. Hemostasis can be divided into two main phases: the primary, cellular phase, and the secondary, humoral phase. The former begins soon after endothelial disruption and determines vasoconstriction, platelet adhe- sion, and formation of a soft aggregate plug [5]. After the injury occurs, there is a temporary local contraction of vascular smooth muscle and the blood flow slows, promoting platelet adhesion and activation. Within a few seconds of the damage, circulating von Willebrand factors attach to the subendothelium at the site of injury and adhere to the glycoproteins on the surface of the platelets. When platelets adhere to the damaged surface, they are activated by contact with collagen-exposing receptors that bind circulating fibrinogen. This leads to the formation of a soft plug of aggregated platelets and fibrinogen. This phase of hemostasis is short lived, and the soft plug can easily be dislodged from the damaged surface. The soft platelet plug is stabilized during secondary hemostasis to form a clot. Platelets actively promote vasoconstriction and the resultant reduc- tion in blood flow, thanks to the secretion of serotonin, prostaglandin, and thromboxane while the coagulation cascade is initiated. The coagulation cascade is a series of dependent reactions involving several plasma proteins, calcium ions, and blood platelets that lead to the conversion of fibrinogen to fibrin. Coagulation factors are synthesized by the liver and are activated only once the cascade process begins. Then each step of the cascade is initiated and completed via a series of sequential and dependent coagulation factor activation reactions. Finally, thrombin converts the soluble plasma protein fibrinogen to the insoluble protein fibrin, while simultaneously converting factor XIII to factor XIIIa. This factor conversion stabilizes the fibrin and results in cross-linking of the fibrin monomers, producing a stable clot (Figure 7.1) [5].

Hemostasis in surgery

There are several options for the surgeon to control bleeding, including mechanical and thermal techniques and devices as well as pharmacother- apies and topical agents. Application of direct pressure or compression at a bleeding site is quite often the first choice to control bleeding. When bleeding is easily identifiable mechanical methods can be successfully used to seal the source of bleeding and include sutures, ligating clips,

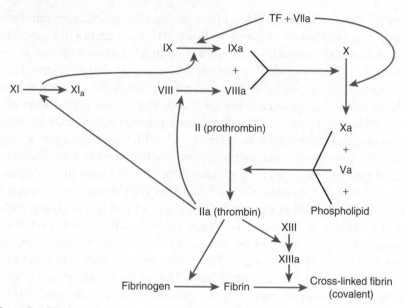

Figure 7.1 Pathways in blood coagulation.

and staples. These methods, however, are not always appropriate in all surgical procedures [6]. This is the case when the source of bleeding is diffuse, oozing or difficult to identify or when the patient has an inherent or surgery-induced coagulopathy. The so-called non-surgical bleedings can be a result of the patient's features such as congenital hypocoagulability, acquired hypocoagulability as in cirrhotic patients, or can derive from operative factors such as hemodilution, acidosis, hypothermia, massive transfusion, as well as from the prior administration of antiplatelet or anticoagulant drugs [7]. These are the cases when cautery and suture ligation are not feasible. When it is not possible to control bleeding even temporary packing has been proposed [8, 9]. For this reason, over the past decades, means such as lasers (CO_2, Argon, and Nd-YAG) and spray-electrocoagulation have been introduced. However, the frequent use of cautery and other thermal techniques can have drawbacks [10]. Thus it may be impossible or extremely difficult to effectively stop blood loss via mechanical or thermal hemostatic techniques. For instance, on bony surfaces, parenchymal tissues, inflamed or friable vessels, or tissues containing multiple and diffuse capillaries, it is quite impossible to reach hemostasis with conventional methods. The use of effective pharmacological methods during surgery can be a useful option or an adjunct to other methods in these situations. Pharmacological methods aim to enhance hemostasis by increasing the natural clotting mechanisms. This may include the use of pharmacological agents, such as epinephrine, desmopressin, topical hemostatic agents, tissue sealants, and tissue adhesives. Topical hemostatic agents can be applied directly to the bleeding site and may prevent continuous unrelenting bleeding throughout the entire procedure and into the postoperative recovery period [11]. Hemostasis using topical agents can also avoid the adverse effects of systemic hemostatic medications, such as hypercoagulation and its side-effects. The flexibility associated with topical agents can also make them an attractive option. In surgical procedures where the amount of blood loss is unpredictable, topical hemostatics can be used sparingly when blood loss is minimal and more liberally during severe bleeding. Furthermore, as hemostasis is attained and maintained at the bleeding site, there may be prolonged benefit with respect to postoperative blood loss.

Safety of hemostatics

Hemostatics are prepared from human protein derived from plasma such as fibrinogen, thrombin and factor XIII. Some products also contain bovine aprotinin [12]. In order to reduce the risk of viral transmission from commercial products, plasma donations undergo a series of procedures to eliminate potential contaminants. This is carried out by careful selection of plasma donors, wide testing of the donation for markers of infection, the elimination of human viruses through different purification systems and, finally, the use of virus-inactivation methods during the preparation of the products.

The selection of the donors is aimed at excluding all those people with certain risk factors such as history or exposure to hepatitis virus or HIV, such as, for instance, people with intravenous drug abuse or high risk sexual behavior. One of the most relevant problems when working with blood-derived products is the potential transmission of pathogens during the so-called window period between the donation time and the seroconversion, when the laboratory tests are able to identify the markers of infection. This risk has gradually decreased and it is now estimated that the per-unit values for transfusion–transmitted HIV and hepatitis C virus in the US are 1 in 1 100 000 and 1 in 250 000, respectively [13].

Plasma derivatives and bovine tissue undergo a variety of procedures during processing, which involve viral inactivation and elimination [12]. In order to reduce the viral copy number and infectivity of certain plasma fractions they undergo a process of plasma fractionation and/or nanofiltration [14]. During viral inactivation, virus infectivity is reduced by disrupting the protein or lipid coat of the virus, if present, and/or by destroying the nucleic acid. This phase has to be reached preserving the molecular integrity of the plasma proteins. Physical inactivation of viruses can be achieved by a number of methods including heat inactivation and ultraviolet or ionizing radiation. Solvent/detergent treatment is a chemical treatment used for viral reduction by some commercial producers of fibrin sealant [14]. However, this kind of procedure is not effective in inactivated non-enveloped viruses such as hepatitis A virus and parvovirus B19, thus the use of heat treatment is used to achieve a high level of safety in the final product [12]. For this reason heat treatment can be implemented, such as pasteurization (aqueous solution for 10 h at 60 °C), dry heat for 72 h at 80 °C, or nanofiltration coupled with dry heat for 1 h at 100 °C [12].

Nowadays the risk of viral transmission through hemostatic products can be considered overcome. Only one case of Parvovirus B19 transmission has been reported in the literature [15]. Manufacturers of plasma products have responded quickly to this recent report and some are already using PCR screening for parvovirus B19 [12]. Still there are concerns about the potential risk of hyper-immunization and bovine spongiform encephalopathy (BSE) contamination from products originating from bovine sources. However, the switch from bovine thrombin to human thrombin in fibrin sealants has increased the safety of these sealants [14].

Topical hemostatics

A great number of topical hemostatic agents are available for the surgeon. It is important to have a global view of each product, because they have different possibilities of usage. So as not to waste time and resources it is compulsory to understand how and when to use each product.

They can be divided into two categories: those that provide their mechanism of action on the clotting cascade in a biologically active manner and those that act passively through contact activation and promotion of platelet aggregation. Passive topical hemostatic agents include collagens, cellulose, and gelatins, while active agents include thrombin and fibrinogen, and products in which they are combined with a passive agent to provide an active overall product [16, 17].

Active agents
This group includes products containing fibrinogen and thrombin. These products are adhesive hemostatics; they accelerate the physiological

hemostatic process with several actions, such as reproducing the final phases of the clotting cascade, platelet adhesion and activation, and concentration of the blood cells in the bleeding site. For these reasons these products can be successfully used in coagulopathic patients. Their adhesive action is due to the polymerization of fibrin monomers, producing a sealing action.

Passive agents

The principle of this class of hemostatics is to provide the structure so as to allow the concentration of platelets and clotting factors, platelet adhesion and activation, and stabilization of the clot. They accelerate the physiological clotting mechanism [18]. Passive topical hemostatic agents include collagens, cellulose, and gelatins [16].

Adhesive hemostatics (fibrin glues)

Fibrin-based products are the most used and aged hemostatic products. Their use as fibrin glues, that is combination of fibrinogen and thrombin, was first seen in WWII when E.P. Cronkite used these glues to facilitate the adhesion of skin grafts in seriously burned soldiers. At that time several side effects arose, mainly due to transmission of hepatitis viruses in some patients. Later the use of bovine-derived thrombin was proposed; however, it was then abandoned because of the onset of serious coagulophathy secondary to auto-antibodies against bovine clotting factors [19]. It was only in 1998 that the Food and Drug Administration approved the first virus-inactivated fibrin glues (Tisseel®, Baxter).

Fibrin glues induce the clot in the site of bleeding taking part to the last phases of coagulation. They are made up by two components, the first is human purified fibrinogen and the second is thrombin. Generally, other plasmatic proteins are added, such as factor XIII, fibronectin, and antifibrinolitic agents such as tranexamic acid and aprotinin. Industrial fibrin sealants are obtained by fractionation of human plasma [17]. Fibrinogen is generally obtained by precipitation from cryoprecipitate or from Cohn fraction I. As described above the products have to be processed by different steps of viral reduction and inactivation by solvent/detergent, vapor heat treatment or pasteurization [17]. Thrombin is generated by the activation of purified human or bovine pro-thrombin, then chromatographic steps and ultrafiltration are needed. Viral inactivation follows the same process as that for fibrinogen.

At the end of the process of manufacturing fibrinogen, the concentration in most products reaches 20 g/l, and the time for the clotting formation, once mixed with thrombin, is 2–10 seconds. Generally these products are successfully able to stop the bleeding, but a potential lack of action could be due to low fibrinogen concentration, and the weakness of the fibrin clot once mixed with fibrinogen [17].

Thrombin, with calcium ions, breaks the fibrinogen chain, leading to the formation of fibrin monomers. These polymerize so as to make jelly-like unstable clot. Factor XIII, activated by thrombin and calcium, strengthens the links among fibrin monomers making a stable, insoluble clot [20], regardless of the coagulation pattern of the patient. In fact, unlike passive agents that require a normal clotting function, the active agents contain thrombin that takes part at the end of the clotting cascade, making its action less susceptible to coagulopathies caused by clotting factor deficiencies or platelet malfunction [6]. All fibrin-based products have hemostatic, adhesive and sealing features. Furthermore, some commercial products have a biostimulant filling action as well as preventing adhesion onset. Fibrin glues can also be used in patients taking anti-aggregant or anti-platelet drugs, in patients with clotting or platelet disorders. Hemostasis velocity depends on thrombin concentration, while the strength of clot is mainly related to fibrinogen concentration. Adhesive and sealing actions are related to the polymerization process of the fibrin monomers forming the plug. Adhesive function is strictly connected to fibrinogen, XIII factor and fibronectine concentration [21]. Filling and biostimuling actions start a few hours after clotting formation because of fibroblast proliferation, granulocyte infiltration, and the subsequent granulation tissue formation [20]. This is the reason why these products have an action also in wound healing, stimulating macrophage proliferation and collagen production at the site of application.

Antifibrinolitic agents are usually added to hemostatic products to increase the stability of the clot. The most commonly used are bovine aprotinin and tranexamic acid. The former is a specific inhibitor of several proteases such as chymotrypsin, elastase, trypsin, urokinase, kallikrein, and plasmin, the last is a synthetic analog of lysine and is a specific inhibitor of plasminogen. It has a low molecular weight and does not interfere with wound healing, but it has potential neurotoxicity.

Fibrin sealants are available commercially for the surgeon; generally they are applied by a double syringe system, which allows the simultaneous application of equal volumes of thrombin and fibrinogen, either through a blunt tip or through a spray tip [17]. The use with the spray device is particularly useful when hemostasis needs to be achieved over wide surfaces (such as live cut margins) and provides a homogeneous application of the product. On the other hand in bleeding sites that are difficult to access the use of the blunt tip is more indicated, so as to apply small amounts of sealant until bleeding has stopped. The application of fibrin glue on the site of bleeding promotes hemostasis and thus reduces the blood loss. Also these sealants are biocompatible and biodegradable and induce neither an inflammatory response nor tissue necrosis [17]. These products are also used as biodegradable carriers that release drugs, such as antibiotics, growth factors or anti-neoplastics in cases of tumors, at the site of application [22].

Surgical settings

Fibrin glues have been successfully used in many surgical procedures and the recent diffusion of mini-invasive surgery such as laparoscopic and robotic surgery, with reduced possibilities as to direct hemostasis, has led to further developments of chemical–pharmacological hemostatic methods.

In general surgery fibrin sealants are widely used for the closure of gastrointestinal fistulas, including anorectal, colorectal, gastrocutaneous, esophagogastrointestinal, intractable complex, pancreatic, perineal, and gastrojejunal fistulas [23]. Even though widely used also in breast cancer surgery, the indication to use fibrin glue for the prevention of seromas is not clear. Authors are discordant; some assert that it is useful to reduce postoperative drainage or seroma formation [24–26], on the other hand some do not support this opinion in terms of cost effectiveness [27, 28]. It has also been successfully used in laparoscopic and laparotomic transabdominal inguinal hernia repair [29, 30], with good results in terms of post-operative pain. Many authors support the use of fibrin glues in the endoscopic treatment of upper gastro-intestinal bleeding [31–37], showing that endoscopic hemostasis with fibrin adhesive is safe and effective especially in patients with impaired hemostasis, as for instance in cirrhotic patients. The application of fibrin sealant in liver surgery is of great interest, as it is a highly vascular organ with a friable cut surface, causing bleeding that may present as oozing, difficult to control with standard surgical hemostatic devices. Fibrin sealant can help control the diffuse bleeding associated with liver surgery [38–40], as well as prevent post-operative biliary leakages.

Several studies have shown that fibrin sealant has been used effectively for hemostasis in patients undergoing cardiovascular and vascular surgery as is the case of fibrin glue as a hemostatic after sternotomy instead of bone wax [41] in the replacement of the ascending aorta [42]; it has also recently been proven as an efficacious hemostatic agent in ePTFE graft placement surgery [43].

Fibrin sealant has recently been used effectively to prevent and to treat cerebrospinal fluid leakage both spontaneous and after neurosurgery [44], it has wide indications in thoracic surgery in the prevention of air leaks [45] and in urologic surgery it is used both as a hemostatic during partial nephrectomy, renal reconstruction after trauma, bladder surgery and as a sealant in the prevention of urinary fistulas [23].

Topical hemostatics (Passive agents)

Topical hemostatics are absorbable agents that can be used alone or in combination with fibrin sealants. Passive topical hemostatic agents are available in different forms of application and devices for the surgeon; this determines their effectiveness [46]. Gauze, sheets, sponges, and fleece are the most used in the operating theatre; however, fleece and powdered forms might be difficult to handle because of their high electrostatic charge, which makes them stick to instruments and gloves, with suboptimal results in terms of hemostasis [16]. The vast variety of products lets each surgeon be confident with one product rather than another. These products include collagen, gelatin and oxidized cellulose. Their mechanism of action is to promote platelet activation and aggregation when directly applied to the bleeding tissue and they can absorb body fluids several times their own weight. Topical hemostatic agents depend on fibrin production to achieve hemostasis; this is the reason why these agents are suitable only for patients who have an intact coagulation cascade [47]. They can be used to control suture bleeding and to achieve hemostasis on the surface of parenchymatous organs; they are able to stop venous or minimal bleeding and should not be used to stop arterial bleeding, whereas fibrin sealants are more appropriate to do so. Topical hemostatic agents differ in biodegradability and their dissolution and absorption depends on the material, the site of implantation and it takes several weeks to be complete [17]; thus when hemostasis is achieved, it is preferable to remove the material in excess from the surgical site. In fact, enzymatic dissolution of the product determines a cell-mediated response by macrophages, causing an inflammatory state. Furthermore, the risks of postoperative bacterial contamination and potential nerve constriction against bony surfaces have to be reported. These products are typically used as first-line agents because of their immediate availability and low associated costs [48].

Collagen-based products

Collagen-based products possess a microfibrillar structure consisting of collagen molecules with hydrochloric acid non-covalently bound to some of the available amino acid groups. The helical structure, and large surface area it provides, are important to achieve hemostasis [49]. These agents are frequently combined with active hemostatics, for instance thrombin, so as to enhance the pro-coagulant action. The collagen product can be applied directly on to the source of bleeding in the form of powder or paste, or using a sponge or fleece. Also these products can be useful in several surgical specialties: general, hepatic, cardiovascular, and orthopedic surgery.

Collagens of animal origin, in particular bovine derived, have the potential to determine immunological events even though the occurrence of allergic reactions is low compared to other common allergies [50].

Cellulose-based products

Oxidized cellulose and oxidized regenerated cellulose have been used for several decades. A number of mechanisms are thought to contribute to their hemostatic action; they mainly induce clotting through contact activation: blood absorption, surface interactions with proteins and platelets, and activation of both the intrinsic and extrinsic pathways [49]. They also have an anti-microbial activity, leading to infection prevention at the site of hemostasis, probably because of the low pH of these agents that may also contribute to hemostasis. Absorption of regenerated oxidized cellulose is thought to require 1–2 weeks and oxidized cellulose 3–4 weeks. It is, however, recommended to use the minimal amount of the product and to remove the product from the site of bleeding once hemostasis is achieved, so as to avoid the potential risk of infection [51]. Furthermore, granulomas developed at the site of hemostasis (without removal of the product) can be difficult to distinguish radiologically from other pathologies causing serious problems in the post-operative period [52–55]. These products can be useful in several surgical specialties: otorhinolaryngology, as well as general, hepatic, cardiovascular, and orthopedic surgery.

Gelatin agents

Gelatin-based hemostatic agents are made from purified pork skin gelatin or bovine-derived gelatin. Their mechanism of action is due to a mechanical matrix that facilitates clotting and can be combined with topical thrombin, as with the collagen-based agents. Gelatin-based agents are available in sponge, powder, and granular forms. Gelatin agents can absorb a large amount of blood and fluids, so as to adjust to irregular wounds and surgical cavities and restrict blood flow and provide a stable surrounding where the clot can form. Gelatin-based products have been reported to induce a better quality clot than collagen based hemostats [56]. Degradation time *in vivo* of two of these agents is typically 4–6 weeks.

These products are practical to use in minimally invasive procedures and can be useful in anorectal surgery, nasal bleeding, neurosurgery, urology, and general surgery.

References

1 Nielsen HJ. Detrimental effects of perioperative blood transfusion. Br J Surg. 1995;82:582–7.
2 Vamvakas EC. Possible mechanisms of allogeneic blood transfusion-associated postoperative infection. Transfus Med Rev. 2002;16:144–60.
3 Lundblad RL, Bradshaw RA, Gabriel D, Ortel TL, Lawson J, Mann KG. A review of the therapeutic uses of thrombin. Thromb Haemost. 2004;91(5):851–860.
4 Adams GL, Manson RJ, Turner I, Sindram D, Lawson JH. The balance of thrombosis and hemorrhage in surgery. Hematol Oncol Clin North Am. 2007;21(1):13–24.
5 Hemostasis. In: Porter RS, ed. The Merck Manuals Online Medical Library. http://www.merck.com/mmpe/sec11/ch134/ch134a.html. November 2005. Accessed February 12, 2012.
6 Oz MC, Rondinone JF, Shargill NS. FloSeal Matrix: new generation topical hemostatic sealant. J Card Surg. 2003;18(6):486–493.
7 Howard BM, Daley AT, Cohen MJ. Prohemostatic Interventions in Trauma: Resuscitation-Associated Coagulopathy, Acute Traumatic Coagulopathy, Hemostatic Resuscitation, and Other Hemostatic Interventions. Semin Thromb Hemost. 2012 Mar 30.
8 Allard MA, Dondero F, Sommacale D, et al. Liver packing during elective surgery: an option that can be considered. World J Surg. 2011 Nov;35(11):2493–8.
9 Di Benedetto F, Tarantino G, D'Amico G, et al. Which is the last stage before packing in elective liver surgery? World J Surg. 2011 Oct;35(10):2360–1;
10 Sabel M, Stummer W. The use of local agents: Surgicel and Surgifoam. Eur Spine J. 2004;13(Suppl 1):S97–S101. Epub May 15, 2004.
11 Bochicchio G, Dunne J, Bochicchio K, Scalea T. The combination of platelet-enriched autologous plasma with bovine collagen and thrombin decreases the need for multiple blood transfusions in trauma patients with retroperitoneal bleeding. J Trauma. 2004;56(1):76–9.
12 Joch C. The safety of fibrin sealants. Cardiovasc Surg. 2003 Aug;11 Suppl 1:23–8.
13 Dodds, RY. Current viral risks of blood and blood products. Annals of Medicine. 2000;32:469–74.
14 Tock B, Drohan W, Hess J, et al. Haemophilia and advanced fibrin sealant technologies. Haemophilia. 1998;4:449–55.
15 Alving BM, Weinstein MJ, Finlayson JS, et al. Fibrin sealant: summary of a conference on characteristics and clinical uses. Transfusion. 1995;35:783–90.
16 Samudrala S. Topical hemostatic agents in surgery: a surgeon's perspective. AORN J. 2008 Sep;88(3).

17 Masci E, Santolieri L, Belloni F, et al. Topical hemostatic agents in surgical practice. Transfus Apher Sci. 2011 Dec;45(3):305–11.

18 Brunicardi FC, Anderson DK, Billiar TR, et al. Hemostasis, surgical bleeding, and transfusion. Schwartz's Principles of Surgery. 8th ed. New York, NY: McGraw-Hill; 2005, p. 93.

19 Seccia M, Panucucci S. Emostatici topici, Adesivi e Sigillanti in Chirurgia. Pisa University Press; 2009.

20 Mosesson MW. Fibrinogen and fibrin polymerization and functions. Blood Coagul Fibrinolysos. 1999;10 (Suppl. 1):S45–8.

21 Siedentop KH, Park JJ, Shah AN, et al. Safety and efficacy of currently available fibrin tissue adhesives. Am J Otolaryngol. 2001 Jul-Aug;22(4):230–5.

22 Tredwell S, Jackson JK, Hamilton D, et al. Use of fibrin sealants for the localized, controlled release of cefazolin. Can J Surg. 2006;49(5):347–52.

23 Albala DM, Lawson JH. Recent clinical and investigational applications of fibrin sealant in selected surgical specialties. J Am Coll Surg. 2006 Apr;202(4):685–97. Epub 2006 Feb 20. Review.

24 Hivelin M, Heusse JL, Matar N, et al. Fibrin sealant decreases postoperative drainage in immediate breast reconstruction by deep inferior epigastric perforator flap after mastectomy with axillary dissection. Microsurgery. 2011 Jan;31(1): 18–25.

25 van Bemmel AJ, van de Velde CJ, Schmitz RF, et al. Prevention of seroma formation after axillary dissection in breast cancer: a systematic review. Eur J Surg Oncol. 2011 Oct;37(10):829–35.

26 Ruggiero R, Procaccini E, Piazza P, et al. Effectiveness of fibrin glue in conjunction with collagen patches to reduce seroma formation after axillary lymphadenectomy for breast cancer. Am J Surg. 2008 Aug;196(2):170–4.

27 Carless PA, Henry DA. Systematic review and meta-analysis of the use of fibrin sealant to prevent seroma formation after breast cancer surgery. Br J Surg. 2006 Jul;93(7):810–9. Review.

28 Cipolla C, Fricano S, Vieni S, et al. Does the use of fibrin glue prevent seroma formation after axillary lymphadenectomy for breast cancer? A prospective randomized trial in 159 patients. J Surg Oncol. 2010 Jun 1;101(7):600–3.

29 Fortelny RH, Petter-Puchner AH, Glaser KS, et al. Use of fibrin sealant (Tisseel/Tissucol) in hernia repair: a systematic review. Surg Endosc. 2012 Jan 26.

30 Fortelny RH, Petter-Puchner AH, May C, et al. The impact of atraumatic fibrin sealant vs. staple mesh fixation in TAPP hernia repair on chronic pain and quality of life: results of a randomized controlled study. Surg Endosc. 2012 Jan;26(1): 249–54.

31 Imhof M, Ohmann C, Roher HD, Glutig H. DUESUC study group. Endoscopic versus operative treatment in high-risk ulcer bleeding patients–results of a randomised study. Langenbecks Arch Surg. 2003;387:327–36.

32 Datta D, Vlavianos P, Alisa A, Westaby D. Use of fibrin glue (Beriplast) in the management of bleeding gastric varices. Endoscopy. 2003;35:675–8.

33 Lin HJ, Hsieh YH, Tseng GY, et al. Endoscopic injection with fibrin sealant versus epinephrine for arrest of peptic ulcer bleeding: a randomized, comparative trial. J Clin Gastroenterol. 2002;35:218–21.

34 Heneghan MA, Byrne A, Harrison PM. An open pilot study of the effects of a human fibrin glue for endoscopic treatment of patients with acute bleeding from gastric varices. Gastrointest Endosc. 2002;56:422–26.

35 Pescatore P, Jornod P, Borovicka J, et al. Epinephrine versus epinephrine plus fibrin glue injection in peptic ulcer bleeding: a prospective randomized trial. Gastrointest Endosc. 2002;55:348–53.

36 Sitter H, Lorenz W, Nicolay U, et al. From clinical effectiveness to everyday practice: implementing findings from a cost effectiveness analysis for endoscopic injection therapy for upper-gastrointestinal bleeding. Eur J Gastroenterol Hepatol. 2003;15:295–304.

37 Tirindelli MC, Greco R, Marchesi F, et al. Fibrin glue for endoscopic gastrointestinal bleeding in patients with impaired haemostasis. Transfus Med. 2008 Jun;18(3):207–8.

38 Schwartz M, Madariaga J, Hirose R, et al. Comparison of a new fibrin sealant with standard topical hemostatic agents. Arch Surg. 2004;139:1148–54.

39 Saif R, Jacob M, Robinson S, et al. Use of fibrin-based sealants and gelatin-matrix hemostats in laparoscopic liver surgery. Surg Laparosc Endosc Percutan Tech. 2011 Jun;21(3):131–41. Review.

40 Berrevoet F, de Hemptinne B. Use of topical hemostatic agents during liver resection. Dig Surg. 2007;24(4):288–93. Epub 2007 Jul 27.

41 Yu L, Gu T, Song L, et al. Fibrin sealant provides superior hemostasis for sternotomy compared with bone wax. Ann Thorac Surg. 2012 Feb;93(2):641–4.

42 Christenson JT, Kalangos A. Autologous fibrin glue reinforced by platelets in surgery of ascending aorta. Thorac Cardiovasc Surg. 2004;52:225–229.

43 Saha SP, Muluk S, Schenk W 3rd,, et al. Use of fibrin sealant as a hemostatic agent in expanded polytetrafluoroethylene graft placement surgery. Ann Vasc Surg. 2011 Aug;25(6):813–22.

44 Daele JJ, Goffart Y, Machiels S. Traumatic, iatrogenic, and spontaneous cerebrospinal fluid (CSF) leak: endoscopic repair. B-ENT. 2011;7 (Suppl 17):47–60. Review.

45 Gonfiotti A, Santini PF, Jaus M, et al. Safety and effectiveness of a new fibrin pleural air leak sealant: a multicenter, controlled, prospective, parallel-group, randomized clinical trial. Ann Thorac Surg. 2011 Oct;92(4):1217–24.

46 Tomizawa Y. Clinical benefits and risk analysis of topical hemostats: a review. J Artif Organs. 2005;8(3):137–42.

47 Davie EW, Kulman JD. An overview of the structure and function of thrombin. Semin Thromb Hemost. 2006;32(Suppl 1):3–15.

48 Schreiber MA, Neveleff DJ. Achieving hemostasis with topical hemostats: making clinically and economically appropriate decisions in the surgical and trauma settings. AORN J. 2011 Nov;94(5):S1–20.

49 Seyednejad H, Imani M, Jamieson T, et al. Topical haemostatic agents. Br J Surg. 2008 Oct;95(10):1197–225.

50 Lynn AK, Yannas IV, Bonfield W. Antigenicity and immunogenicity of collagen. J Biomed Mater Res B Appl Biomater. 2004;71(2):343–54.

51 Gao HW, Lin CK, Yu CP, Yu MS, Chen A. Oxidized cellulose (SurgicelTM) granuloma mimicking a primary ovarian tumor. Int J Gynecol Pathol. 2002;21:422–3.

52 Azmy AF. Oxidized cellulose haemostat mimicking a possible recurrence of neuroblastoma. BJU Int. 2001;88:295–6.

53 Somani BK, Kasthuri RS, Shave RM, Emtage LA. Surgicel granuloma mimicking a renal tumour. Surgery. 2006;139:451.

54 Kothbauer KF, Jallo GI, Siffert J, Jimenez E, Allen JC, Epstein FJ. Foreign body reaction to hemostatic materials mimicking recurrent brain tumor. Report of three cases. J Neurosurg. 2001;95:503–6.

55 Sandhu GS, ElexpuruCamiruaga JA, Buckley S. Oxidized cellulose (Surgicel) granulomata mimicking tumour recurrence. Br J Neurosurg. 1996;10:617–19.

56 Szpalski M, Gunzburg R, Sztern B. An overview of blood-sparing techniques used in spine surgery during the perioperative period. Eur Spine J. 2004; 13(Suppl 1):S18–S27.

CHAPTER 8

Intraoperative strategies for transfusion-free medicine

Joseph D. Tobias

Department of Anesthesiology and Pain Medicine, Nationwide Children's Hospital, Columbus, OH, USA

Introduction

Perioperative transfusions account for greater than half of the more than 20 million units of blood and blood products that are administered each year in the United States. Therefore many of the techniques to limit the need for allogeneic blood products have focused on the intraoperative period when the greatest blood loss may occur. Given these data, it appears that effective intraoperative strategies may provide the greatest avenue for the overall decrease in the need for allogeneic blood products. Furthermore when considering the acuity of illness of these patients and the additional impact that the surgical procedure imposes on homeostasis, avoidance of perioperative transfusions may greatly alter patient outcomes including the incidence of nosocomial infections, duration of postoperative mechanical ventilation, length or stay and even mortality [1].

Of the surgical procedures recognized as being associated with significant blood loss, cardiothoracic, hepatic and major orthopedic procedures especially those involving the hip, pelvis and spine lead the list with estimated losses that may exceed one-half to an entire blood volume [2]. During these procedures, as blood is lost and replaced with allogeneic blood, ongoing blood loss may be exacerbated by the development of disturbances in coagulation function related to the dilution of normal coagulation factors, alterations in acid-base status, hypothermia or disseminated intravascular coagulation (DIC). Although in most circumstances, the administration of blood and/or blood products including fresh frozen plasma (FFP), cryoprecipitate, and platelet concentrates can be used to effectively correct hemoglobin concentrations and coagulation

Transfusion-Free Medicine and Surgery, Second Edition. Edited by Nicolas Jabbour.
© 2014 John Wiley & Sons, Ltd. Published 2014 by John Wiley & Sons, Ltd.

function, there is a growing body of evidence which demonstrates a growing list of the potential adverse effects of the administration of allogeneic blood products including the transmission of infectious diseases, immunosuppression, transfusion-related acute lung injury, transfusion reactions, and graft-versus-host disease [3–5]. Although improved laboratory testing has significantly decreased the risk of transmitting infectious diseases including the human immunodeficiency virus and hepatitis with blood products, there is also a growing body of evidence that demonstrates the potential deleterious effects of the immunosuppressive effects of allogeneic transfusion [6–8]. This latter effect may be particularly problematic during the perioperative period and may impact on the incidence of perioperative infections, tumor recurrence in patients with oncologic diseases, and even mortality. Recent evidence is also mounting regarding the potential dangers of transfusion-related acute lung injury (TRALI) and its impact on critically ill patients [8]. In fact, the two most common causes of acute mortality related to allogeneic transfusion are now postulated to include a clerical error resulting in a hemolytic transfusion reaction and TRALI. Additional problems which may be more common with non-red cell containing components include volume overload (transfusion associated cardiac overload or TACO), anaphylactoid reactions, and alterations in serum ionized calcium, which may lead to hypotension, cardiovascular compromise, and even cardiac arrest [9].

Given these and other concerns, there remains significant interest in avoiding or limiting the need for allogeneic blood products especially during the perioperative period and in critically ill patients. The following chapter reviews several of the potential options for limiting allogeneic blood product use during the perioperative period. Techniques to be reviewed include:

1 General considerations such as the optimization of preoperative coagulation function, correction of preoperative anemia, and intraoperative anesthetic technique including fluid therapy, proper patient positioning, and maintenance of normothermia;

2 Autologous transfusion therapy including preoperative donation or intraoperative collection using acute normovolemic hemodilution (ANH) with or without the use of erythropoietin as well as intraoperative and postoperative blood salvage;

3 Pharmacologic manipulation of the coagulation cascade with anti-fibrinolytic agents, desmopressin (DDAVP), recombinant coagulation factors (VII and XIII) or novel agents undergoing phase II and III trials;

4 Controlled hypotension.

Although, many of these techniques are effective alone, in many instances, the performance of major surgical procedures without the use of allogeneic blood products can only be accomplished by combining several of these techniques. In addition to the previously noted benefits of limiting the use of allogeneic blood products, the added benefit may be a reduction in cost given the price tag involved with the obtainment, preparation, and delivery of blood products. Although the safety of blood products has increased with increased screening for infectious agent, these processes further increase the cost of blood products. As such, as we evaluate new techniques to limit the use of allogeneic blood products, the cost of these techniques in relationship to the cost of blood products must be considered. In line with this, the techniques outlined in this chapter can only be cost effective if they are focused on the populations that are most likely to require allogeneic blood products. For the operating room setting, this can be accomplished by selecting procedures during which more than 25–40% of patients require transfusion.

General considerations

Effective preoperative evaluation and preparation of the patient are essential not only for safe anesthesia practice, but also to limit allogeneic blood product use. Patients presenting for major surgery may have chronic medical conditions that affect coagulation function. For example, patients with scoliosis presenting for posterior spinal fusion may have associated cerebral palsy and static encephalopathy at times complicated by seizure disorders. The chronic administration of anticonvulsant agents including phenytoin and carbamazepime may adversely affect coagulation function. Additionally, in these patients or chronically ill elderly patients, nutritional issues and poor intake of vitamin K may predispose to chronic low levels of vitamin K dependent coagulation factors resulting in chronic coagulation dysfunction. Preoperative screening of coagulation function and simple measures such as the administration of vitamin K (oral or intramuscular) may alleviate such problems. Other associated medications may also affect platelet function. Patients with chronic orthopedic problems and pain frequently use non-steroidal anti-inflammatory agents (NSAIDs) that may affect platelet function. Although acetylsalicylic acid irreversibly inhibits cyclo-oxygenase and platelet function for the life of the platelet, NSAIDs result in reversible inhibition of platelet function that is dependent on the plasma concentration and hence the half-life of the NSAID. Discontinuation of most NSAIDs for 2–5 days prior to surgery will result in return of normal platelet function.

More importantly, hidden perioperative concerns may be present from undisclosed herbal medications related to their effects on coagulation function. In particular, garlic, ginkgo biloba, and ginseng may lead to increased perioperative bleeding. It has been estimated that up to 70% of the patients will fail to disclose their herbal medicine use during routine preoperative assessment. According to the Dietary Supplement Health and Education Act of 1994, herbal medications are classified as dietary supplements and therefore, these agents are exempt from the safety and efficacy requirements and regulations that prescription and over-the-counter drugs must fulfill including preclinical animal studies, premarketing controlled clinical trials, or postmarketing surveillance. In fact, in order to have these drugs removed from the market, they must be proven to be unsafe. These issues further emphasize the importance of thorough questioning of patients during preoperative visit and a full disclosure to the patients regarding the potential risks of such medications [10].

Perhaps one of the most important and most effective means of limiting the need for perioperative transfusion is the identification and treatment of preoperative anemia. In a prospective evaluation of 230 consecutive patients over a 15-month period undergoing spinal surgery, four preoperative independent predictors were identified to be associated with need for allogeneic transfusion [11]. These included age older than 50 years (adjusted odds ratio = 4.9), preoperative hemoglobin level less than 12 gm/dL (adjusted odds ratio = 6.9, fusion of more than two levels (adjusted odds ratio = 6.7), and the performance of a transpedicular osteotomy (adjusted odds ratio = 19.9). Chronic anemia is generally multifactorial in etiology with most patients remaining asymptomatic. It is present in up to 75% of patients presenting for elective surgery with iron deficiency and chronic disease as the cause of anemia in a high proportion of these patients. In addition to increasing the need for allogeneic blood products, preoperative anemia has also been shown to be a risk factor for postoperative morbidity and mortality [12, 13]. Considering the evidence supporting that both anemia and red blood cell transfusions are associated with increased morbidity and mortality during the perioperative period, a strategy to minimize both conditions may improve patient outcomes significantly. An effective means for the diagnosis and treatment of anemia in patients scheduled to undergo elective surgery has been may reviewed and advocated by the Network for Advancement of Transfusion Alternatives [14–16]. The preoperative evaluation includes a complete blood cell count, ferritin, vitamin B_{12}, and red blood cell folate levels.

The latter two (vitamin B_{12} and folate deficiencies) are more common in older patients. As such, patients over 65 years of age and those at risk for nutritional deficiencies should be evaluated. Deficiencies in either vitamin B_{12} or folate can be treated successfully with oral medications. Low ferritin invariably points to iron deficiency, which can be treated with either oral or intravenous iron therapy [15, 16]. The treatment of anemia of chronic disease may be more complex, requiring the use of an erythrocyte stimulating agent such as erythropoietin. Once the cause of anemia is identified, therapy should be initiated and follow-up studies obtained to demonstrate an effective response prior to embarking on elective surgical procedures.

Intraoperative issues can also impact on blood loss including choice of anesthetic technique (see below for a full discussion of controlled hypotension), fluid therapy, temperature control, and patient positioning. Although control of intraoperative blood pressure and use of controlled hypotension is a significant factor in intraoperative blood loss, other aspects of the anesthetic technique may also impact on the need for allogeneic blood transfusions. A simple maneuver, whenever feasible, is to maintain appropriate patient positioning. This can be as simple as elevating the head of the bed for head and neck procedures or appropriate positioning on the surgical table during prone orthopedic cases to maximize abdominal decompression. Both of these techniques can aid decreasing venous tone and limiting surgical bleeding.

Interestingly, some studies suggest that modification of the anesthetic technique may also impact on intraoperative blood loss. In a prospective trial of adolescents undergoing posterior spinal fusion, decreased blood loss was noted with the pre-incisional administration of lumbar intrathecal morphine [17]. Estimated blood loss (mL/kg) in patients receiving 0, 2, and 5 µg/kg of intrathecal morphine was 41 ± 23, 34 ± 19, and 14 ± 10 ($p < 0.05$ versus other two groups) respectively in the three groups.

Maintenance of normothermia is also of paramount importance in controlling blood loss, decreasing requirements for allogeneic blood products, decreasing postoperative infections, and shortening hospital stay [18, 19]. Core body temperature below $34\,°C$ has been shown to be a risk factor for the development of coagulopathy in trauma patients while even mild hypothermia has been shown to increase blood loss during hip arthroplasty [19–21]. The importance of the maintenance of intraoperative normothermia is illustrated by Widman et al. who demonstrated the thermogenic effect of the infusion of an amino acid solution during hip arthroplasty in adults during spinal anesthesia [22]. In those patients receiving the amino acid solution, the pre-anesthesia temperature increased by $0.4 \pm 0.2\,°C$ while it was unchanged in the control group. At the completion of the surgical procedure, temperature had decreased by $0.4 \pm 0.3\,°C$ in patients receiving the amino acid infusion and by $0.9 \pm 0.4\,°C$ in control patients. Blood loss was $702 \pm 344\,mL$ in the control group and $516 \pm 272\,mL$ ($p < 0.05$) in patients that received the amino acid infusion. Although the technique is innovative and demonstrates the benefits of intraoperative temperature control, it is also cumbersome and costly. In most anesthetic suites, maintenance of normothermia is provided by a combination of warming the room prior to the patient's arrival, maintenance of a warm environment until the patient is anesthetized, positioned and draped plus the use of forced air warming blankets and blood/fluid warmers to warm intravenous fluids. In the adult population, preoperative warming with the use of specialized robes and forced air warmer devices are becoming more popular [23]. The latter may be especially useful in the elderly patient who may be at risk for perioperative hypothermia

The choice of intraoperative fluid administration may affect coagulation function thereby impacting on blood loss. During intraoperative care or the use of replacement fluid for ANH (see below), various non-blood fluids including crystalloids and colloids are administered. During ANH, blood is removed, replaced with isotonic fluids and saved for reinfusion at a later time thereby resulting in the dilution of red blood cells, plasma proteins and platelets. As such, it may be assumed that coagulation would be adversely impacted do to the dilution of coagulation factors and platelets. However, the opposite effect occurs due to the dilution of proteins with anti-coagulatory effects such as anti-thrombin III [24]. A 25–30% hemodilution with replacement by isotonic crystalloids results in an augmentation of coagulation function.

Colloids used for volume expansion and blood replacement may also adversely affect coagulation function. There are three colloids routinely used intraoperatively including albumin, gelatins, and starches. Albumin and gelatins are generally considered to have no effect on or to augment coagulation function [25]. However, a limited number of other studies have suggested a decrease in factor VIII/von Willebrand factor complex beyond what would be expected for the degree of hemodilution provided as well as reduced quality of the clot formed with the administration of gelatins [26, 27]. Future studies are needed to define the clinical significance of this effect; however, in most clinical circumstances, the clinical impact is limited.

In the United States and many countries, the hydroxyethyl starches are the most commonly administered colloid during the perioperative period.

These agents are classified based on their molecular weight as well as the molar substitution (the percentage of the glucose units on the starch molecule contain hydroxyethyl units). The latter generally ranges from 25–50%. These fluids are further characterized by their concentration in the solution and the fluid in which they are diluted (Ringer's lactate or normal saline) [28]. Medium or high molecular weight hydroxyethyl starches (HES) with a high molar substitution alter coagulation function through their effects on von Willebrand factor. The latter is particularly relevant when these fluids are administered in doses exceeding 20–25 mL/kg [29]. The newest generation of hydroxyethyl starches (tetrastarches) with a lower molecular weight and molar substitution (0.4) that have been introduced into clinical practice have been shown to have a limited effect on platelet function [30].

Postoperative care can also have a significant impact on limiting the need for perioperative allogeneic blood products. Simple measures should as limitation of blood work and obtaining the minimal volume required for laboratory analysis is mandatory especially in young infants and children as studies have demonstrated significant waste and the drawing of excessive volumes for routine laboratory panels [31]. Education of the entire perioperative team is necessary as unnecessary laboratory tests may be ordered out of habit and transfusions administered during off-hours by less experienced members of the surgical team. The use of a computerized ordering system with alerts based on current evidence for transfusion practices has been shown to decrease transfusions [32].

Autologous blood

There are three means of obtaining autologous blood for transfusion:
1 acute normovolemic hemodilution (ANH)
2 preoperative autologous donation,
3 perioperative salvage of shed blood.

Acute normovolemic (isovolemic) hemodilution

ANH involves phlebotomy and blood collection, which is performed in the operating room generally after the induction of anesthesia [33]. The removed blood is replaced with either crystalloid or colloid to maintain euvolemia. The latter is ensured by monitoring vital signs and at times, measures of end-organ oxygen delivery (see below). Hemodilution decreases the hematocrit of blood shed during surgery, thereby limiting the mass of red blood cells lost, and provides autologous blood with active coagulation factors and platelets for reinfusion at the completion of the case. The degree of hemodilution is defined by the final hematocrit that is achieved. Moderate hemodilution is defined as a final hematocrit between 25% and 30%; severe hemodilution, which is not routinely employed is defined as a hematocrit between 10% and 20%.

In general, the technique should be employed when the anticipated blood loss is 1000 to 2000 mL or greater in adults. In children, ANH may be considered if the blood loss is expected to be greater than 50% of the estimated blood volume. Despite the relative safety of this technique, there are absolute and relative contraindications to its use (Table 8.1) [33]. To ensure that an adequate volume of blood can be removed to make the technique effective, the initial hematocrit should generally be ≥36%. Any type of ongoing disturbance in coagulation function is one contraindication to ANH, as replacement of blood with asanquinous fluid further dilutes coagulation factors and platelets. Renal insufficiency or failure is also a relative contraindication since diuresis of the fluids after the reinfusion of blood may be impaired. Other relative contraindications include severe pulmonary disease, cirrhosis, severe hypertension, significant cerebrovascular disease or any concurrent illness, which may not allow the patient to tolerate the lower hematocrit or may preclude the increase in cardiac output to compensate for it. In the absence of co-morbid features, age should not be considered a contraindication except that the technique is generally not indicated in infants less than 6 months of age as the compensatory mechanisms for anemia may not be developed at this age. An increase in oxygen delivery cannot be provided by increasing stroke volume and the presence of fetal hemoglobin with a leftward shift of the oxy-hemoglobin dissociation curve impairs oxygen release at the tissue level.

Hemodilution can be performed in an awake or anesthetized patient in the operating room immediately preceding surgery. The quantity of blood to be withdrawn can be calculated, using the patient's current blood volume (BV), initial hematocrit (H_1), and the final desired hematocrit

Table 8.1 Relative contraindications to acute normovolemic hemodilution.

Inherited or acquired coagulation defect
Renal failure
Severe pulmonary disease
Severe hypertension
Underlying cardiovascular disease
Significant cerebrovascular disease
Infants less than 6 months of age

(H_E). The volume of blood to be withdrawn = BV × (H_1 − H_E)/H_{AV} where H_{AV} = the average of H_1 and H_E. Blood is collected in standard blood bank collection bags containing anticoagulant (usually citrate phosphate dextrose). Alternatively, in smaller patients, the blood can be drawn into a syringe with the appropriate amount of anticoagulant added. It is imperative to measure the amount of blood withdrawn so that adequate volume resuscitation may be performed. This can be performed by weighing the bag to determine the volume of blood removed or removal of the blood into a syringe in aliquots with subsequent placement into the bag. The blood can be withdrawn from a central line, arterial cannula or peripheral IV cannula. When deciding upon the site of blood withdrawal, it should be remembered that given the viscosity of blood, short catheters with a large bore are most effective for rapid blood removal. As the blood is withdrawn, colloid or crystalloid may be used for volume replacement (see below). Continuous monitoring of blood pressure via an intra-arterial catheter may be helpful during the procedure, but is not mandatory. As blood is withdrawn, fluids are administered for replacement using either colloid in a 1:1 or crystalloid in a 3:1 ratio. Classic teaching suggests that heart rate and blood pressure should be monitored to identify inadequate fluid replacement and hypovolemia. However, our experience suggests that in the presence of general anesthesia, the HR response is blunted and generally not effective in identifying hemodynamic issues except in the extreme state. We have demonstrated the potential utility of monitoring end oxygenation using near infrared spectroscopy as a means of ensuring that the removal of the autologous blood is well tolerated [34, 35]. The technique also allows one to limit the amount of replacement fluid which is useful when ANH is used prior to cardiac surgery and cardiopulmonary bypass. If significant amounts of colloid or crystalloid are administered during the process for these patients, the secondary dilution that occurs with the prime of CPB circuit may result in a hematocrit that is too low thereby necessitating the administration of blood.

A central venous catheter, while not necessary in all patients, may be indicated to assess volume status and oxygen delivery depending on the patient's underlying status. Once the blood is collected, it may be kept at room temperature for up to 4 to 6 hours. If the blood is not to be reinfused within 6 hours, it should be refrigerated and used within 24 hours. Refrigeration will decrease or inactivate platelet function and eliminate one of the benefits of the fresh autologous blood. It is preferable to reinfuse the blood after surgical blood loss has been controlled. The order of units to be reinfused is opposite the order in which they were removed such that the last unit salvaged is the first unit reinfused. The first unit salvaged is given last because it will have the highest hematocrit and concentration of clotting factors and platelets.

As with resuscitation measures in general, there is controversy at to whether volume replacement for ANH should include crystalloids or colloids. Crystalloid is administered in a 3:1 volume ratio relative to the amount of whole blood removed. Only isotonic fluids should be used such as normal saline, lactated Ringer's, or Plasmalyte™. The advantages of crystalloid are that it can be easily diuresed and is inexpensive. However, because the entire volume does not remain in the intravascular space, a 3:1 replacement ratio should be used. With crystalloids, colloid oncotic pressure (COP) will not be maintained, and tissue edema may result with a compromise of oxygen delivery (see below).

Korosue et al. compared the effects of hemodilution with crystalloid (lactated Ringer's) or colloid (low molecular weight dextran) in dogs subjected to focal cerebral ischemia and found improved neurologic outcome in animals that received the colloid solution [36]. They attributed this to a reduction of COP by the crystalloid solution and concluded that a decrease in COP would lead to edema formation in the area of focal ischemia. However, since lactated Ringer's is not an isotonic fluid, it reduces osmolarity, which may also augment edema formation in ischemic brain. Therefore, the same outcome may not occur with true isotonic fluids such as normal saline. While different investigators have advocated one fluid over another for specific reasons, some of which are supported by laboratory or animal investigations, no clear-cut benefit on postoperative outcome has been demonstrated with any particular crystalloid or with colloid as opposed to crystalloid.

In the general practice of ANH, colloids are infused as a 1:1 replacement for blood. Thus less volume is required while COP is maintained. Most colloids have a half-life longer than 4 hours and may not be rapidly diuresed from the body, therefore, there is a theoretical risk of hypervolemia and fluid overload if the salvaged blood is reinfused rapidly during a time when there is no ongoing blood loss [37]. Given this concern, some authorities have suggested that the replacement colloid should be a short-acting product such as pentastarch which has a half-life of less than 4 hours.

Both albumin and high molecular weight HES have half-lives greater than 24 hours. Albumin is prepared from pooled human plasma in a process that eliminates the risk of disease transmission. The chances of adverse effects are minimal, but it is expensive. Hetastarch, a high-molecular-weight polysaccharide of the HES family, can have an adverse effect on hemostasis when infused in volumes greater than 20–25 mL/kg [38]. Pentastarch, a HES with a lower molecular weight than hetastarch, has less effect on hemostasis [39]. Given their adverse effect profile, neither dextran 70 nor dextran 40 have a role in ANH [40].

Although the purpose of hemodilution is a decrease in the hematocrit with a corresponding decrease in the loss of red cell mass during intra-operative bleeding in addition to the salvage of autologous blood with active platelets and coagulation factors for infusion at a later time, there are several physiologic consequences of the technique. Any alteration in the relation between the red cell mass and the plasma volume will alter microcirculatory flow and blood viscosity. Blood viscosity is influenced by shear rates and hematocrit. The ratio of shear stress (force required to move a fluid) to shear rate (rate at which a fluid flows) defines viscosity. For example, fluids with a higher viscosity require a higher shear stress (force) to move. Most fluids are Newtonian in that they have a constant viscosity regardless of the velocity of the flow. Therefore, a change in force causes a proportional change in flow rate. Blood is not a Newtonian fluid because changes in flow rate will produce a change in viscosity and therefore not a linear increase in flow velocity.

Viscosity also changes disproportionately to changes in hematocrit. A change in hematocrit is followed by an exponential increase or decrease in blood viscosity. The shear rate determines the rate of change. The lower the shear rate, the greater the rate of change in viscosity. Viscosity is shear-dependent down to a hematocrit of 25% to 30%. As a result of these factors, hemodilution has the most significant effect at moderate hemodilution to a hematocrit of 25 to 30%. Hemodilution to lower hematocrits does not result in a further reduction of viscosity or shear rate and therefore does not help in increasing flow to and through the microcirculation.

The initial effect of isovolemic hemodilution with a reduction in the hematocrit is a reduction of the arterial oxygen content of the blood. Compensatory mechanisms to maintain adequate oxygen delivery include increased cardiac output, increased oxygen extraction at the tissue level, and a rightward shift of the oxyhemoglobin dissociation curve. Increased cardiac output is due primarily to an increase in stroke volume without significant changes in heart rate. An increase in heart rate during ANH should be considered a sign of hypovolemia or inadequate anesthesia. The primary factor responsible for the increased stroke volume is increased venous return due to reduced whole-blood viscosity and improved microcirculatory flow [41, 42]. The increased venous return is reflected by an elevation of left ventricular (LV) end-diastolic pressure [43]. The reduced viscosity of the blood also results in a reduction of the systemic vascular resistance thereby reducing afterload and improving left ventricular ejection [44, 45]. Myocardial contractility increases, most likely because of activation of cardiac sympathetic fibers. Bowens and colleagues demonstrated, in anesthetized dogs, that the increase in cardiac output, due to isovolemic hemodilution, remains stable over a prolonged period of time without adverse hemodynamic consequences [46]. The increase in cardiac output does not require an intact autonomic system as it occurs even in dogs following cardiac denervation or β-adrenergic blockage [47].

As arterial oxygen content and delivery decline, the oxygen extraction ratio increases. In the resting state, peripheral oxygen extraction does not increase until the hematocrit decreases to less than 20% to 25% [48]. This relationship holds true provided that hypovolemia does not occur. In the presence of hypovolemia, the arteriovenous oxygen difference will widen even at a hematocrit greater than 20–25%. Although a decrease in the mixed venous oxygen generally occurs at a hematocrit of 15–20%, more severe degrees of hemodilution may be tolerated in the presence of normal cardiovascular reserve. Van Woerkins and colleagues [42] demonstrated a constant mixed venous PO_2 and oxygen saturation in dogs down to a mean hematocrit of 9.3 ± 0.3% with an exchange of 50 mL/kg of blood. In this animal model, cardiac output doubled resulting in increased flow to all organs except the liver and adrenals. The greatest increase in flow occurred to the heart and brain. The increased flow rates and cardiac output maintained oxygen delivery down to a hematocrit of 9%.

In a cohort of eight pediatric patients with a mean age of 12 years, Fontana et al. demonstrated no short-term adverse effects with hemodilution to a mean hemoglobin of 3.0 grams/dL [49]. Mixed venous oxygen saturation decreased from a mean of 90.8% to 72.3% while oxygen extraction increased from 17.3% to 44.4%. Although this extreme degree of hemodilution is not recommended in clinical practice, it demonstrates the significant compensatory processes that occur with severe hemodilution. The caveat is that the patients in this study were anesthetized which likely impacted their metabolic demands.

The compensatory mechanisms to maintain oxygen delivery during hemodilution may not be possible in patients with underlying cardiorespiratory dysfunction. The absolute value of hematocrit (lowest tolerable hematocrit) at which a decrease in the mixed venous oxygen tension occurs will also be influenced by the use of anesthetic agents and neuromuscular blocking agents. Although these agents decrease peripheral oxygen consumption, they also may blunt the compensatory cardiovascular mechanisms. Van der Linden et al. demonstrated that there was a marked blunting of the cardiac output response during hemodilution when animals were anesthetized with high dose halothane (2 MAC) or ketamine compared to low dose regimens (1 MAC halothane) [50, 51].

A decrease in oxygen affinity, demonstrated by a rightward shift of the oxyhemoglobin dissociation curve, is an additional compensatory mechanism that maintains tissue oxygen delivery during hemodilution. This mechanism, which facilitates oxygen release from hemoglobin, does not become operative until the hematocrit reaches 20% [52]. The mechanism responsible for the shift is an increase in 2,3-diphosphoglycerate (2,3-DPG) in erythrocytes. Sunder-Plassman and coworkers [52] found a decrease in oxygen affinity in dogs during hemodilution to a mean hematocrit of 10% and demonstrated a linear relation between hemoglobin oxygen affinity and 2,3-DPG levels. The effect reaches maximum values within 90 minutes after hemodilution.

Van Woerkins et al. demonstrated an additional compensatory mechanism, the redistribution of regional blood flow [42]. The redistribution of flow is dependent on the metabolic demands of the various tissue beds. They noted increased flow to all organs except the liver and adrenal glands, with the heart and brain receiving the most delivery. When considering the coronary bed, the increased flow is disproportionately greater when compared with the increase in cardiac output. In dogs, Holtz et al. demonstrated a 220% increase in cardiac output while coronary blood flow increased by 650 [53]. This disparity results from a greater reduction in coronary vascular resistance than in flow.

The changes in myocardial oxygen consumption are dependent on the level of hemodilution. Jan and Chien demonstrated that myocardial oxygen consumption and coronary sinus oxygen saturation remained constant between a hematocrit of 60% down to 20% [54]. When the hematocrit declined below 20%, myocardial oxygen consumption declined and coronary sinus oxygen saturation began to increase. The authors inferred from these data that there was myocardial ischemia with impairment of oxygen extraction at a hematocrit less than 20%. Conflicting data were published by Van Woerkins and colleagues who found that myocardial oxygen consumption increased down to a hematocrit of 9% in anesthetized pigs [42]. Because coronary blood flow and oxygen delivery increased, the myocardial oxygen extraction ratio remained constant. The authors concluded that increased myocardial blood flow was responsible for an increase in oxygen delivery, which met the metabolic demands of the myocardium.

The distribution of coronary blood flow during isovolemic hemodilution has also been a subject of controversy. Two separate investigations demonstrated the distribution of flow away from the endocardium during hemodilution to a hematocrit of 15% [55, 56]. However, others observed that coronary blood flow remained unchanged between the endocardium and epicardium with hemodilution to a hematocrit of 7% [57]. Although the data are conflicting, if there is a redistribution of flow away from the endocardium it could theoretically expose the patient to ischemia despite the global increase in myocardial blood flow and apparent preservation of myocardial oxygen delivery.

Despite laboratory evidence demonstrating the preservation of coronary blood flow and myocardial oxygen delivery, alterations in flow may be observed in certain pathophysiologic states. Simple tachycardia with the resultant reduced perfusion time and increased oxygen consumption may result in ischemia. The presence of coronary artery stenosis when combined with isovolemic hemodilution may also lead to myocardial ischemia. Geha and Baue examined this issue in dogs with hemodilution to hematocrits of 20% followed by graded coronary occlusion [58]. With 50% occlusion of the left anterior descending (LAD) artery, there was no decrease in myocardial function, no evidence of ischemia, and an increase in coronary blood flow. However, when the occlusion was increased to 67%, there was impaired flow with ischemia. Tachycardia did not occur, although there was a 7% increase in heart rate with hemodilution to a hematocrit of 20%. Further animal work has demonstrated that the critical level of isovolemic hemodilution in the presence of a critical stenosis of a coronary vessel is between a hematocrit of 15% and 25% [59]. Other factors that may compromise coronary blood flow include decreased mean arterial pressure (MAP) and left ventricular hypertrophy (LVH). Therefore, the minimal safe hematocrit in patients with compromised cardiac function is defined as the hematocrit at which coronary blood flow can no longer increase sufficiently to meet myocardial demand. The authors concluded that identification of this level clinically may be difficult. While hemodilution appears safe in patients with normal myocardial function, problems may arise in the presence of compromised cardiovascular function or alterations in coronary anatomy, especially if combined with tachycardia, decreased perfusion pressure, or decreases in the hematocrit to less than 20%. Given these data and those previously outlined from animal studies, it is logical to suggest that extremes of hemodilution should be avoided in patients with compromised cardiovascular status (abnormal LV function, clinically significant coronary artery disease).

Isovolemic hemodilution also leads to a redistribution of flow to other organ beds including the cerebral circulation with cerebral blood flow (CBF) being inversely proportional to the degree of hemodilution or the hematocrit. Todd et al. evaluated the effects of hemodilution with 6% hetastarch in Sprague-Dawley rats [60]. Both CBF and cerebral blood volume increased inversely with the reduction is hematocrit. They also noted that although the increases paralleled each other, there was not a consistent relationship between these two parameters. Therefore, arteriolar vasodilation is not the only factor responsible for the observed increase in CBF. Other suggested mechanisms include capillary recruitment, nitric oxide release or an increase in postarteriolar volume [61].

There is less information concerning the effects of hemodilution outside the cardiovascular system and central nervous system (CNS). Reduced viscosity, as a result of a reduction in erythrocyte and fibrinogen content, results in improved microcirculatory flow in various organs with a more even distribution of tissue PO_2. Sunder-Plassman and others demonstrated this phenomenon by continuously measuring tissue PO_2 in the liver, kidneys, pancreas, small intestine, and skeletal muscle during isovolemic hemodilution to a hematocrit of 20% [52]. They observed a more homogenous distribution of flow as evidenced by an equilibration of the tissue PO_2 throughout the tissue beds. They concluded that microcirculatory flow improved oxygenation to the peripheral tissues with an equal increase in all organ beds. At a hematocrit of 15%, a less homogenous redistribution of flow has been noted. Fan et al. demonstrated that, despite a significant increase in cardiac output, greater increases in coronary and cerebral blood flow occurred compared with smaller increases in renal and hepatic blood flow [62]. Renal oxygen extraction has been shown to remain constant despite reductions in oxygen delivery and flow redistribution to the inner renal cortex [63]. Hepatic and gastrointestinal blood flow are preserved [64]. Utley et al., using a canine model with a hematocrit of 25% ± 2% and non-pulsatile CPB, noted no deleterious effects on end-organ perfusion including the gastrointestinal system [65].

Clinical applications of isovolemic hemodilution

Various studies have demonstrated the efficacy of ANH as a means of limiting the need for perioperative homologous blood transfusions. Laks et al. reported their experience with ANH during hip arthroplasty [45]. ANH was used to reduce the hematocrit to less than 30%. Cardiac output increased, while both the oxygen delivery and the arteriovenous oxygen difference decreased with no change in tissue oxygen consumption. No evidence of metabolic acidosis was noted. Additional studies have demonstrated the efficacy of ANH during scoliosis surgery in the pediatric population [66, 67]. Haberkern and Dangel combined hemodilution to a hematocrit of 20% to 25% with mild hypothermia and controlled hypotension [54]. They reported a 75% decrease in the need for homologous blood. No adverse effects were noted.

ANH has also been used for patients of the Jehovah's Witness faith when undergoing cardiac surgery. Because of the continuity of flow maintained between the patient and the CPB circuit, many patients consider this an acceptable technique. Stein et al. reported their experience with ANH during cardiac surgery for children of Jehovah's Witnesses [68]. The patients ranged in age from 1.5 to 17 years and in weight from 9.1 to 63 kg. Asanquinous priming of the CPB circuit was used combined with moderate to deep hyperthermia. There was a decrease of the hematocrit to a mean of 17.9%. One death occurred related to persistent pulmonary hypertension. No adverse sequelae related to the technique were noted, although no direct measurement of regional blood flow/oxygen delivery was performed. Although the hematocrits were as low as 10% during CPB, the authors recommended maintaining a value of 20% when discontinuing CPB to maintain myocardial oxygen delivery and function. Following rewarming, prior to separation from CPB, ultrafiltration can be instituted to remove excess crystalloid and raise the hematocrit.

The literature holds no definitive answer regarding the minimal safe hematocrit for hemodilution. The degree of hemodilution should be based on the patient's ability to compensate hemodynamically to maintain tissue perfusion and oxygen delivery. Patients with myocardial dysfunction may not have sufficient cardiac reserve to tolerate a reduction of the hematocrit to 20%. The presence of valvular disease, poor ventricular function, and coronary artery disease must be evaluated to determine the lowest tolerable hematocrit. Neonates and infants are generally not good candidates for ANH as they are incapable of increasing stroke volume to compensate for the decrease oxygen content of the blood and the presence of fetal hemoglobin shifts the oxy-hemoglobin dissociation curve to the left thereby further impeding oxygen delivery to the tissues.

In patients without cardiac disease, tissue oxygenation is well maintained at a hematocrit of 20% provided that euvolemia is maintained and the fractional concentration of oxygen is increased. An additional factor that helps to maintain the oxygen supply to demand ratio is a decrease in peripheral oxygen use due to anesthetic and neuromuscular blocking agents. The prevention of factors that increase oxygen consumption, such as pain, shivering, and fever, may alter the balance during emergence from anesthesia and the postoperative period. Robertie and Gravlee have published guidelines for transfusion thresholds based on the available clinical and basic science research [48]. These recommendations are based on assumptions concerning hematocrit and cardiac output that are needed to maintain adequate oxygen content and delivery. In patients that are ASA class I, a hemoglobin of 6 gm/dL (or a hematocrit of 18%) may be acceptable during ANH. This level may even be tolerated postoperatively, as long as the course remains uncomplicated. ASA class II and many class III patients will tolerate hemodilution to 24%; however, patients with coronary artery disease, myocardial dysfunction, or those with increased metabolic demands (fever, pain, agitation) may require higher hematocrits. Patients who are unable to increase cardiac output and regional blood flow (those with congenital, valvular, or ischemic cardiac disease) may require a minimum hematocrit as high as 30%. Regardless of the patient's status, intraoperative monitoring for coronary ischemia and decreased end-organ perfusion is required. In many patients, this can be done non-invasively with ECG monitoring, observation of heart rate, monitoring of urine output, and intermittent assessment of acid-base status. When more extreme degrees of ANH are used or when the patient has associated co-morbid features, invasive hemodynamic monitoring should be considered.

ANH may also be used as an alternative to preoperative autologous donation. In a prospective trial of adult patients undergoing radical retropubic prostatectomy, ANH was shown to be equally as effective as preoperative autologous donation in avoiding allogeneic blood products and maintaining postoperative hemoglobin values while avoiding the costs of preoperative autologous donation, which were three times that of ANH [69]. ANH may be combined with erythropoietin therapy as a means of increasing the preoperative hematocrit and augmenting the amount of blood that can be removed. There is also research interest in the combination of ANH with artificial oxygen carriers or blood substitutes, a technique known as "augmented ANH".

Preoperative autologous donation

Although the potential for the preoperative donation of autologous blood was first suggested by Fantus in 1937 when he founded the first blood bank in the United States [70], it was not until the 1980s that autologous transfusion programs gained widespread clinical use during the heightened awareness of the risks of infectious disease transmission with allogeneic blood products. Various benefits of the preoperative donation of autologous blood have been demonstrated including reduced exposure to allogeneic blood, the availability of blood for patients with rare phenotypes, a reduction of blood shortages, and the avoidance of transfusion-induced immunosuppression [71, 72]. In rare cases, it may even be an option for patients who refuse allogeneic transfusions based on religious beliefs. Despite these benefits, the overall use of autologous donation continues to decrease in the United States and throughout the world related to improved availability of other less costly techniques of blood salvage and the recognition that adverse effects related to clerical errors may still occur (see below).

The criteria for autologous donation are less stringent than those for allogeneic donors [73, 74]. Patients with absolute contraindications to allogeneic donation such as known malignancies and infections such as HIV or hepatitis may participate. Although earlier programs had age restrictions, many institutions have programs which allow autologous donation in children younger than 2 years and adults older than 80 years [75–78]. Patients who weigh 50 kg or more may donate a standard unit of blood (approximately 450 to 500 mL), whereas patients weighing less than 50 kg donated proportionately smaller volumes.

The technique of blood collection is the same as for allogeneic donation except that the blood is generally kept as whole blood and not separated into its components. A patient's hematocrit is checked prior to each donation to ensure that it is greater than 33%. Patients are placed on iron supplementation with the initiation of donation. Donations may be made every 3 days, but the usual practice is to donate one unit per week. The last unit should be donated at least 3 days prior to surgery and preferably up to one week to allow the hematocrit to increase and for plasma proteins to normalize intravascular volume prior to the surgical procedure. Blood is collected in bags with standard anticoagulants (CPD-A or citrate-phosphate-dextrose-adenine) for blood storage, having shelf lives of 35 to 42 days.

Although it has been reported that complications requiring hospitalization were 12 times more frequent after autologous than after allogeneic donation [79], the autologous and allogeneic donors differed in age and first time donor status. First time donors have been shown to have a higher rate of adverse reactions and were more common in the autologous group. Autologous predonation has relatively few contraindications (Table 8.2). The presence of bacteremia is an absolute contraindication due to the obvious concerns of reinfection during transfusion. Severe or unstable angina necessitating hospitalization, severe aortic stenosis, anemia, severe pulmonary diseases, hemodynamic instability, or limited cardiac reserve due to other lesions have been suggested as contraindications to preoperative donation [80]. However, these contraindications have been challenged by several authors with the demonstration of successful donation even in the presence of co-morbid conditions [81]. In a cohort of

Bacteremia
Angina or underlying cardiovascular disease
Aortic stenosis
Pulmonary disease
Anemia
Pregnancy (1st and 3rd trimesters)
Severe end-organ (renal or hepatic disease)

Table 8.2 Relative contraindications to preoperative autologous donation.

patients with end-stage cardiac or pulmonary disease who were awaiting organ transplantation, 65% of those awaiting cardiac transplantation were able to donate 1 to 8 units of blood [81]. The exposure to homologous blood products decreased from 88% in the non-donors to 54% in the donors. Of the 24 lung-transplant candidates, 63% predonated and had a homologous blood exposure rate of 45% versus 100% for those who were ineligible for donation. No serious complications were noted. These studies demonstrated the possibility of autologous donation even in the so-called "high risk" groups and its efficacy in reducing the need for homologous transfusion.

Age should generally not be considered a barrier to autologous predonation. Goodnough et al. reported that autologous blood accounted for 95% of the transfusion requirements in 1672 patients undergoing elective spinal surgery, 60% of whom were older than 60 years [82]. Autologous donation has also been used in pregnant women, diagnosed with placenta previa, without adverse effects on either the mother or the fetus [83, 84]. However, autologous donation should be limited to the second trimester to avoid spontaneous abortions (in the first trimester) and preterm labor (in the third trimester).

The limiting factor in autologous predonation is frequently anemia despite effective iron supplementation [85]. This has been attributed to inadequate erythropoietin levels. To facilitate predonation, supplementation with erythropoietin has been attempted [86]. Patients who had received erythropoietin (600 unites/kg twice a week) were able to donate 5.4 units compared to 4.1 units in the placebo group. The investigators suggested that erythropoietin may be a useful adjunct in autologous predonation (see below for a full discussion of the perioperative applications of erythropoietin in avoiding allogeneic transfusions).

A major issue with predonation of autologous blood is the cost and inconvenience to the patient with the need for repeated visits to the donation center. These issues become of greater importance given the reports that a significant percentage of predonated autologous blood is discarded (30–50%) [87, 88]. If autologous blood is going to be crossed over for use in the general population, the allogeneic donation criteria must be applied. Despite the differences in the criteria for autologous and allogeneic donation, up to 30% of autologous blood could be used. Autologous blood should not be given merely because it is available. The same criteria used for the transfusion of homologous blood are generally recommended when transfusing autologous blood. Because of the risks for incorrect identification and possible bacterial contamination, it is prudent to avoid transfusion unless indicated.

Intraoperative blood salvage

The intraoperative collection and reinfusion of shed blood, was first used in the nineteenth century [89]. The technique is now used routinely during cardiac, trauma, vascular, orthopedic, and gynecologic surgery. There are currently several devices available from different manufacturers for both intraoperative and postoperative blood salvage [90]. The blood can either be unprocessed (anticoagulated and reinfused) or processed (anticoagulated, washed with saline, and then reinfused).

Semicontinuous flow devices are used most commonly for the intraoperative collection of shed blood. They are also the most complex to use as they involve the processing of the salvaged blood. The disposable equipment consists of a blood aspirator and anticoagulation assembly, a reservoir with filter, a centrifuge bowl, a waste bag, and tubing. The double-liner aspiration set includes an anticoagulation line so that either heparin or citrate can be combined with the aspirated blood at a controlled rate. The anticoagulated blood is collected into a disposable reservoir containing a filter. The filtered blood is then pumped into a bowl, centrifuged and washed with saline, and pumped into a reinfusion bag. There are different sized bowls for pediatric and adult patients so that even small quantities of blood can be processed allowing these devices to be used in infants and children. During washing, the majority of the white blood cells, platelets, clotting factors, free plasma hemoglobin, and anticoagulant should be removed. The entire process takes approximately 3–10 minutes. The red blood cell suspension has a hematocrit of approximately 55–75%.

The second type of device used for intraoperative salvage, otherwise known as the canister collection technique, includes a rigid canister with a sterile, disposable liner. Blood is aspirated from the wound and anticoagulated in a similar manner to that of semicontinuous flow devices. The blood can either be washed (processed) prior to infusion or reinfused without washing (unprocessed). Functioning platelets and coagulation factors are present if the blood is left unwashed; however, there is an increased risk for adverse effects due to cellular debris, free hemoglobin, and fragmented blood components (see below).

The third type of collection is a single-use, self-contained rigid plastic reservoir that provides unprocessed blood for reinfusion. Citrate, the anticoagulant, is placed in the container of a fixed quantity prior to use. Once the container is full, it is reinfused. This apparatus can also be used for postoperative blood collection and reinfusion. The surgical drains are connected to the canister and every 4 hours, the blood is reinfused and a new canister is attached to the surgical drains. Coagulation factors and platelets are present in the blood.

The indications for intraoperative blood salvage include anticipated loss of greater than 20% of the patient's blood volume or a surgical procedure in which more than 10% of the patients require allogeneic transfusions. Conventional salvage devices have bowls with a capacity of 125 mL and wash the blood in increments of approximately 300 mL thus mandating that this amount of blood is lost before any of the shed blood can be returned to the patient, thereby rendering these machines ineffective in smaller patients. However, new technology with smaller bowls allow for use of this technology with blood loss of only 100 mL. Alternatively, newer devices, which allow for the continuous washing and return of shed blood are now available. These devices allow for the immediate processing of shed blood and therefore may be used even with blood loss of less than 100 mL thereby making them effective even in neonates and infants. Despite the small volumes, the washed blood maintains a consistent quality and hematocrit.

Intraoperative blood salvage is most cost-effective when large volumes of blood are harvested, such as in liver transplantation and major vascular surgery [91, 92]. For the semicontinuous devices which allow processing of blood, the cost includes both the disposable and non-disposable items. Disposable items (tubing, bowl, separator, reservoir, suction assembly tubing, and anticoagulant) cost approximately $350-$500 plus the initial cost of the device ($20 000 to $40 000). Despite this, salvaged blood still tends to be less expensive than allogeneic blood.

Reported contraindications to the intraoperative blood salvage are usually related to the contamination of the collected blood with infectious or noninfectious agents (Tables 8.3 and 8.4). The latter is especially true of topical hemostatic agents. Salvage of blood during cancer surgery is controversial. Although there is concern regarding dissemination of tumor cells since washing does not remove the malignant cells. There have been reports regarding the use of intraoperative blood salvage in patients undergoing surgery for urologic malignant disease without adverse effects [93]. No difference in prognosis or outcome has been

Table 8.3 Absolute Contraindications for intraoperative cell salvage.

Bacterial contamination of the surgical site
Presence of amniotic fluid
Presence of local hemostatic agents (see
   Table 8.4)
Oncologic surgery

Table 8.4 Common hemostatic agents and their use with intra-operative cell salvage (ICS).

Agent	Type	Source	Use with ICS	Precautions
AVITENE	Collagen (powder and web)	Med-Chem	No	Flush wound with large amount of saline after product activated before resuming ICS
COLLOSTAT	Collagen powder	Vitaphore	No	Flush wound with large amount of saline after product activated before resuming ICS
COLLOSTAT	Collagen matrix sponge	Vitaphore	Yes	Avoid direct aspiration into ICS suction
GELFOAM	Gelatin powder	Upjohn	No	Flush wound with large amount of saline after product activated before resuming ICS
GELFOAM	Gelatin sponge	Upjohn	No	Flush wound with large amount of saline after product activated before resuming ICS
HELISTAT	Absorbable collagen sponge	Colla-tec, Inc.	Yes	Avoid direct aspiration into ICS suction
HEMOPAD	Non-woven collagen pad	Astra	No	Flush wound with large amount of saline after product activated before resuming ICS
INSTAT	Collagen sponge	J&J	No	Flush wound with large amount of saline after product activated before resuming ICS
SURGICEL	Collagen fabric	J&J	Yes	Avoid direct aspiration into ICS suction
THROMBOGEN	Bovine thrombin spray	J&J	Yes	Avoid direct aspiration into ICS suction
THROMBOSTAT	Bovine thrombin spray	Park Davis	Yes	Avoid direct aspiration into ICS suction

demonstrated in oncologic surgery patients in whom cell salvage was used when compared to those in whom it was not used. Other suggested modalities in oncologic surgery to treat salvaged blood prior to reinfusion include the use of leukocyte depletion filters to remove, or irradiation to inactivate, cancer cells.

Intraoperative blood salvage should not be used if there is a risk of bacterial contamination from bowel contents or an infected wound (Table 8.3). Aspiration of protamine or other hemostatic agents, for example, thrombin, is not recommended because of the risks for initiating systemic coagulation [94]. Wound irrigants, debris, and amniotic fluid should not be salvaged since these agents may also initiate intravascular coagulation [95]. The reinfusion of salvaged blood from an ectopic pregnancy is considered acceptable.

Other complications related to blood salvage include air and fat embolism, hemolysis with hemoglobinuria, pulmonary dysfunction, renal dysfunction, coagulopathy, electrolyte disturbances, and sepsis (Table 8.5) [96–98]. Although air embolism is uncommon except with improper use of the devices, there are reports of fatal air embolism when the blood was reinfused under pressure [99]. Avoidance of pressurized retransfusion and de-airing of the infusion bag should eliminate this complication.

Hemolysis may occur if the suction level is too high or if the aspiration method causes excessive mixing of air with blood. Free hemoglobin may be released during salvage and washing because of erythrocyte damage. Free hemoglobin levels exceeding 100 to 150 mg/dL may lead to hemoglobinuria and acute renal failure, as the binding capacity of haptoglobin is saturated and free hemoglobin is filtered in the renal tubules. Although there are reports of free hemoglobin levels of 350 mg/dL in salvaged blood and mild creatinine elevations, alterations in renal function are rare [100, 101]. If adequate diuresis is maintained, hemoglobin can be excreted without adverse effects on renal function. Simple bedside

Table 8.5 Potential complications of cell salvage.

Infection
Disseminated intravascular coagulopathy (DIC)
Hemolysis
Pulmonary dysfunction
Air or fat embolism

monitoring for free hemoglobin in the urine is relatively quick and easy, as the urine will be positive for blood by dipstick yet no red blood cells will be seen under microscopic examination. Diuresis should be maintained until the urine is free of hemoglobin.

Reinfusion of fragmented cellular components and debris may lead to activation of the eicosanoid or kininogen system with systemic vasodilation and hemodynamic compromise. The fragments may also act as microemboli and contribute to pulmonary dysfunction [102–104]. Given these concerns, the blood should be reinfused through a 40 μm filter to remove this debris. Coagulopathy is one of the most common adverse effects associated with intraoperative blood salvage. The incidence and severity of the coagulopathy increases with the volume of blood that is reinfused. Coagulopathy may be related to one of several factors including qualitative or quantitative platelet defects, dilution of coagulation factors, or the initiation of disseminated intravascular coagulation (DIC). Several coagulation factors including factors I, V, VIII, and X are decreased in salvaged blood. While the dilution of platelets and coagulation factors is the most common cause of coagulopathy, residual anticoagulant may also interfere with the coagulation cascade. Improper washing and centrifuge techniques may lead to the infusion of excessive amounts of heparin or citrate. Monitoring of coagulation function (prothrombin time/partial thromboplastin time, activated clotting time, or thromboelastogram) may be indicated when large volumes of salvaged blood are used or when clinical bleeding is noted.

Aside from coagulation disturbances, excessive quantities of citrate may lead to disturbances of calcium homeostasis. Hypocalcemia is uncommon except with massive blood loss (greater than 3000 to 4000 mL) or liver failure. With hepatic insufficiency, citrate metabolism may be slowed, leading to the excessive binding of calcium. Additional metabolic consequences may also occur with intraoperative blood salvage. Washing with saline and removal of bicarbonate can lead to a dilutional metabolic acidosis as well as the dilution of other electrolytes with hypomagnesaemia and hypocalcemia [105]. Electrolyte and acid-base disturbances may be limited by using a balanced electrolyte solution instead of saline to wash the red blood cells prior to reinfusion. Periodic monitoring of serum electrolytes and acid-base status is necessary when large volumes of blood are salvaged.

Mechanical problems with the cell-saver devices or human error may impart some degree of risk to health care providers. If the tubing from the cell saver to the reservoir bag is inadvertently clamped, high pressure in the tubing will cause it to disconnect and spray blood throughout the operating room. Such problems mandate that personnel involved in the use of cell saver devices be educated and familiar with the equipment prior to operating these devices. Many institutions use the perfusionist staff to operate the devices. Although this ensures a certain level of education and competency with such devices, the cost of such personnel may make the cost of the technology prohibitive.

Pharmacologic agents for blood conservation

Following surgical trauma, the body's inherent defense mechanisms of coagulation play a vital role in forming a platelet-fibrin plug thereby halting further hemorrhage. Although generally effective, pharmacologic agents may be used to pharmacologically boost the body's ability to accomplish this task.

DDAVP

DDAVP or deamino-8-D-arginine vasopressin is a synthetic analogue of vasopressin initially used in the treatment of diabetes insipidus [106]. DDAVP is produced by the deamination of the hemicysteine at position 1 of the natural hormone thereby protecting the molecule from peptidase degradation. A second modification, D-arginine substitution for L-arginine at position 8 decreases the cardiovascular effects of the molecule [107]. These alterations result in a more potent and prolonged antidiuretic activity with effects limited to the V_2 vasopressin receptor and limited activity at the V_1 vasopressin receptor. As a result, there are no effects on the smooth muscle of the uterus or the gastrointestinal tract. The in vivo half-life is 55–60 minutes.

DDAVP promotes hemostasis by augmenting the release of factor VIII and von Willebrand factor (vWF) from endothelial cells [108, 109]. Factor VIII, a glycoprotein, accelerates the activation of factor X by activated factor IX. Hemostatic functions of vWF include increasing platelet adherence to vascular subendothelium, formation of molecular bridges between platelets to increase aggregation, protection of factor VIII in plasma from proteolytic enzymes, and stimulation of factor VIII synthesis. DDAVP is not effective in patients with severe forms of hemophilia or von Willebrand's disease. Such patients have impaired production of either factor VIII or vWF and therefore cannot release these compounds in response to DDAVP. Even in the normal host, tachyphylaxis may occur in response to DDAVP because of depletion of vWF stores.

The recommended dose of DDAVP is 0.15 to 0.3 μg/kg administered intravenous over 15 to 20 minutes the morning of surgery. Levels of factor VIII and vWF increase to 3–5 times those of baseline. Administration over 20 to 30 minutes avoids systemic hypotension since the agent can cause systemic vasodilation. The agent may also be given subcutaneously or intranasally with plasma levels achieved within 1 hour [110, 111]. Both routes produce plasma concentrations of factor VIII and vWF that are equivalent to those seen with intravenous administration.

Untoward effects of DDAVP include decreased free water clearance from antidiuretic hormone activity, hypotension, and at least the theoretical potential for an increased incidence of perioperative thrombotic events. The latter remains at least a theoretical concern of any agent that augments the natural coagulation system. Hyponatremia is uncommon following a single dose and is generally seen only when excessive free water is administered perioperatively. Hypotension results from endothelial-cell release of prostacyclin when DDAVP is administered rapidly. This can be avoided by slow administration (15 min or longer). Although there are anecdotal reports of thrombotic complications, prospective studies in adults undergoing coronary artery bypass grafting have indicated no difference in the perioperative myocardial infarction rates between patients who received DDAVP and control groups [112, 113].

Desmopressin has been used as adjuvant therapy in the treatment of von Willenbrand's disease and hemophilia A, as well as for the correction of platelet dysfunction associated with uremia, cirrhosis, and aspirin therapy [114, 115]. Although it has also been suggested as a potential agent to decrease blood loss in major surgical procedures in patients with normal platelet function; as the studies listed below will demonstrate, the results regarding its efficacy have been conflicting. The preoperative administration of DDAVP to adults with normal preoperative hemostatic function who were undergoing spinal fusion reduced blood loss by 32.5% and reduced the need for erythrocyte transfusion by 25.6% [116]. When administered following the reversal of heparin with protamine after CPB, blood loss was approximately half that of the placebo group [112]. However, more recent prospective, randomized trials in spinal surgery have demonstrated no benefit of the preoperative administration of DDAVP [117, 118], while Seear et al. demonstrated no difference in blood loss in children undergoing cardiac surgery with the use of DDAVP [119]. Furthermore, a meta-analysis of studies in cardiac surgery demonstrated no effect of DDAVP during routine cardiac surgery; however, there was a significant reduction in blood loss during high-risk surgery including repeat surgery or patients with a history of recent aspirin intake [120, 121].

Antifibrinolytic agents

With the activation of the coagulation cascade, protective mechanisms are also activated to control the thrombotic process and the production of fibrin. One of these processes is the fibrinolytic cascade which results from the conversion of plasminogen to plasmin. Pharmacologic blockade of the fibrinolytic pathway is feasible and is a frequent adjunct to control bleeding in various types of surgical procedures. Although generally considered together, the agents formerly used for this process, aprotinin and the two lysine analogues [epsilon-aminocaproic acid (EACA), and tranexamic acid (TA)] have different mechanisms of action. In the arena of cardiac surgery, aprotinin was generally considered the favorite agent. Numerous randomized trials and observational studies demonstrated its efficacy in reducing blood loss in cardiac and orthopedic surgery [122–126].

Despite its efficacy, there were lingering concerns regarding its potential effects on renal function. Renal toxicity is postulated to result from aprotinin's strong affinity for renal tissue and subsequent accumulation in proximal tubular epithelial cells and/or of its inhibition of serine proteases (kallikrein-kininogen system). Histopathologic examination of renal tissue following high-dose aprotinin administration reveals obstructed proximal convoluted tubules and swollen tubular epithelial cells. These issues were finally demonstrated in a relatively conclusive manner in the Blood Conservation Using Antifibrinolytics in a Randomized Trial (BART) study [127]. The BART study was the only large, randomized trial comparing aprotinin, TXA, and EACA. It was terminated early because of a consistent trend demonstrating higher mortality in the patients receiving aprotinin. Although controversy still exists with other trials demonstrating conflicting reports, aprotinin has been removed from the market and is no longer available for clinical use.

TXA and EACA are gamma aminocarboxylic acid analogues of lysine. During normal coagulation function, plasminogen is converted to plasmin that inhibits fibrin formation. EACA and TA bind to the lysine moiety that binds plasminogen to fibrinogen, thus displacing it from the fibrinogen surface and inhibiting fibrinolysis. EACA and TA also prevent plasmin degradation of platelet glycoprotein 1b receptors, thus preserving platelet function. These agents have found greatest applications in surgeries associated with activation of the fibrinolytic systems including cardiac, hepatic, and prostate surgery. A recent meta-analysis of the available trials of the anti-fibrinolytic agents including EACA, TA, and aprotinin demonstrated a decrease in the exposure to allogeneic blood products in patients receiving these agents as well as a decrease in the incidence of postoperative bleeding and the need for surgical re-exploration following cardiac surgery in adult patients [121].

One of the major problems with evaluating the efficacy of the lysine analogues is the wide variability in dosing regimens among the studies. Although oral preparations of EACA and TXA are available, for perioperative use these agents are administered intravenously. TXA is generally considered to be 10 times as potent as EACA and yet some studies have used equivalent dosing schemes. Ninety percent of EACA is excreted in the urine within 4–6 hours of administration while 90% of TXA is present in the urine after approximately 24 hours. In general, EACA is administered as an intravenous loading dose of 100–150 mg/kg followed by an infusion of 10–15 mg/kg/hr. However, the variability in tranexamic acid dosing in the literature is much more significant with loading doses varying from 10 to 100 mg/kg and infusions varying from 1 to 10 mg/kg/hr.

With the use of the lysine analogues, several studies involving various types of surgical procedures have shown significant reductions in blood loss. Beneficial effects on blood loss and the need for allogeneic transfusions have been demonstrated in the orthopedic surgical population. Florentino-Pineda et al. evaluated the efficacy of EACA (100 mg/kg followed by 10 mg/kg/hr) in 28 adolescents undergoing postoperative spinal fusion [128]. The anesthetic technique including the use of controlled hypotension was consistent between the two groups. Patients receiving EACA had decreased intraoperative blood loss (988 ± 411 mL versus 1405 ± 670 mL, p = 0.024) and decreased transfusion requirements (1.2 ± 1.1 units versus 2.2 ± 1.3 units, p = 0.003). Similar findings were reported by Neilipovitz et al. in their study of 40 adolescents undergoing posterior spinal fusion [129]. Patients who received TXA (10 mg/kg followed by 1 mg/kg/hr) had decreased total blood transfused (cell saver plus allogeneic packed red blood cells) of 1253 ± 884 mL versus 1784 ± 733 mL (p = 0.045). However, the amount of allogeneic blood transfused between the two groups did not reach statistical significance (874 ± 790 mL versus 1254 ± 542 mL, p = 0.08). Three randomized controlled trials in adults undergoing orthopedic surgical procedures demonstrated a significant decrease in transfusion requirements in patients receiving TXA [130–132]. Similar effects have been demonstrated in hepatic transplantation [133], prostatectomy [134], and cardiac surgery [135, 136]. Although several studies demonstrate decreased blood loss and transfusion requirements with the antifibrinolytic agents, these results are not universal. Other investigators have demonstrated no benefit of using TXA or EACA in cardiac surgery and orthopedic surgery in oncology patients [137, 138].

More recently, in the pediatric population, some additional insight has been provided into appropriate dosing regimens. As noted previously, although generally considered to be 7–10 times as potent as EACA, TXA dosing regimens have at times been equivalent on a mg per mg basis. In 43 children ranging in age from 2 months to 6 years, TXA was compared to placebo during craniosynostosis surgery [139]. TXA, administered as a loading dose of 50 mg/kg followed by an infusion of 5 mg/kg/hr resulted in significantly lower perioperative blood loss (65 versus 119 ml/kg, p < 0.001) and lower mean blood transfusion requirements (33 versus 56 mL/kg, p = 0.006). TXA also reduced the exposure to units of blood products (median of 1 versus 3, p < 0.001). The authors additionally measured TXA plasma concentrations during the infusion and found that the plasma concentrations were greater the reported threshold for inhibition of fibrinolysis (10 μg/mL) and for plasmin-induced platelet activation (16 μg/mL). A subsequent study, also performed in pediatric patients undergoing craniosynostosis surgery, demonstrated similar efficacy in reducing allogeneic blood product use when using TXA administered as a loading dose of 15 mg/kg followed by an infusion of 10 mg/kg/hr [140].

Adverse effects of EACA and TXA may be related either to their effects on coagulation or the route of excretion. Since these agents are cleared by the kidneys, thrombosis of the kidneys, ureters, or lower urinary tract may occur if urologic bleeding is present. Both EACA and TA may be associated with nausea, vomiting, diarrhea and hypotension with rapid intravenous administration. Of primary concern with any agent that inhibits the fibrinolytic system is the potential to increase the incidence of postoperative thrombotic events such as deep venous thrombosis, stroke, or myocardial infarction (MI). Ovrum et al. reported 5 cases of postoperative MI in patients receiving TA during cardiac bypass [137]. However, the majority of the other prospective, randomized trials have demonstrated no increased incidence of such problems when comparing the EACA or TXA group to placebo patients. Also of note, is the recognition of the potential for seizures with the administration of TXA especially in adults having cardiac surgery that involves an open chamber (valve replacement) [141]. In a cohort of 8929 adult patients having cardiac surgery, seizures were more common in patients receiving TXA doses in excess of 100 mg/kg [142].

Recombinant factor VIIa

Factor VII plays a key role in both the extrinsic and the intrinsic coagulation cascade. Factor VII is activated after contact with tissue factor that is exposed at the site of tissue injury. Activated factor VII can then directly activate factor IX of the intrinsic cascade. Activated factor IX with activated factor XIII can then activate factor X. Alternatively through the extrinsic cascade, activated factor VII can directly activate factor X. Activated factor

X can then enter the common cascade leading to the conversion of pro-thrombin to thrombin and subsequent fibrin formation.

Recombinant DNA technology provides the means for the production of pharmacologic quantities of various coagulation factors including factor VII. In 1988, a patient with hemophilia and inhibitors against factor VIII who was undergoing knee surgery was the first patient to be treated with recombinant factor VIIa (rFVIIa). To date, the majority of experience in both the adult and pediatric population with the use of rFVIIa has been in the treatment of patients with hemophilia who have developed auto-antibodies against factor VIII (inhibitors) thereby making subsequent infusions of factor VIII ineffective. In this scenario, rFVIIa has been shown to effectively control bleeding.

Following its efficacy in the hemophilia population, there has been an increasing body of clinical experience with rFVIIa in the non-hemophiliac population with coagulation disturbances of various etiologies. In many of these cases, although anecdotal, rFVIIa has been used to control life-threatening hemorrhage when other modalities including the administration of platelets, cryoprecipiate, and FFP failed [143–146]. Scenarios have included the perioperative period including patients undergoing cardiovascular, thoracic, hepatic, intra-abdominal, and orthopedic procedures [147–150]. Friederich et al. evaluated the effects of rFVII given prior to the start of retropubic prostatectomy in patients with normal preoperative coagulation function [151]. Patients were randomized to receive placebo, rFVIIa (20 µg/kg) or rFVIIa (40 µg/kg) prior to surgical incision. Median perioperative blood loss was 2688 mL, 1235 mL, and 1089 ml respectively (p = 0.001) in the three groups. Seven of twelve placebo patients required allogeneic RBC transfusions compared to no patients who received 40 µg/kg of rFVIIa. The authors also noted a decreased surgical time (180 minutes in control patients versus 126 minutes and 120 minutes in the two rFVIIa groups, p = 0.014).

The greatest off-label use of rFVIIa has been in the arena of cardiac surgery where it appears that its use has increased exponentially to treat refractory hemorrhage after CPB and cardiac surgeries. Although much of the evidence is gathered from nonrandomized studies, case reports, and case series, the evidence from these reports suggests that rFVIIa administered may control hemorrhage after cardiac surgery. However, it is evident that the data from randomized trials are conflicting. In adults, a prospective randomized trial that compared rFVIIa with placebo after CPB and reversal of heparin in complex noncoronary cardiac surgery reported a significant decrease in allogeneic blood product use with no difference in adverse outcomes [152]. In contrast, a randomized study in the pediatric population showed no decrease in bleeding or transfusion requirements in patients who received rFVIIa [153].

To date, there are limited data on which to base a recommendation for the widespread, prophylactic use of rFVIIa in patients with normal coagulation function. Additional prospective, randomized trials are needed to evaluate the efficacy of this agent in diminishing perioperative blood loss. However, rFVIIa may be effective when there is ongoing life-threatening bleeding and the coagulopathy has not responded to standard therapy (FFP, platelets, cryoprecipiate); time is not available to wait for blood typing, thawing, and administration of FFP; there are concerns regarding the potential hemodynamic effects of FFP; or religious issues preclude the use of blood products. Recombinant FVIIa can be quickly reconstituted from powder with a small volume of sterile water and administered intravenously over 2–3 minutes.

The initial clinical experience suggested that adverse effects with rFVIIa were limited with only a low incidence of thrombotic complications [154, 155]. In the majority of these cases, the patients had several other risk factors for perioperative thromboembolic complications. As rFVIIa requires tissue factor for activation and tissue factor is released only with vascular damage, the risk of excessive thrombogenesis should be limited [156]. However, recent data have suggested at least a trend toward a higher rate of thrombotic complications when rFVIIa is used in adults having cardiac surgery. A meta-analysis of five clinical trials with a total of 298 patients revealed a statistically nonsignificant decrease in the need for surgical reexploration for bleeding and equivalent mortality [157]. However, there was a trend toward increased stroke. Additionally concern was raised by a recent clinical trial evaluating the dose-escalating safety and efficacy of rFVIIa in postoperative cardiac surgical patients with refractory bleeding [158]. The patients were randomized to receive placebo, rFVIIa 40 μg/kg, or rFVIIa 80 μg/kg. With either dose of rFVIIa, although there was significantly less bleeding rates (p = 0.03) and decreased need for allogeneic transfusion (p = 0.01), there was also a non-significant increase in serious adverse thrombotic events. Additionally, since rFVIIa does not correct other factor deficiencies, the coagulopathy may recur once the rFVIIa is cleared. Therefore, other therapies may be needed to correct other coagulation function. These additional therapies may include repeat dosing of rFVIIa, administration of FFP or vitamin K.

Miscellaneous agents

Various other procoagulant agents have been used in a limited number of investigation trials in various clinical scenarios, generally the adult cardiac surgical population. Many of these agents are still in preliminary trials and their efficacy and potential adverse effect profile have yet to be determined. Factor XIII is necessary for crosslinking of fibrin monomers to form a stable fibrin clot.

Low endogenous levels of factor XIIIa have been associated with increased blood loss after neurosurgical procedures and coronary artery bypass grafting in adults. There is currently a recombinant form of factor XIII available for clinical use. Dose ranging from 25 to 50 IU/kg restore factor XIII to preoperative levels with no significant increase in thrombotic events [159]. The current literature suggests that factor XIII is only useful in patients with documented low levels prior to its administration [160]. Prophylactic administration to patients with normal levels does not appear to decrease blood loss or transfusion requirements.

Prothrombin complex concentrates (PCCs) contain vitamin K-dependent coagulation factors (II, VII, IX, and X). PCCs are generally considered the agent of choice for the rapid reversal of oral anticoagulants such as coumadin in the setting of life-threatening bleeding or the need for emergent surgery. These agents have also been used in various life-threatening bleeding scenarios in patients with hepatic failure and coagulation disturbances of various etiologies [161]. In such cases, reports of success are merely anecdotal with limited evidence-based medicine on which to suggest their use. The recommended dose of PCC to reverse anticoagulation in an adult varies from 1000 to 1500 IU. When used in combination with rFVIIa, mortality from thrombotic events has been reported and therefore the simultaneous administration of these two agents is not recommended.

Another coagulation factor that is consumed by CPB is fibrinogen. CPB leads to degranulation of platelets and consumption of clotting factors including fibrinogen. Although generally treated with the administration of cryoprecipitate as a rich source of fibrinogen, a fibrinogen concentration is now available in certain countries. Its primary use has been in the adult cardiac surgical population as the data clearly demonstrate that cardiac surgery is the most common indication for cryoprecipitate transfusion with up to 10% of patients receiving fibrinogen replacement through the administration of cryoprecipitate [162]. Although the small preliminary clinical studies have suggested that prophylactic administration of fibrinogen concentrates in a dose of approximately 2 grams may decrease bleeding after coronary artery bypass grafting surgery, larger trials are necessary to establish the safety and efficacy of such therapy.

Human recombinant erythropoietin

Although not used as a procoagulant agent, human recombinant erythropoietin (HRE) is a pharmacologic agent that continues to play a significant role in bloodless surgery. HRE was originally used in the management of chronic anemia related to renal failure or to treat marrow failure related to cancer chemotherapy. HRE is a glycoprotein, produced by the kidney in response to tissue hypoxia. It stimulates erythropoiesis by the bone marrow leading to dose-dependent increases in reticulocyte count, hemoglobin, and hematocrit. Recombinant technology allows the production of the hormone in a form that is indistinguishable from the endogenous hormone. Following intravenous administration, it undergoes biphasic clearance and has a distribution half-life of 4.4 hours. Intravenous administration results in higher plasma levels than intramuscular or subcutaneous administration. HRE is used in various scenarios throughout the perioperative process including its simple administration to treat a preoperative low hemoglobin value, its use to augment the efficacy of autologous donation, to increase the hemoglobin and therefore the yield of ANH, and during the postoperative period to stimulate erythropoiesis and speed recovery from anemia [164].

One of the problems when evaluating the studies concerning HRE is that there are considerable inconsistencies in regard to the dose, frequency, duration of therapy, timing, and even route of administration (intravenous versus subcutaneous). In the perioperative period, twice weekly subcutaneous dosing of erythropoietin is a common means of administration. Serum iron levels must be sufficient for erythropoiesis to be augmented and therefore, oral iron supplementation is frequently used with erythropoietin therapy. In rare instances, intravenous iron therapy may be necessary. Despite such issues, the potential benefits of such therapy are illustrated by a recent study which demonstrated that even a single preoperative dose of 500 IU/kg resulted in a decreased percentage (56% versus 86%) of patients requiring allogeneic blood product use in adult cardiac surgery patients with preoperative anemia [165].

Adverse effects are more common in patients with chronic renal insufficiency and include hypertension, hypertensive encephalopathy, seizures, myocardial infarction, cerebrovascular accident, hyperkalemia, thrombosis, and malaise. It remains unclear as to whether these adverse effects are due to the primary disease, erythropoietin therapy, or to a combination of the two. However, in light of this, it should be remembered that erythropoeitin-stimulating agents are approved by the Food and Drug Administration (FDA) to treat chronic anemia related to renal disease or cancer. A second indication is to reduce allogeneic blood transfusions in patients scheduled to undergo elective noncardiac, nonvascular surgeries. The FDA also clearly states that "Epogen is not indicated for use in patients undergoing cardiac and vascular surgery." Additionally, although approved as noted above, the FDA has also issued a warning in the prescribing information stating that erythropoietin-stimulating agents increase the risk of death, myocardial infarction, stroke, venous thromboembolism, thrombosis of vascular access, and tumor progression and recurrence [166]. These adverse events have occurred predominantly in the nonsurgical population following repeated doses of HRE over a longer timeframe than would generally be used for a surgical procedure. And yet, a higher incidence of postoperative deep vein thrombosis (4.7% with HRE vs. 2.1% with placebo) has been reported in at least one randomized trial of spine surgery patients who received preoperative HRE (600 IU/kg subcutaneous weekly for 3 weeks before surgery without prophylactic anticoagulation) [167].

Controlled hypotension

Controlled hypotension (also referred to as deliberate or induced hypotension) is the intentional or planned reduction of the systolic blood pressure to 80–90 mmHg, the mean arterial pressure (MAP) to 50–65 mmHg or a 30% reduction of the MAP from its baseline value. The latter definition being relevant for the pediatric-aged patient whose baseline MAP may be within the 50–65 mmHg range at baseline. Although the primary application of controlled hypotension is to limit intraoperative blood loss, an additional benefit may be improved visualization of the surgical field.

Controlled hypotension (CH) was first described by Cushing in 1917. In 1947, Gardner described the use of arteriotomy and removal of 1600 mL of blood to reduce systolic blood pressure and limit intraoperative blood loss. Gilles in 1948 described the first use of regional anesthesia (subarachnoid blockade) as an alternative to phlebotomy-induced hypotension. With the introduction of short-acting ganglionic blocking agents in the 1950s and continuous vasodilator infusions in the 1960s, the popularity and feasibility of CH increased. In 1966, Eckenhoff and Rich performed the first controlled study of CH and demonstrated a 50% reduction in blood loss by lowering the MAP to 55–65 mmHg [168] Other studies have provided additional evidence of the efficacy of CH, especially during major orthopedic procedures including total hip arthroplasty and spine surgery, with reported reductions of intraoperative blood loss of up to 50% [169].

With any decrease in MAP, there is a concern of the potential for a decrease in end-organ perfusion and tissue hypoxia. The theory behind CH lies in the autoregulatory function of the arteriolar bed in end-organ tissues so that with a decrease in MAP, perfusion and blood flow are maintained. Although a full review of the literature and discussion of this matter is beyond the scope of this chapter, this issue has been addressed by several studies, which have demonstrated the maintenance of end-organ perfusion and tissue oxygenation during CH with several different pharmacologic agents [170–172]. The interest and enthusiasm for controlled hypotension for spinal surgery has also waned recently given concerns regarding its role in visual disturbances following spinal surgery [173, 174]. Although the exact etiology of such problems has not been elucidated, its recent increased occurrence or at least recognition has led to a decrease in the use of CH in some clinical arenas.

An additional question that has been raised regarding CH is whether it is the reduction in MAP or cardiac output that determines intraoperative blood loss. Sivarajan et al. randomized patients to sodium nitroprusside or trimethaphan for CH [175]. Although cardiac output increased in patients receiving nitroprusside when compared to trimethaphan, no difference in blood loss was noted between the two groups thereby demonstrating that it is the control of MAP not cardiac output that determines blood loss.

Advances in drug therapy have provided the clinician with several pharmacologic options for CH. While it is now generally accepted that it is the reduction in MAP and not cardiac output that is the primary determinant of intraoperative blood loss, there remains some controversy as to which of the many available agents is optimal for CH. In fact, it is likely that any of a number of agents can be used. The available agents can be divided into those used by themselves (primary agents) and those used to limit the dose requirements and therefore the adverse effects of other agents (adjuncts or secondary agents). Primary agents include regional anesthetic techniques (spinal and epidural anesthesia), the inhalational anesthetic agents (halothane, isoflurane, sevoflurane), the nitrovasodilators (sodium nitroprusside and nitroglycerin), trimethaphan, prostaglandin E1 (PGE1), and adenosine. The calcium channel blockers and beta adrenergic antagonists have been used as both primary agents as well as adjuncts to other agents. The pharmacologic agents used primarily as adjuncts or secondary agents include the angiotensin converting enzyme inhibitors (e.g., captopril, enalaprilat) and alpha$_2$ adrenergic agonists such as clonidine. These agents and their uses have been reviewed elsewhere, as such, only a few of the more commonly used agents will be discussed [176].

Sodium nitroprusside (SNP)

Given its availability for decades and its titration by continuous infusion, SNP has been one of the agents used most commonly for CH. SNP is a direct-acting, non-selective peripheral vasodilator that primarily dilates resistance vessels leading to venous pooling and decreased systemic vascular resistance. It has a rapid onset of action (approximately 30 seconds), a peak hypotensive effect within two minutes with a return of blood pressure to baseline values within three minutes of its discontinuation. SNP releases nitric oxide (formerly endothelial-derived relaxant factor), which activates guanylate cyclase leading to an increase in the intracellular concentration of cyclic guanosine monophosphate (cGMP). Cyclic GMP decreases the availability of intracellular calcium through one of two mechanisms: decreased release from the sarcoplasmic reticulum into smooth muscle or increased uptake by the sarcoplasmic reticulum. The net result is decreased free cytosolic calcium and vascular smooth muscle relaxation. Adverse effects include rebound hypertension, coronary steal, increased intracranial pressure, increased intrapulmonary shunt with ablation of hypoxic pulmonary vasoconstriction, platelet dysfunction and cyanide toxicity. Direct peripheral vasodilation results in baroreceptor-mediated sympathetic responses with tachycardia and increased myocardial contractility. The renin-angiotensin system and sympathetic nervous system are also activated. The result is tachycardia and increased cardiac output, which may offset the initial drop in MAP and require the addition of beta adrenergic antagonist to control the tachycardia. Plasma catecholamine and renin activity may remain elevated after discontinuation of SNP resulting in rebound hypertension.

An additional potential issue with SNP is the possibility of inducing coronary ischemia through a coronary steal phenomena. The dilatation of normal coronary arteries in non-ischemic areas of the myocardium may lead to an intracoronary steal with decreased oxygen delivery to areas supplied by diseased vasculature that is unable to vasodilate in response to SNP. Since myocardial oxygen extraction is already maximal, increased coronary blood flow from the accumulation of metabolic vasodilator substances is the primary mechanism responsible for meeting increased oxygen demands. As blood pressure decreases, coronary blood flow is maintained by vasodilatation of coronary vessels. In patients with coronary artery disease and stenosis, vasodilatation may be incomplete. Therefore, ischemia may occur with a decrease in MAP to 50 to 60 mm Hg. The potential for ischemia may be further increased by tachycardia and a decreased diastolic blood pressure induced by SNP.

SNP is a direct cerebral vasodilator, which may lead to increased cerebral blood flow and cerebral blood volume. Although the clinical consequences of this are minimal in patients with normal intracranial compliance, increased intracranial pressure may occur in patients with reduced intracranial compliance. A similar effect may be seen with any of the direct acting vasodilating agents. SNP may also have deleterious effects on the pulmonary vasculature and respiratory function. Hypoxic pulmonary vasoconstriction (HPV) acts as a protective mechanism to shunt blood away from unventilated alveoli thereby maintaining the matching of ventilation with perfusion. SNP may interfere with HPV leading to increased pulmonary shunting. These effects may be further magnified by preoperative pulmonary parenchymal disease, intraoperative positioning, and positive pressure ventilation. Despite these effects, the clinical consequences are generally minimal in patients with normal preoperative respiratory function.

Platelet function may be altered during SNP administration due to inhibition of thrombasthenin, a smooth muscle-like protein leading to a defect in platelet aggregation. Hines and Barash infused SNP in 19 cardiac surgery patients to maintain a MAP of 80 mm Hg prior to cardiopulmonary bypass [177]. Infusion rates greater than 3 µg/kg/min (or a total dose of 16 mg in adults) decreased platelet aggregation with a prolongation of the bleeding time. ADP-aggregation studies demonstrated a 33% reduction in aggregation. Despite the alteration in laboratory evaluation of platelet function, clinical bleeding did not occur. Therefore, the clinical consequences of this phenomenon are thought to be minimal in patients with normal platelet function. Additional concerns with SNP administration are the possibility of cyanide and thiocyanate accumulation. Cyanide is a breakdown product of SNP as each molecule of SNP contains five molecules of cyanide. During metabolism by the rhodinase enzyme system of the liver, free cyanide is released. The plasma concentrations of both cyanide and thiocyanate are proportional to the total dose of SNP. Following metabolism of SNP, cyanide may either be converted to thiocyanate by the rhodinase system, combine with methemoglobin to produce cyanomethemoglobin, or bind with cytochrome oxidase. The latter may result in deleterious physiologic effects through the impairment of the electron transport system and oxidative phosphorylation. Cyanide has a high affinity for cytochrome oxidase and if conversion to thiocyanate is slow or inadequate, cellular hypoxia and metabolic acidosis may result. Clinical signs of cyanide toxicity include an elevated mixed venous oxygen tension or a significant increase in infusion requirements over time (tachyphylaxis). The risks of toxicity can be decreased by limiting the total dose of SNP as well as the duration of the infusion. Increased cyanide levels are more common with the acute administration of more than 5 to 8 µg/kg/min or prolonged (more than 24 hours) infusion rates greater than 2 µg/kg/min. As cyanide metabolism occurs primarily in the liver, patients with altered hepatic function may be at increased risk for toxicity. Toxicity is also more common in patients with dietary deficiency of vitamin B_{12} or sulfur. The latter compound is required for the hepatic conversion of cyanide to thiosulfate. Metabolism by the rhodinase system produces thiocyanate that is then excreted by the kidneys. Thiocyanate toxicity may occur in the presence of prolonged therapy or renal failure. Symptoms of toxicity include skeletal muscle weakness, mental confusion, seizures and nausea. Symptoms generally occur with plasma concentrations greater than 10 mg/dl. Thiocyanate may also alter thyroid function leading to hypothyroidism due to the inhibition of iodine uptake into the thyroid gland.

Calcium channel antagonists

Nicardipine is a calcium channel antagonist of the dihydropyridine class that vasodilates the systemic, cerebral, and coronary vasculature with limited effects on myocardial contractility and stroke volume. Unlike SNP, nicardipine does have some intrinsic negative chronotropic effects that may limit the rebound tachycardia. Like other direct acting vasodilators, nicardipine and the other calcium channel antagonists may increase intracranial pressure. Bernard et al. compared the efficacy of SNP versus nicardipine in 20 patients during isoflurane anesthesia for spinal surgery [178]. An initial dose of nicardipine of 6.2 ± 0.9 mg was required to achieve a MAP of 55–60 mm Hg. Infusion requirements varied from 3 to 5 mg/hour to maintain a similar MAP. The decrease in MAP was associated with a decrease in pulmonary and systemic vascular resistance, increased cardiac output, and decreased arteriovenous oxygen content. Unlike SNP, no change in arterial oxygenation was seen with nicardipine suggesting that it may have minimal effects on hypoxic pulmonary vasoconstriction. The efficacy of nicardipine compared favorably with that of SNP. One problem that was noted with nicardipine was prolonged hypotension following discontinuation of the infusion. Hypotension persisted for a mean of 43 minutes with a range of 27–88 minutes following discontinuation of the infusion. No untoward consequences of the prolonged effect were noted. A follow-up study of Bernard et al. compared SNP to nicardipine for controlled hypotension during hip arthroplasty in 24 patients [179]. Similar cardiovascular changes were noted with nicardipine dose requirements of 1–3 μg/kg/min following the initial titration dose of 4.7 ± 1.5 mg. Once again, hypotension persisted for 10–20 minutes following discontinuation of the infusion as opposed to the rebound hypertension that was seen following discontinuation of the SNP infusion.

In the pediatric adolescent population, patients undergoing spinal fusion for scoliosis were randomized to SNP or nicardipine for controlled hypotension during posterior spinal fusion in 20 pediatric patients [180].

Patients who received nicardipine had decreased blood loss when compared with SNP (761 ± 199 mL versus 1297.5 ± 264 mL, p < 0.05). Time to restoration of blood pressure back to baseline upon discontinuation of the infusion was significantly longer with nicardipine than with SNP (26.8 ± 4.0 minutes versus 7.3 ± 1.1 minutes, p < 0.001).

Summary

Increasing evidence has demonstrated the potential adverse effects associated with the use of allogeneic blood products. These effects may have significant deleterious effects on patients that may impact on cost and length of hospitalization and in specific circumstances even mortality. Many of the major surgical procedures can result in significant blood loss and the need for allogeneic blood transfusions. Intraoperative options to limit the need for allogeneic blood product administration include:

1 general considerations including optimization of preoperative coagulation function, correction of preoperative anemia, use of a lower transfusion trigger in patients without co-morbid conditions, proper patient positioning, and maintenance of normothermia;

2 autologous transfusion therapy including preoperative donation with the use of erythropoietin, intraoperative collection using acute ANH and perioperative blood salvage;

3 pharmacologic manipulation of the coagulation cascade with epsilon amino caproic acid, TXA, and potentially rFVIIa, and

4 controlled hypotension.

Although many of these techniques are effective alone, the combination of several of these techniques can potentially lead us to the goal of performing major surgical procedures without the use of allogeneic blood products. Many of the techniques, such as autologous donation, ANH, and controlled hypotension, have been proven in several studies to be effective. Studies regarding the efficacy of the various pharmacologic agents may not be as compelling or there are conflicting reports regarding their efficacy. Since the technology of artificial blood products (see Chapter 12 for a full discussion of these agents), which may limit the need for allogeneic transfusion, may take years yet to perfect, use of the techniques described in this chapter should be considered as part of a multi-disciplinary comprehensive approach to provide bloodless surgery.

References

1 Gilliss BM, Looney MR, Gropper MA. Reducing noninfectious risks of blood transfusion. Anesthesiology. 2011;115:635–49.

2 Guay J, Haig M, Lortie L, et al. Predicting blood loss in surgery for idiopathic scoliosis. Can J Anaesth. 1994;41:775–81.

3 Goodnough LT, Bercher ME, Kanter MH, et al. Transfusion medicine: First of two parts - blood transfusion. New Engl J Med. 1999;340:438–47.

4 Parshuram C, Doyle J, Lau W, et al. Transfusion-associated graft versus host disease. Pediatr Crit Care Med. 2002;3:57–62.

5 Schriemer PA, Longnecker DE, Mintz PD. The possible immunosuppressive effects of perioperative blood transfusion in cancer patients. Anesthesiology. 1988;68:422–8.

6 Taylor RT, Manganaro L, O'Brien J, et al. Impact of allogeneic packed red blood cell transfusion on nosocomial infection rates in the critically ill patient. Crit Care Med. 2002;30:2249–54.

7 Carson JL, Altman DG, Duff A, et al. Risk of bacterial infection with allogeneic blood transfusion among patients undergoing hip fracture repair. Transfusion. 199;39:694–700.

8 Stubbs JR. Transfusion-related acute lung injury, an evolving syndrome: the road of discovery, with emphasis on the role of the Mayo Clinic. Transfus Med Rev. 2011;25:66–75.

9 Cote CJ, Drop LJ, Hoaglin DC, et al. Ionized hypocalcemia after fresh frozen plasma administration to thermally injured children. Anesth Analg. 1988;67:152–60.

10 Ang-Lee MK, Moss J, Yuan CS. Herbal medicines and perioperative care. JAMA. 2001;286:208–16.

11 Lenoir B, Merckx P, Paugam-Burtz C, Dauzac C, Agostini MM, Guigui P, Mantz J. Individual probability of allogeneic erythrocyte transfusion in elective spine surgery: the predictive model of transfusion in spine surgery. Anesthesiology. 2009;110:1050–60.

12 Kulier A, Levin J, Moser R, et al. Impact of preoperative anemia on outcome in patients undergoing coronary artery bypass graft surgery. Circulation. 2007;116:471–9.

13 Beattie WS, Karkouti K, Wijeysundera DN, Tait G. Risk associated with preoperative anemia in noncardiac surgery: a single-center cohort study. Anesthesiology. 2009;110:574–81.

14 Hare GM, Baker JE, Pavenski K. Assessment and treatment of preoperative anemia: Continuing Professional Development. Can J Anaesth. 2011;58:569-81.

15 Munoz M, Garcia-Erce JA, Cuenca J, et al. On the role of iron therapy for reducing allogeneic blood transfusion in orthopaedic surgery. Blood Transus. 2012;10:8–22.

16 Goodnough LT, Maniatis A, Earnshaw P, et al. Detection, evaluation, and management of preoperative anaemia in the elective orthopaedic surgical patient: NATA guidelines. Br J Anaesth. 2011;106:13–22.

17 Gall O, Aubineau JV, Berniere J, et al. Analgesic effect of low-dose intrathecal morphine after spinal fusion in children. Anesthesiology. 2001;94:447–52.

18 Kurz A, Sessler DI, Lenhardt R. Study of Wound Infection and Temperature Control Group. Perioperative normothermia to reduce the incidence of surgical-wound associated infection and shorten hospitalization. N Engl J Med. 1996;334:1209–15.

19 Schmied H, Kurz A, Sessler D, et al. Mild hypothermia increases blood loss and transfusion requirements during total hip arthroplasty. Lancet. 1996;347:289–92.

20 Cosgriff N, Moore EE, Sauaia A, et al. Predicting life-threatening coagulopathy in the massively transfused trauma patient: hypothermia and acidosis revisited. J Trauma. 1997;42:857–61.

21 Winkler M, Akca O, Birkenberg B, et al. Aggressive warming reduces blood loss during hip arthroplasty. Anesth Analg. 2000;91:978–84.

22 Widman J, Hammarqvist F, Sellden E. Amino acid infusion induces thermogenesis and reduces blood loss during hip arthroplasty under spinal anesthesia. Anesth Analg. 2002;95:1757–62.

23 Cobbe KA, Di Staso R, Duff J, Walker K, Draper N. Preventing inadvertent hypothermia: comparing two protocols for preoperative forced-air warming. J Perianesth Nurs. 2012;27:18–24.

24 Ruttmann TG, James MF, Viljoen JF. Haemodilution induces a hypercoagulable state. Br J Anaesth. 1996;76:412–14.

25 Karoutsos S, Nathan N, Lahrimi A, et al. Thromboelastogram reveals hypercoagulability after administration of gelatin solution. Br J Anaesth. 1999;82:175–7.

26 de Jonge E, Levi M, Berends F, et al. Impaired haemostais by intravenous administration of a gelatin-based plasma expander in human subjects. Thromb Haemost. 1998;79:286–90.

27 Mardel SN, Saunders FM, Allen H, et al. Reduced quality of clot formation with gelatin-based plasma substitutes. Br J Anaesth. 1998;80:204–7.

28 Westphal M, James MF, Kozek-Langenecker S, Stocker R, Guidet Bertrand, Van Aken H. Hydroxyethyl starches: Different products – different effects. Anesthesiology. 2009;111:187–202.

29 Ruttmann TG, James MFM, Aronson I. In vivo investigation into the effects of haemodilution with hydroxyethyl starch (200/0.5) and normal saline on coagulation. Br J Anaesth. 1998;80:612–6.

30 Raja SG, Akhtar S, Shahbaz Y, Masood A. In cardiac surgery patients does Voluven impair coagulation less than other colloids? Interact Cardiovasc Thorac Surg. 2011;12:1022–7.

31 Valentine S, Bateman S. Identifying factors to minimize phlebotomy-induced blood loss in the pediatric intensive care unit. Pediatr Crit Care Med. 2012;13:22–7.

32 Adams ES, Longhurst CA, Pageler N, et al. Computerized physician order entry with decision support decreases blood transfusion in children. Pediatrics 2011;127:e1112–9.

33 Weber TP, Hartlage AG, Aken HV, Booke M. Anaesthetic strategies to reduce perioperative blood loss in paediatric surgery. Eur J Anaesth. 2003;20:175–81.

34 Tobias JD. Assessment of cerebral oxygenation using near infrared spectroscopy during isovolemic hemodilution in pediatric patients. J Clin Monitor Comput. 2011;25:171–4.

35 Dewhirst E, Winch P, Naguib A, Galantowicz M, Tobias JD. Cerebral oximetry values during preoperative phlebotomy to limit allogeneic blood use in patients undergoing cardiac surgery. J Cardiothor Vasc Anesth (in press).

36 Korosue K, Heros RC, Ogilvy CS, et al. Comparison of crystalloids and colloids for hemodilution in a model of focal cerebral ischemia. J Neurosurg. 1990;73:576–84.

37 Davies MJ. The role of colloids in blood conservation. Int Anesthesiol Clin. 1990;28:205–9.

38 Stump DC, Strauss RG, Henricksen RA, et al. Effects of hydroxy-ethyl starch on blood coagulation, particularly factor VIII. Transfusion. 1985;28:349–54.

39 Strauss RG, Stansfield C, Henriksen RA, Villhauer PJ. Pentastarch may cause fewer effects on coagulation than hetastarch. Transfusion. 1988;28:257–60.

40 Renck H, Ljungstrom KG, Resberg B, et al. Prevention of dextran-induced anaphylactic reactions by hapten inhibition. Acta Chir Scand. 1983;149:349–53.

41 Glick G, Plauth WH, Braunwald E. Role of the autonomic nervous system in the circulatory response to acutely induced anemia in unanesthetized dogs. J Clin Invest. 1964;43:2112–24.

42 Van Woerkins J, Trouborst A, Duncker DJ. Catecholamines and regional hemodynamics during isovolemic hemodilution alone and in combination with adenosine-induced controlled hypotension. J Appl Phys. 1992;72:760–76.

43 Guyton AC, Richardson TQ. Effect of hematocrit on venous return. Circ Res. 1961;9:157–65.

44 Crystal GJ, Rooney MW, Salem MR. Regional hemodynamics and oxygen supply during isovolemic hemodilution alone and in combination with adenosine-induced controlled hypotension. Anesth Analg. 1988;67:211–8.

45 Laks H, Pilon RN, Klovekorn WP, et al. Acute normovolemic hemodilution: effects on hemodynamics, oxygen, transport, and lung water in anesthetized man. Surg Forum. 1974;180:103–9.

46 Bowens C, Spahn DR, Frasco PE, et al. Hemodilution induces stable changes in global cardiovascular and regional myocardial function. Anesth Analg. 1993;76:1027–32.

47 Tarnow J, Eberlein HJ, Hess E, et al. Hemodynamic interactions of hemodilution anaesthesia, propranolol pretreatment and hypovolemia. I: Systemic Circulation. Basic Res Cardiol. 1979;74:109–22.

48 Robertie PG, Gravlee GP. Safe limits of isovolemic hemodilution and recommendation for erythrocyte transfusion. Int Anesthesiol Clin. 1990;28:197–203.

49 Fontana JL, Welborn L, Mongan PD, et al. Oxygen consumption and cardiovascular function in children during profound intraoperative normovolemic hemodilution. Anesth Analg. 1995;80:219–25.

50 Van der Linden P, De Hert S, Mathieu N, et al. Tolerance to acute hemodilution: Effect of anesthetic depth. Anesthesiology. 2003;99:97–104.

51 Gillies IDS. Anemia and anaesthesia. Br J Anaesth. 1974;46:589-602.

52 Sunder-Plassman L, Kessler M, Jesch F. Acute normovolemic hemodilution: changes in tissue oxygen supply and hemoglobin-oxygen affinity. Bibl Haematol. 1975;41:44–53.

53 Holtz J, Bassenge E, von Restoriff W, et al. Transmural differences in myocardial blood flow and in coronary dilatory capacity in hemodiluted conscious dogs. Basic Res Cardiol. 1976;71:36–46.

54 Jan KM, Chien S. Effect of hematocrit variations on coronary hemodynamics and oxygen utilization. Am J Physiol. 1977;233:H106–13.

55 Messmer K. Hemodilution. Surg Clin North Am. 1975;55:659–78.

56 Buckberg G, Brazier J. Coronary blood flow and cardiac function during hemodilution. Bibl Haematol. 1975;41:173–5.

57 Crystal GJ. Coronary hemodynamic responses during acute hemodilution in canine hearts. Am J Physiol. 1988;254:H525-31.

58 Geha AS, Baue AE. Graded coronary stenosis and coronary flow during acute normovolemic anemia. World J Surg. 1978;2:645–52.

59 Spahn DR, Smith LR, McRae RL, Leone BJ. Effects of acute isovolemic hemodilution and anesthesia on regional function in left ventricular myocardium with compromised coronary blood flow. Acta Anaesthesiol Scand. 1992;36:628–36.

60 Todd MM, Weeks JB, Warner DS. Cerebral blood flow, blood volume and brain tissue hematocrit during isovolemic hemodilution with hetastarch in rats. Am J Physiol. 1992;263:H75–82.

61 Pohl U, Busse R. Hypoxia stimulates release of endothelial-derived relaxant factor. Am J Physiol. 1989;256:H1595–600.

62 Fan FC, Chen RY, Schuessler GB, et al. Effects of hematocrit variations on regional hemodynamics and oxygen transport in the dog. Am J Physiol. 1980;238:H545–52.

63 Kessler M, Messmer K. Tissue oxygenation during hemodilution. Bibl Haematol. 1975;41:16–33.

64 Biernat S, Kulig A, Lepert R, et al. Pathomorphologic and histochemical changes in the liver during hemodilution. Am J Surg. 1974;128:24–30.

65 Utley JR, Wachtel C, Cain RB, et al. Effects of hypothermia, hemodilution and pump oxygenation on organ water content, blood flow, oxygen delivery and renal function. Ann Thorac Surg. 1981;31:121–33.

66 Olsfanger D, Jedeikin R, Metser H, et al. Acute normovolemic hemodilution and idiopathic scoliosis surgery: effects on homologous blood requirements. Anesth Intensive Care. 1993;21:429–31.

67 Haberken M, Dangel P. Normovolemic hemodilution and intraoperative autotransfusion in children: experience with 30 cases of spinal fusion. Eur J Pediatr Surg. 1991;1:30–55.

68 Stein JI, Gombotz H, Rigoler B, et al. Open heart surgery in children of Jehovah's Witnesses: extreme hemodilution on cardiopulmonary bypass. Pediatr Cardiol. 1991;12:170–4.

69 Monk TG, Goodnough LT, Brecher ME, et al. A prospective randomized comparison of three blood conservation strategies for radical prostatectomy. Anesthesiology. 1999;91:24–33.

70 Fantus B. Blood preservation. JAMA. 1937;109:128–31.

71 Stehling L. Autologous transfusion. Int Anesthesiol Clin. 1990;28:190–6.

72 Mann M, Sacks HJ, Goldfinger D. Safety of autologous blood donation prior to elective surgery for a variety of potentially "high risk" patients. Transfusion. 1983;23:229–32.

73 Scott WJ, Rede R, Castleman B. Efficacy, complications and cost of a comprehensive blood conservation program for cardiac operations. J Thorac Cardiovasc Surg. 1992;103:1001–7.

74 Owings DV, Kruskall MS, Therier RL, et al. Autologous blood donations prior to elective cardiac surgery: safety and effect on subsequent blood use. JAMA. 1989;262:1963–8.

75 DePelma L, Luban NLC. Autologous blood transfusion in pediatrics. Pediatrics. 1990;85:125–8.

76 Klimber IW. Autotransfusion and blood conservation in oncologic surgery. Semin Surg Oncol. 1989;5:286–92.

77 Tate DE, Friedmen RJ. Blood conservation in spinal surgery: review of current techniques. Spine. 1992;17:1450–6.

78 Silvergleid DJ. Safety and effectiveness of predeposit autologous transfusion in preteen and adolescent children. JAMA. 1987;257:3403–4.

79 Popovsky MA, Whitaker B, Arnold NL. Severe outcomes of allogeneic and autologous blood donation: Frequency and characterization. Transfusion 1995;35: 734–7.

80 Haugen R, Hill G. A large scale autologous blood program in a community hospital. JAMA. 1987;257:1211–4.

81 Goldfinger D, Capen S, Czer L, et al. Safety and efficacy of preoperative donation of blood for autologous use by patients with end-stage heart or lung disease who are awaiting organ transplantation. Transfusion. 1993;33:336–40.

82 Goodnough LT, Marcus RE. Effect of autologous blood donation in patients undergoing elective spine surgery. Spine 1992;17:172–5.

83 McVay PA, Hoag RW, Hoag MS, et al. Safety and use of autologous blood donation during the third trimester of pregnancy. Am J Obstet Gynecol. 1989;160:1479–88.

84 Davis R. Banked autologous blood for caesarean section. Anaesth Intensive Care. 1979;7:358–61.

85 Goodnough L, Wasmen J. Limitations to donating adequate autologous blood prior to elective surgery. Arch Surg. 1989;124:494–6.

86 Goodnough L, Rudnick S, Price TH, et al. Increased preoperative collection of autologous blood with recombinant human erythropoietin therapy. NEJM. 1989;321:1163–8.

87 Goh M, Kleer CG, Kielczewski P, et al. Autologous blood donation prior to anatomical radical retropubic prostatectomy: Is it necessary? Urology 1997;49:569–73.

88 AuBuchon JP. Autologous transfusion and directed donations: current controversies and future directions. Transfus Med Rev. 1989;3:290–306.

89 Duncan J. On reinfusion of blood in primary and other amputations. Br Med J. 1886;1:192–7.

90 Rubens FD, Boodhwani M, Lavalee G, et al. Perioperative red blood cell salvage. Can J Anaesth. 2003;50:S31–40.

91 Gardner A, Gibbs M, Evans C, et al. Relative cost of autologous red cell salvage versus allogeneic red cell transfusion during abdominal aortic aneurysm repair. Anaesth Intens Care. 2000;28:646–9.

92 Solomon MD, Rutledge ML, Kane LE, et al. Cost comparison of intraoperative autologous versus homologous transfusion. Transfusion. 1988;28:379–82.

93 Dale RF, Kipling RM, Smith MF, et al. Separation of malignant cells during autotransfusion. Br J Surg. 1988;75:581–4.

94 Robicseck F, Duncan GD, Born GVR, et al. Inherent dangers of simultaneous application of microfibrillar collagen hemostat and blood saving devices. J Thorac Cardiovasc Surg. 1986;92:766–8.

95 Murray DJ, Gress K, Weinstein SL. Coagulopathy after reinfusion of autologous scavenged red blood cells. Anesth Analg. 1992;75;125–9.

96 Wheeler TJ, Tobias JD. Complications of autotransfusion with salvaged blood. J Post Anesthesia Nurs. 1994;9:150–2.

97 Bull MH, Bull BS, Van Arsdell GS, Smith LL. Clinical implications of procoagulant and leukoattractant formation during intraoperative blood salvage. Arch Surg. 1988;123:1073–6.

98 O'Riordan WD. Autotransfusion in the emergency department of a community hospital. JACEP. 1977;6:233–7.

99 Linden JV, Kaplan HS, Murphy MT. Fatal air embolism due to perioperative blood recovery. Anesth Analg. 1997;84:422–6.

100 Symbas PN. Extraoperative autotransfusion from hemothorax. Surgery. 1978;84:722–7.

101 Litwin MS, Relihan M, Olsen RE. Pulmonary microemboli associated with massive transfusion. Ann Surg. 1975;181;51–7.

102 Mattox KL. Autotransfusion in the emergency department. JACEP. 1975;4:218–22.

103 Horst HM, Dlugos S, Fath JJ, et al. Coagulopathy and intraoperative blood salvage. J Trauma. 1992;32:646–53.

104 Halpern NA, Alicea M, Seabrook B, et al. Cell saver autologous transfusion: Metabolic consequences of washing blood with normal saline. J Trauma. 1996;41:407-15.

105 Halpern NA, Alicea M, Seabrook B, et al. Isolyte S, a physiologic multielectrolyte solution, is preferable to normal saline to wash cell saver salvaged blood: Conclusions from a prospective, randomized study in a canine model. Crit Care Med. 1997;25:2031–8.

106 Richardson DW, Robinson HG. Desmopressin. Ann Intern Med. 1985;103:228–34.

107 Mannucci PM. Desmopressin: a non-transfusional form of treatment for congenital and acquired bleeding disorders. Blood. 1088;72:1449–55.

108 Horrow JC. Desmopressin and antifibrinolytics. Int Anesthesiol Clin. 1990;28:230–5.

109 Salva KM, Kim HC, Nahum K, et al. DDAVP in the treatment of bleeding disorders. Pharmacotherapy. 1988;8:94–9.

110 Mannucci PM, Vicenti V, Alberca I, et al. Intravenous and subcutaneous administration of desmopressin. (DDAVP) to hemophiliacs: pharmacokinetics and factor VIII responses. Thromb Haemost. 1987;58:1037–9.

111 Lethagen S, Harris AS, Sjorin E, Nilsson IM. Intranasal and intravenous administration of desmopressin: effect on F VIII/vWF, pharmacokinetics and reproducibility. Thromb Haemostasis. 1987;58:1033–6.

112 Salzman EW, Weinstein MJ, Weintraub RM, et al. Treatment with desmopressin acetate to reduce blood loss after cardiac surgery. NEJM. 1986;314:1402–6.

113 Czer LSC, Bateman TM, Gray RJ, et al. Treatment of severe platelet dysfunction and hemorrhage after cardiopulmonary bypass: reduction in blood product usage with desmopressin. J Am Coll Cardiol. 1987;9:1139–47.

114 Mannucci PM, Remuzzi G, Pusineri F, et al. Desamino-8-D-Arginine vasopressin shortens the bleeding time in uremia. NEJM. 1983;308:8–12.

115 Mannucci PM, Vicente V, Vianello L, et al. Controlled trial of a desmopressin in liver cirrhosis and other conditions associated with a prolonged bleeding time. Blood. 1986;67:1148–53.

116 Kobrinsky NL, Letts RM, Patel LR, et al. 1-Desamino-8-D-Arginine vasopressin (desmopressin) decrease operative blood loss in patients having Harrington rod spinal fusion surgery. Ann Intern Med. 1987;107:446–50.

117 Theroux MC, Corddry DH, Tietz AE, et al. A study of desmopressin and blood loss during spinal fusion for neuromuscular scoliosis: A randomized, controlled, double-blinded study. Anesthesiology. 1997;87:260–7.

118 Alanay A, Acaroglu E, Oxdemir O, et al. Effects of deamino-8-D-arginine vasopressin on blood loss and coagulation factors in scoliosis surgery. Spine 1999;9:877–82.

119 Seear MD, Wadsworth LD, Rogers PC. The effect of desmopressin acetate (DDAVP) on postoperative blood loss after cardiac operations in children. J Thorac Cardiovasc Surg. 1989;98:217–9.

120 Laupacis A, Fergusson D. Drugs to minimize perioperative blood loss in cardiac surgery: meta-analysis using perioperative blood transfusion as the outcome. The international study of perioperative transfusion (ISPOT) investigators. Anesth Analg. 1997;85:1258–67.

121 Levi M, Cromheecke ME, de Jonge E, et al. Pharmacological strategies to decrease excessive blood loss in cardiac surgery: a meta-analysis of clinically relevant end-points. Lancet 1999;354:1940–7.

122 Royston D, Taylor KM, Sapsford RN, Bidstup BP. Effect of aprotinin on need for blood transfusion after repeat open-heart surgery. Lancet. 1987;2:1289–91.

123 Urban MK, Beckman J, Gordon M, et al. The efficacy of antifibrinolytics in the reduction of blood loss during complex adult reconstructive spine surgery. Spine. 2001;26:1152–7.

124 Capdevila X, Calvet Y, Biboulet P, et al. Aprotinin decreases blood loss and homol-ogous transfusions in patients undergoing major orthopedic surgery. Anesthesiology. 1998;88:50–7.

125 Janssens M, Joris J, David JL, et al. High-dose aprotinin reduces blood loss in patients undergoing total hip replacement surgery. Anesthesiology. 1994;80: 23–9.

126 Bidstrup BP, Harrison J, Royston D, et al. Aprotinin therapy in cardiac operations: a report on use in 41 cardiac centers in the United Kingdom. Ann Thorac Surg. 1993;55:971–6.

127 Fergusson DA, Hébert PC, Mazer CD, and the BART Investigators. A compari-son of aprotinin and lysine analogues in high-risk cardiac surgery. N Engl J Med. 2008;29;358:2319–31.

128 Florentino-Pineda I, Blakemore LC, Thompson GH, et al. The effect of epsilon aminocaproic acid on perioperative blood loss in patients with idiopathic scoliosis undergoing posterior spinal fusion. Spine. 2001;26:1147–51.

129 Neilipovitz DT, Murto K, Hall L, et al. A randomized trial of tranexamic acid to reduce blood transfusion for scoliosis surgery. Anesth Analg. 2001;93:82–7.

130 Hippala S, Strid L, Wennerstrand MI, et al. Tranexamic acid reduces perioperative blood loss associated with total knee arthroplasty. Br J Anaesth. 1995;74:534–7.

131 Hippala S, Strid LJ, Wennerstrand MI, et al. Tranexamic acid radically decreases blood loss and transfusions associated with total knee arthroplasty. Anesth Analg. 1997;84:839–44.

132 Benoni G, Fredin H. Fibrinolytic inhibition with tranexamic acid reduces blood loss and blood transfusion after knee arthroplasty: a prospective, randomized double blind study of 86 patients. J Bone Joint Surg Br. 1996;78:434–40.

133 Boylan JF, Klinck JR, Sandler AN, et al. Tranexamic acid reduces blood loss, transfusion requirements and coagulation factor use in primary orthotopic liver transplantation. Anesthesiology 1996;85:1043–8.

134 Sack E, Spaet TH, Gentile R, et al. Reduction of prostatectomy bleeding by epsilon-aminocaproic acid. New Engl J Med. 1962;266:541–64.

135 DelRossi AJ, Cernaianu AC, Botros S, et al. Prophylactic treatment of postperfusion bleeding using EACA. Chest. 1989;96:27–30.

136 Horrow JC, Hlavecek J, Strong MD, et al. Prophylactic tranexamic acid decreases bleeding after cardiac operations. J Thorac Cardiovasc Surg. 1990;99:70–4.

137 Ovrum E, Holen EA, Abdelnoor M, et al. Tranexamic acid is not necessary to reduce blood loss after coronary artery bypass operations. J Thorac Cardiovasc Surg. 1993;105:78–83.

138 Amar D, Grant FM, Zhang H, et al. Antifibrinolytic therapy and perioperative blood loss in cancer patients undergoing major orthopedic surgery. Anesthesiology. 2003;98:337–42.

139 Goobie SM, Meier PM, Pereira LM, et al. Efficacy of tranexamic acid in pediatric craniosynostosis surgery: a double-blind, placebo-controlled trial. Anesth Analg. 2011;114:862–71.

140 Dadure C, Sauter M, Bringuier S, et al. Intraoperative tranexamic acid reduces blood transfusion in children undergoing craniosynostosis surgery. Anesth Analg. 2011;114:856–61.

141 Manji RA, Grocott HP, Leake J, et al. Seizures following cardiac surgery: the impact of tranexamic acid and other risk factors. Can J Anaesth. 2012;59:6–13.

142 Kalavrouziotis D, Voisine P, Mohammadi S, Dionne S, Dagenais F. High-dose tranexamic acid is an independent predictor of early seizure after cardiopulmonary bypass. Ann Thorac Surg. 2012;93:148–54.

143 Wells PS. Safety and efficacy of methods for reducing perioperative allogeneic transfusion: A critical review. Am J Therap. 2002;9:377–88.

144 Kalicinski P, Kaminski A, Drewniak T, et al. Quick correction of hemostasis in two patients with fulminant liver failure undergoing liver transplantation by recombinant activated factor VII. Transplant Proc. 1999;31:378–9.

145 Tobias JD, Berkenbosch JW. Synthetic factor VIIa concentrate to treat coagulopathy and gastrointestinal bleeding in an infant with end-stage liver disease. Clin Pediatr. 2002;41:613–6.

146 Tobias JD, Groeper K, Berkenbosch JW. Preliminary experience with the use of recombinant factor VIIa to treat coagulation disturbances in pediatric patients. South Med J. 2003;96:12–6.

147 Martinowitz U, Kenet G, Segal E, et al. Recombinant factor VII for adjunctive hemorrhage control in trauma. J Trauma. 2001;51:431–9.

148 Hendriks HGD, Meijer K, de Wolf JT, et al. Reduced transfusion requirements by recombinant factor VIIa in orthotopic liver transplantation. Transplantation. 2001;71:402–5.

149 Murkin JM. A novel hemostatic agent: the potential role of recombinant activated factor VII in anesthetic practice. Can J Anaesth. 2002;49:S21–6.

150 Tobias JD. Synthetic factor VIIa to treat dilutional coagulopathy during posterior spinal fusion in two children. Anesthesiology. 2002;96:1522–5.

151 Friederich PW, Henny CP, Messelink EJ, et al. Effect of recombinant activated factor VII on perioperative blood loss in patients undergoing retropubic prostatectomy: a double-blind place-controlled randomized trial. Lancet. 2002;36: 201–5.

152 Diprose P, Herbertson MJ, O'Shaughnessy D, et al. Activated recombinant factor VII after cardiopulmonary bypass reduces allogeneic transfusion in complex non-coronary cardiac surgery: Randomized double-blind placebo-controlled pilot study. Br J Anaesth. 2005;95:596–602.

153 Ekert H, Brizard C, Eyers R, et al. Elective administration in infants of low-dose recombinant activated factor VII (rFVIIa) in cardiopulmonary bypass surgery for congenital heart disease does not shorten time to chest closure or reduce blood loss and need for transfusions: A randomized, double-blind, parallel group, placebo-controlled study of rFVIIa and standard haemostatic replacement therapy versus standard haemostatic replacement therapy. Blood Coagul Fibrinolysis. 2006;17:389–95.

154 Roberts HR. Recombinant factor VIIa (NovoSeven) and the safety of treatment. Semin Hematol. 2001;38(Suppl 12):48–50.

155 Roberts HR. Clinical experience with activated factor VII: focus on safety aspects. Blood Coag Fibrin. 1998;9:S115–8.

156 Gallisti S, Cvrin G, Muntean W. Recombinant factor VIIa does not induce hypercoagulability in vitro. Thromb Haemost. 1999;81:245–9.

157 Zangrillo A, Mizzi A, Biondi-Zoccai G, et al. Recombinant activated factor VII in cardiac surgery: A meta-analysis. J Cardiothorac Vasc Anesth. 2009;23:34–40.

158 Gill R, Herbertson M, Vuylsteke A, et al. Safety and efficacy of recombinant activated factor VII: A randomized placebo-controlled trial in the setting of bleeding after cardiac surgery. Circulation. 2009;120:21–7.

159 Levy JH, Gill R, Nussmeier NA, et al. Repletion of factor XIII following cardiopulmonary bypass using a recombinant A-subunit homodimer A preliminary report. Thromb Haemost. 2009;102:765–71.

160 Gödje O, Gallmeier U, Schelian M, Grünewald M, Mair H. Coagulation factor XIII reduces postoperative bleeding after coronary surgery with extracorporeal circulation. Thorac Cardiovasc Surg. 2006;54:26–33.

161 Stuklis RG, O'Shaughnessy DF, Ohri SK. Novel approach to bleeding in patients undergoing cardiac surgery with liver dysfunction. Eur J Cardiothorac Surg. 2001;19:219–20.

162 Alport EC, Callum JL, Nahirniak S. Cryoprecipitate use in 25 Canadian hospitals: Commonly used outside of the published guidelines. Transfusion. 2008;48:2122–7.

163 Rahe-Meyer N, Solomon C, Winterhalter M, et al. Thromboelastometry-guided administration of fibrinogen concentrate for the treatment of excessive intraoperative bleeding in thoracoabdominal aortic aneurysm surgery. J Thorac Cardiovasc Surg. 2009;138:694–702.

164 Meneghini L, Zadra N, Anloni V, et al. Erythropoietin therapy and acute preoperative normovolemic haemodilution in infants undergoing craniosynostosis surgery. Paediatr Anaesth. 2003;13:392–6.

165 Yoo YC, Shim JK, Kim JC, et al. Effect of single human erythropoietin injection on transfusion requirements in preoperatively anemic patients undergoing valvular heart surgery. Anesthesiology. 2012;115:929–37.

166 Lippi G, Franchini M, Favaloro EJ. Thrombotic complications of erythropoiesis-stimulating agents. Semin Thromb Hemost. 2010;36:537–49.

167 Stowell CP, Jones SC, Enny C, Langholff W, Leitz G. An open-label, randomized, parallel-group study of perioperative epoetin alfa versus standard of care for blood conservation in major elective spinal surgery: Safety analysis. Spine. 2009;34:2479–85.

168 Eckenhoff JE, Rich JC. Clinical experiences with deliberate hypotension. Anesth Analg. 1966;45:21–8.

169 Sollevi A. Hypotensive anesthesia and blood loss. Acta Anaesth Scand. 1988;89(Suppl):39–43.

170 Sperry RJ, Monk CR, Durieux ME, et al. The influence of hemorrhage on organ perfusion during deliberate hypotension in rats. Anesthesiology. 1992;77:1171–7.

171 Seyde WC, Longnecker DE. Cerebral oxygen tension in rats during deliberate hypotension with sodium nitroprusside, 2-chloroadenosine or deep isoflurane anesthesia. Anesthesiology. 1986;64:480–5.

172 Ringaert KRA, Mutch WAC, Malo LA. Regional cerebral blood flow and response to carbon dioxide during controlled hypotension with isoflurane anesthesia in the rat. Anesth Analg. 1988;67:383–8.

173 American Society of Anesthesiologists Task Force on Perioperative Visual Loss. Practice advisory for perioperative visual loss associated with spine surgery: an updated report by the American Society of Anesthesiologists Task Force on Perioperative Visual Loss. Anesthesiology. 2012;116:274–85.

174 Lee LA, Roth S, Posner KL, Cheney FW, Caplan RA, Newman NJ, Domino KB. The American Society of Anesthesiologists Postoperative Visual Loss Registry: analysis of 93 spine surgery cases with postoperative visual loss. Anesthesiology. 2006;105:652–9.

175 Sivarajan M, Amory DW, Everett GB, et al. Blood pressure, not cardiac output, determines blood loss during induced hypotension. Anesth Analg. 1980;59:203–6.

176 Tobias JD. Controlled hypotension in children: a critical review of available agents. Paediatr Drugs. 2002;4:439–53.

177 Hines R, Barash P. Infusion of sodium nitroprusside induces platelet dysfunction in vitro. Anesthesiology. 1989;70:611–5.

178 Bernard JM, Passuti N, Pinaud M. Long term hypotensive technique with nicardipine and nitroprusside during isoflurane anesthesia for spinal surgery. Anesth Analg. 1992;72:179–85.

179 Bernard JM, Pinaud M, Francois T, et al. Deliberate hypotension with nicardipine or nitroprusside during total hip arthroplasty. Anesth Analg. 1991;73:341–5.

180 Hersey SL, O'Dell NE, Lowe S, et al. Nicardipine versus nitroprusside for controlled hypotension during spinal surgery in adolescents. Anesth Analg. 1997;84:1239–44.

CHAPTER 9

Post-operative management in transfusion-free medicine and surgery in the ICU

Jean-Louis Vincent

Department of Intensive Care, Erasme Hospital, Université libre de Bruxelles, Brussels, Belgium

Introduction

As many as 30% of intensive care unit (ICU) patients receive a transfusion at some point during their ICU stay [1–4], the rationale being that blood transfusion can help restore and maintain oxygen delivery. However, decisions regarding when and how much to transfuse are largely subjective, with little objective evidence to support any particular global transfusion trigger. Until relatively recently, cut-off values of a hemoglobin (Hb) concentration of <10 g/dl or a hematocrit <30% were widely used as transfusion triggers, although studies in patients who refuse blood transfusions have shown that most deaths related to anemia occur only when the Hb concentration falls below much lower levels [5]. With concerns about possible negative effects of transfusion, particularly disease transmission and immunosuppression, the rising costs and limited availability of blood products, and results from several studies suggesting that more restrictive transfusion protocols were at least as good as, and possibly better than more liberal approaches to transfusion [1, 2, 6, 7], many intensivists have re-evaluated the traditional transfusion triggers and there has been a move toward reducing transfusions wherever possible.

In this chapter, we will briefly discuss the impact of blood transfusion on oxygen transport, the concept of "optimal" Hb with currently suggested transfusion thresholds, strategies to reduce iatrogenic blood loss, and clinical strategies to reduce oxygen consumption.

Transfusion-Free Medicine and Surgery, Second Edition. Edited by Nicolas Jabbour.
© 2014 John Wiley & Sons, Ltd. Published 2014 by John Wiley & Sons, Ltd.

Anemia in the ICU

Anemia is common in the ICU patient [1, 2, 4, 8], and its etiology is varied. Causes can be broadly divided into those due to blood loss, those due to reduced RBC production, and those due to increased RBC destruction (hemolysis or sequestration); although in reality many ICU patients with anemia will have a mixture of these conditions. Hemorrhage is perhaps the most common cause of anemia occurring intra- and post-operatively in the ICU patient. However, whereas gastrointestinal hemorrhage or post-traumatic and post-surgical hemorrhage are usually clearly apparent, other less obvious forms of hemorrhage, for example, intramuscular, retroperitoneal, or intrapleural hemorrhage, occurring as complications of various ICU interventions including central venous catheterization and liver biopsy, may be less easily detected.

An important, and often neglected, cause of blood loss, which may contribute to transfusion requirements especially in the ICU patient, is repeated blood sampling [8]. Early observational studies of phlebotomy in ICUs in the United States and Europe reported average blood sampling volumes of 41.1–66.1 mL/day [9–11]. In the ABC study [1], the mean volume per blood draw was 10.3 mL, with an average total daily volume of 41.1 mL. There was a significant positive correlation between organ dysfunction and the number of blood draws and the total amount of blood drawn per day, possibly placing the sickest patients at increased risk for worse anemia and the attendant risks of transfusion [1]. Nguyen et al. reported that in 91 ICU patients the average number of blood samples per day was 11.7 ± 4.7, and the total volume of blood taken per day for laboratory studies was 40.3 ± 15.4 mL [8]. More recently, Branco et al. noted an increase in the mean number of laboratory tests requested in trauma patients admitted to the ICU between 2004 and 2009 (from 65 ± 56 vs. 83 ± 72, $p < 0.001$), and in the total amount of blood sampled during the hospital stay (from 330 ± 351 mL in 2004 to 436 ± 346 mL in 2009, $p = 0.048$), although patient demographics and disease severity were similar in the two time periods [12].

In the study by Nguyen et al., Hb concentrations in non-bleeding ICU patients declined by at least 0.5 g/dL/day during the first 3 days of an ICU stay and continued to decline for patients with sepsis and higher severity of illness [8]. In patients who stayed longer than three days on the ICU, the fall in Hb was greater over the first three days than for subsequent days (0.66 ± 0.84 g/dl/day vs. 0.12 ± 0.29 g/dl/day, $p < 0.01$), and after the third day was directly related to the severity of disease as assessed by the APACHE II and SOFA scores [8]. Interestingly, in

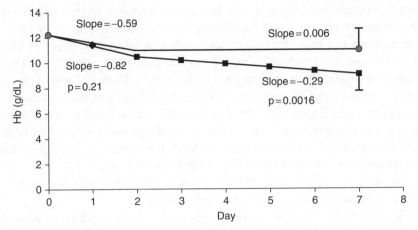

Figure 9.1 Changes in hemoglobin concentrations over time in septic (bottom line), and non-septic (top line) patients. Reproduced from [8] with permission.

non-septic patients, the fall in Hb concentration levelled out after the third ICU day, whereas in septic patients, Hb concentrations continued to decrease (Figure 9.1). The reasons suggested by the authors for this difference between septic and non-septic patients include increased blood taking and invasive procedures in these sicker patients, and decreased red cell survival and a blunted erythropoietin (EPO) response as a result of the active inflammatory response to infection [8].

Role of transfusion in resuscitation

The function of Hb is, in essence, to carry oxygen around the body and release it where it is (most) needed. The characteristics of Hb allow it to take on oxygen in the lungs and unload it at the tissue level. The oxygen carrying capacity of Hb is represented by the familiar sinusoidal oxyHb dissociation curve. The amount of oxygen delivered to the tissues (DO_2) is the product of the cardiac output (CO) and the arterial oxygen content (CaO_2).

$$DO_2 = CaO_2 \times CO$$

Generally, the majority of oxygen is transported on Hb and the CaO_2 thus approximates to the Hb saturation. Increasing the concentration of Hb would thus be expected to increase DO_2 as has been demonstrated in several studies [13–15], and is the basic rationale behind blood transfusion. However, while blood transfusion increases Hb concentration and DO_2, this does not necessarily mean that oxygen uptake (VO_2) and hence oxygen availability to the tissues is increased. Indeed, relatively few studies have evaluated the effect of blood transfusion on oxygenation parameters and those that have, have shown no consistent effect on VO_2 [13–16]. The relationship "increased Hb = improved oxygenation" is thus not quite as simple as one might initially expect. First, the ability of Hb to download oxygen may vary in different disease processes, with, for example, microcirculatory factors such as RBC deformability and altered oxygen extraction capabilities, influencing the transfer of oxygen from Hb in sepsis. Second, for transfused blood, the duration of storage prior to transfusion may limit the ability of Hb to deliver oxygen [17]. Third, by increasing viscosity, a rise in Hb could potentially restrict microcirculatory flow and limit the ability of Hb to reach the tissues.

Severe anemia, however, carries its own risks, including delayed wound healing and increased incidence of cardiac arrhythmias, and is associated with worse outcomes [4, 18, 19]. The problem is thus to determine at which point the risks of transfusion are outweighed by the risks of anemia – the so-called transfusion trigger. In recent years the optimal cut-off for transfusion in critically ill patients has come under intense debate. A randomized controlled trial conducted between 1994 and 1997 showed that a more restrictive transfusion protocol (transfusions given when the Hb concentration decreased below 7.0 g/dl and Hb concentrations maintained at 7.0–9.0 g/dl), was at least as effective and possibly more so than a more conservative approach (transfusions given when the Hb concentration fell below 10.0 g/dl and Hb concentrations maintained at 10.0–12.0 g/dl) [6]. Although overall 30-day mortality was similar in the two groups, the rates were significantly lower with the restrictive transfusion strategy among patients who were less acutely ill (APACHE II score of ≤20), and among younger patients (less than 55 years of age), except for patients with clinically significant cardiac disease. An observational study in Europe, the ABC study, conducted several years later in 1999, also noted that transfused ICU patients had higher mortality rates than patients who were not transfused [1], even when organ dysfunction scores were taken into account. In this study, a transfusion during the ICU stay increased the risk of death by a factor of 1.37 (95% CI: 1.02–1.84). In a systematic review of 45 observational studies reporting the impact of transfusions on patient outcome, Marik and Corwin identified RBC transfusion as an independent predictor of death (pooled OR from 12 studies: 1.7 [95% CI 1.4-1.9]), infectious complications (pooled OR from 9 studies: 1.8 [1.5–2.2]) and ARDS (pooled OR from 6 studies: 2.5 [1.6–3.3]) [20]. Nevertheless, in another observational study in Europe (the SOAP study), conducted along the same lines as the ABC study but several years later in 2002, failed to demonstrate any increased mortality rates [3]. These apparently conflicting results may be related to the favorable effects of deleukocytation which was only used regularly by 46% of ICUs in the ABC study, but is now instituted routinely in most European hospitals.

Patients undergoing cardiac surgery have particularly high transfusion rates, with some studies reporting that as many as 85% of such patients received a blood transfusion postoperatively [21]. However, blood transfusions in cardiac surgery patients have also been associated with worse outcomes [22, 23], and a recent randomized controlled study in more than 500 patients undergoing cardiac surgery with cardiopulmonary bypass reported that a perioperative restrictive transfusion strategy (to maintain a hematocrit at least 24%) was associated with similar morbidity/mortality outcomes compared to a more liberal strategy (to maintain a hematocrit of at least 30%) [7]. Moreover, independent of the transfusion strategy, the number of transfused RBC units was an independent risk factor for clinical complications or death at 30 days (hazard ratio 1.21 for each additional unit transfused; 95% confidence interval 1.1–1.4, $P = .002$). Rather than using a fixed transfusion trigger for all patients, individual patient characteristics, including age and the presence of coronary artery disease, need to be taken into account to estimate a patient's likelihood of benefitting from transfusion [24].

Monitoring the adequacy of oxygenation

One of the challenges in assessing the need for transfusion is that we are hampered by the lack of a good means of measuring and monitoring tissue oxygenation, in particular regional oxygenation, which is believed to be an important factor in the development of multiple organ failure. The need for transfusion will vary according to the individual patient and depending on the underlying etiology of the shock, but as yet there is no precise means of determining when the desired goal, i.e., restored and adequate tissue oxygenation, has been reached. Thus, although measurable global oxygenation parameters may be apparently normal, regional oxygenation may remain impaired [25].

Proposed markers to assess the adequacy of oxygenation include CO, mixed (SvO_2) or central ($ScvO_2$) venous oxygen saturation, and blood lactate levels. Regional methods include gastric tonometry and, more recently, orthogonal polarization spectral (OPS)/sidestream dark field (SDF) or near infra-red spectroscopy (NIRS) techniques, but these remain experimental at present.

Cardiac output

With a pulmonary artery catheter (PAC) in place, CO can be estimated by the thermodilution method. CO can be monitored almost continuously using specially adapted PACs, equipped with a thermal filament positioned some 20 cm from the catheter tip. Concerns have been raised about the safety of the PAC and, increasingly, less invasive methods are being used although these all have their limitations [26].

The CO can be said to represent total body blood flow, but offers no information on the blood flow reaching individual organs. In addition, CO is very variable according to individual characteristics and oxygen requirements; for example, in sepsis a "normal" or even high CO may be insufficient because of the increased oxygen requirements caused by the sepsis process. CO must, therefore, never be interpreted as an isolated parameter but in the light of other factors, including SvO_2.

SvO₂

SvO_2 is the oxygen saturation of Hb in the mixed venous blood, and must be measured in the pulmonary artery. From the Fick equation, VO_2 is the product of the CO and the arteriovenous oxygen difference. If the amount of oxygen dissolved in the blood is ignored, the equation can be rearranged to:

$$SvO_2 = SaO_2 - [VO_2/(CO \times 13.9 \times Hb)$$

where SaO_2 is the arterial oxygen saturation (13.9 is a constant value related to the amount of oxygen bound to 1g Hb, multiplied by 10 to correspond with a VO_2 in ml/min). In the critically ill patient, a normal SvO_2 is considered to be about 70%. If the patient is not anemic or hypoxemic, the SvO_2 reflects the relationship between CO and VO_2. However, both anemia and hypoxemia are common in ICU patients, and SvO_2 must be seen as complementing rather than replacing CO data.

If a PAC is not in place, central venous oxygen saturation ($ScvO_2$) has been suggested as a surrogate marker of SvO_2 [27]. Importantly, whichever measure is used, SvO_2 or $ScvO_2$, values should be interpreted in combination with markers of perfusion and oxygenation including CO and blood lactate levels.

O₂ER

An increase in tissue oxygen demands can be met by an increase in CO, in oxygen extraction or in both. In the normal, healthy individual increased oxygen demands are met by combined increases in both CO and oxygen extraction. In the critically ill patient, various processes such as sepsis can increase tissue oxygen demands, and if the CO is unable to respond adequately, tissue oxygen extraction will increase disproportionately to meet the patient's oxygen demands, with a resultant fall in the SvO_2. As DO_2 falls, oxygen extraction increases to maintain oxygen demand until this compensatory mechanism becomes insufficient and VO_2 starts to fall (VO_2/DO_2 dependency) with resulting inadequate tissue oxygenation.

The O_2ER is the ratio of oxygen demand to delivery and is simple to calculate and independent of Hb concentration.

$$O_2ER = VO_2/DO_2 = (SaO_2 - SvO_2)/SaO_2$$

Plotting consecutive data points on a graph of cardiac index (CI) against O_2ER, and relating them to isopleths of VO_2 can be used to identify whether a patient has reached the point of VO_2/DO_2 dependency. The diagram can also be used to interpret CO values in various groups of patients and to evaluate a patient's response to treatment. In anemic patients, tolerance to anemia is due to increases in CI and O_2ER, which maintain VO_2. While a high CI in an anemic patient may appear adequate, their cardiac response may nevertheless be inadequate for the degree of anemia. The relationship between CI and O_2ER can help interpret the cardiac index in such situations [28]. In patients with anemia and normal cardiac function, a CI/O_2ER ratio <10 suggests an inadequate CI that is due either to hypovolemia or to altered myocardial function (Figure 9.2); if there is no evidence of altered cardiac function in these patients, it is likely that they are hypovolemic [28].

Blood lactate

As tissue oxygenation becomes inadequate and VO_2 becomes DO_2 dependent, anaerobic metabolism begins to play an increasingly important role and blood lactate levels rise. While other causes of hyperlactatemia, including prolonged seizures, alcohol intoxication, extensive neoplastic disease, etc., must be excluded, these are rare and a blood lactate level greater than 2 mEq/l suggests inadequate tissue perfusion and oxygenation [29]. Hyperlactatemia has been clearly associated with a poorer prognosis in various groups of critically ill patients, even in sepsis where other causes of hyperlactatemia may be present in addition to tissue hypoxia [29–31]. Importantly, serial blood lactate levels are of greater significance than any individual value [32].

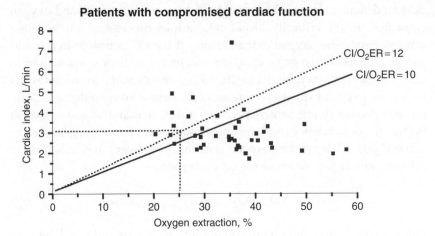

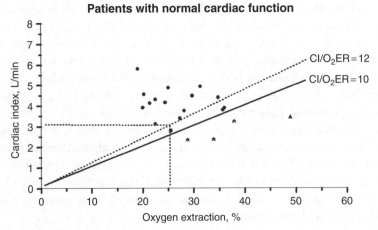

Figure 9.2 Relationship between CI and O_2ER in patients with compromised (upper panel) and normal (lower panel) cardiac function. *three patients with concomitant hypovolemia, Δ = one patient with severe myocardial depression due to sepsis. Adapted from [28] with permission.

Regional markers of tissue oxygenation

All of the above measures provide an indication of the global adequacy of tissue oxygenation, but no indication of local perfusion or oxygenation. In an attempt to provide more local data, gastric tonometry was developed and calculation or measurement of gastric intramucosal pH (pHi) or PCO_2 has been extensively studied. However, while these measures have been shown to correlate with outcome [33, 34], studies targeted at correcting these variables have shown no beneficial effects of such an approach on survival [34, 35]. More recently, other techniques of monitoring the microcirculation have become available, including OPS/SDF and NIRS methods. In a small study of patients with severe sepsis, RBC transfusion did not globally affect NIRS- or SDF-derived variables, but muscle oxygen consumption improved in patients with low baseline values [36]. Similarly, Sakr and colleagues reported that although blood transfusion was associated with increased Hb concentrations in patients with severe sepsis, microvascular perfusion, as assessed by OPS imaging, was only significantly altered in patients with altered perfusion at baseline [25]. In critically ill patients requiring transfusion, NIRS-derived variables were altered only in patients with altered values at baseline [37]. In patients with trauma also, transfusion was associated with an improvement in perfusion in those with relatively altered baseline values as assessed by SDF imaging [38]. Nevertheless, these techniques remain experimental at present and no prospective studies have demonstrated improved outcomes with microcirculation-targeted therapies.

Reducing transfusion requirements

In all patients, and especially those who refuse a blood transfusion, for example Jehovah's Witness (JW) patients, attempts must clearly be made to minimize blood loss, including iatrogenic loss. Pre-operative optimization of oxygenation and red cell mass, and control of coagulation will help reduce the need for post-operative transfusion. Techniques to limit intra-operative blood loss, including normovolemic hemodilution, controlled hypotensive anesthesia, meticulous hemostasis, and red cell salvaging devices, have been dealt with in another chapter. The post-operative management of these patients may include other specific strategies to maximize DO_2 and minimize VO_2, although there are few data, other than case reports and series, on the actual benefits of these strategies in anemic ICU patients.

Reducing phlebotomy losses

Various strategies to limit phlebotomy losses have been suggested [39, 40], including the use of smaller (pediatric) sampling tubes [41, 42], blood conservation devices [43], reduced volumes of discarded blood [44], and educational programs [45, 46]. In a before/after study, introduction of guidelines for laboratory testing in a surgical ICU, which included a list of the tests to be obtained daily, the need to discuss laboratory testing at daily patient's rounds, and the need to provide a written order for all tests, was associated with a 37% decrease in the number of laboratory tests performed which was correlated linearly with the number of red cell transfusions given [46]. In a randomized controlled study, phlebotomy-associated blood loss was reduced by over 80% in patients randomized to a conservative phlebotomy group (use of pediatric phlebotomy tubes and return of discard volume to patient) compared to a standard group [47]. Physicians need to be aware not only of the risks of iatrogenic blood loss and measures by which the volumes involved can be reduced, but also need to be challenged to rationalize their requests for blood samples.

Minimizing oxygen consumption

Deliberate mild hypothermia has been used to reduce oxygen consumption in JW patients, with a proposed target core temperature of 30–32 °C [48]. Although VO_2 is reduced, blood viscosity is, however, increased, which may compromise DO_2, and hemodilution is thus often employed simultaneously. Neuromuscular blockade with sedation, intubation and mechanical ventilation can also reduce VO_2. Neuromuscular blockade may be of particular use in the shivering patient as shivering can increase VO_2 considerably; however, the effects of neuromuscular blockade on VO_2 are not consistent in all patients [49]. In addition, prolonged paralysis and excessive sedation have their own risks including an increased incidence of polyneuropathy.

Increasing CO and DO_2

Intravascular volume and CO must be maintained optimal to ensure adequate tissue perfusion and oxygenation. As DO_2 is the product of CO and the arterial oxygen content, strategies to improve DO_2 can also include an increase in CO and dissolved oxygen. Importantly, attempts to increase CO and DO_2 to "supranormal" levels with combinations of fluids, transfusions and vasoactive agents, have been largely unsuccessful in mixed groups of critically ill patients [50, 51], although may have a place in specific patient groups [52], stressing the need for full assessment and evaluation of each patient with treatment titrated to the individual.

Hyperbaric oxygen therapy can improve tissue DO_2 and has been used in severely anemic JW patients [53], although the potential benefit of such therapy must be weighed against the logistic problems and risks of this treatment modality, which include oxygen toxicity and barotrauma.

Hb-based oxygen carriers may have a place in the post-operative management of some patients to increase DO_2 [54], and with recombinant technology are acceptable to most JW patients [55, 56]. However, there have been concerns about adverse effects [57], increased risks of myocardial infarction in particular, and these products need to be more closely evaluated before they can be widely administered in the ICU setting [58, 59].

Erythropoietin

Under normal conditions, about 1% of circulating RBCs are renewed each day, but following acute blood loss, the rate of erythropoiesis can increase up to tenfold. The principal regulator of erythropoiesis is the hormone EPO. Endogenous EPO stimulates the production and maturation of erythroid progenitor cells, and causes the premature release of a variety of cells, including reticulocytes, from the marrow. The most potent stimuli for EPO release are anemia and hypoxia. In the critically ill patient, the normal EPO response may be blunted [60], contributing to the anemia seen in these patients. These findings led to the suggestion that EPO may be useful in the prevention of anemia in critically ill patients. Several early randomized controlled studies in adult ICU patients, suggested that EPO was associated with a reduced need for transfusion and an increase in Hb concentration compared to placebo [61, 62]. In a more recent and larger study [63], 1460 medical, surgical, or trauma patients were randomized to receive placebo or epoetin alfa (40 000 U) administered weekly for a maximum of 3 weeks. In this study, EPO was not associated with reduced transfusions, but the Hb concentration at day 29 was higher in the EPO group than in the placebo group. Mortality tended to be lower at day 29 and day 140 in patients who received EPO, particularly in trauma patients [63, 64]. However, EPO was associated with a significant increase in the incidence of thrombotic events compared to placebo (hazard ratio, 1.41; 95% CI, 1.06 to 1.86) [63]. Further study is required to determine the role, if any, in critically ill patients, but its routine use is not currently recommended [65].

Other factors

Normal erythrocyte development depends on adequate supplies of iron, folate, and vitamin B12, and nutritional supplements of these products must be given routinely in critically ill patients. In a randomized, double-blind, placebo-controlled trial, Pieracci et al. observed a significant reduction in RBC transfusions (30 vs. 45%) in 97 anemic surgical patients treated with oral ferrous sulfate 325 mg three times a day [66]. There were no differences in the incidence of infections (47 vs. 49%), antibiotic days, lengths of ICU stay or mortality rates (9.4% vs. 9.9%; p = 0.62) between groups. The results of this study are encouraging but need confirmation in larger multicenter randomized trials. Vitamin C may also help by improving iron absorption.

Conclusion

Anemia is common in the critically ill patient, perhaps particularly after surgery, and is associated with worse outcomes. However, strategies can be employed to limit the development of anemia including minimizing iatrogenic blood loss and oxygen consumption. Exogenous erythropoietin, iron, and Hb-based oxygen carriers may have a place in transfusion-free surgery, but further study is needed to determine their precise role.

References

1 Vincent JL, Baron JF, Reinhart K, et al. Anemia and blood transfusion in critically ill patients. JAMA. 2002;288:1499–1507.

2 Corwin HL, Gettinger A, Pearl RG, et al. The CRIT Study: Anemia and blood transfusion in the critically ill–current clinical practice in the United States. Crit Care Med. 2004;32:39–52.

3 Vincent JL, Sakr Y, Sprung C, et al. Are blood transfusions associated with greater mortality rates? Results of the Sepsis Occurrence in Acutely Ill Patients study. Anesthesiology. 2008;108:31–9.

4 Sakr Y, Lobo S, Knuepfer S, et al. Anemia and blood transfusion in a surgical intensive care unit. Crit Care. 2010;14:R92.

5 Viele MK, Weiskopf RB. What can we learn about the need for transfusion from patients who refuse blood? The experience with Jehovah's Witnesses. Transfusion. 1994;34:396–401.

6 Hebert PC, Wells G, Blajchman MA, et al. A multicenter, randomized, controlled clinical trial of transfusion requirements in critical care. Transfusion Requirements in Critical Care Investigators, Canadian Critical Care Trials Group. N Engl J Med. 1999;340:409–17.

7 Hajjar LA, Vincent JL, Galas FR, et al. Transfusion requirements after cardiac surgery: the TRACS randomized controlled trial. JAMA. 2010;304:1559–1567.

8 Nguyen BV, Bota DP, Melot C, et al. Time course of hemoglobin concentrations in nonbleeding intensive care unit patients. Crit Care Med. 2003;31:406–10.

9 Smoller BR, Kruskall MS. Phlebotomy for diagnostic laboratory tests in adults. Pattern of use and effect on transfusion requirements. N Engl J Med. 1986;314:1233–5.

10 Tarpey J, Lawler PG. Iatrogenic anaemia? A survey of venesection in patients in the intensive therapy unit. Anaesthesia. 1990;45:396–8.

11 von Ahsen N, Muller C, Serke S, et al. Important role of nondiagnostic blood loss and blunted erythropoietic response in the anemia of medical intensive care patients. Crit Care Med. 1999;27:2630–39.

12 Branco BC, Inaba K, Doughty R, et al. The increasing burden of phlebotomy in the development of anaemia and need for blood transfusion amongst trauma patients. Injury. 2012;43:78–83.

13 Lorente JA, Landin L, De Pablo R, et al. Effects of blood transfusion on oxygen transport variables in severe sepsis. Crit Care Med. 1993;21:1312–18.

14 Casutt M, Seifert B, Pasch T, et al. Factors influencing the individual effects of blood transfusions on oxygen delivery and oxygen consumption. Crit Care Med. 1999;27:2194–200.

15 Suttner S, Piper SN, Kumle B, et al. The influence of allogeneic red blood cell transfusion compared with 100% oxygen ventilation on systemic oxygen transport and skeletal muscle oxygen tension after cardiac surgery. Anesth Analg. 2004;99: 2–11.

16 Napolitano LM, Kurek S, Luchette FA, et al. Clinical practice guideline: red blood cell transfusion in adult trauma and critical care. J Trauma. 2009;67:1439–42.

17 Almac E, Ince C. The impact of storage on red cell function in blood transfusion. Best Pract Res Clin Anaesthesiol. 2007;21:195–208.

18 Carson JL, Duff A, Poses RM et al. Effect of anaemia and cardiovascular disease on surgical mortality and morbidity. Lancet. 1996;348:1055–60.

19 Mudumbai SC, Cronkite R, Hu KU, et al. Association of admission hematocrit with 6-month and 1-year mortality in intensive care unit patients. Transfusion. 2011;51:2148–59.

20 Marik PE, Corwin HL Efficacy of red blood cell transfusion in the critically ill: a systematic review of the literature. Crit Care Med. 2008;36:2667–2674.

21 Snyder-Ramos SA, Mohnle P, Weng YS, et al. The ongoing variability in blood transfusion practices in cardiac surgery. Transfusion. 2008;48:1284–99.

22 Koch CG, Li L, Duncan AI, et al. Morbidity and mortality risk associated with red blood cell and blood-component transfusion in isolated coronary artery bypass grafting. Crit Care Med. 2006;34:1608–16.

23 Surgenor SD, Kramer RS, Olmstead EM, et al. The association of perioperative red blood cell transfusions and decreased long-term survival after cardiac surgery. Anesth Analg. 2009;108:1741–6.

24 Vincent JL. Indications for blood transfusions: Too complex to base on a single number? Ann Intern Med. 2012;157:71–2.

25 Sakr Y, Chierego M, Piagnerelli M, et al. Microvascular response to red blood cell transfusion in patients with severe sepsis. Crit Care Med. 2007;35:1639–44.

26 Vincent JL, Rhodes A, Perel A, et al. Clinical review: Update on hemodynamic monitoring–a consensus of 16. Crit Care. 2011;15:229.

27 Rivers EP, Ander DS, Powell D. Central venous oxygen saturation monitoring in the critically ill patient. Curr Opin Crit Care. 2001;7:204–11.

28 Yalavatti GS, De Backer D, Vincent JL. Assessment of cardiac index in anemic patients. Chest. 2000;118:782–7.

29 De Backer D. Lactic acidosis. Intensive Care Med. 2003;29:699–702.

30 Nichol AD, Egi M, Pettila V, et al. Relative hyperlactatemia and hospital mortality in critically ill patients: a retrospective multi-centre study. Crit Care. 2010;14:R25.

31 Jansen TC, van Bommel J, Schoonderbeek FJ, et al. Early lactate-guided therapy in intensive care unit patients: a multicenter, open-label, randomized controlled trial. Am J Respir Crit Care Med. 2010;182:752–61.

32 Nichol A, Bailey M, Egi M, et al. Dynamic lactate indices as predictors of outcome in critically ill patients. Crit Care. 2011;15:R242.

33 Levy B, Gawalkiewicz P, Vallet B, et al. Gastric capnometry with air-automated tonometry predicts outcome in critically ill patients. Crit Care Med. 2003;31:474–80.

34 Palizas F, Dubin A, Regueira T, et al. Gastric tonometry versus cardiac index as resuscitation goals in septic shock: a multicenter, randomized, controlled trial. Crit Care. 2009;13:R44.

35 Gomersall CD, Joynt GM, Freebairn RC et al. Resuscitation of critically ill patients based on the results of gastric tonometry: a prospective, randomized, controlled trial. Crit Care Med. 2000;28:607–14.

36 Sadaka F, Aggu-Sher R, Krause K et al. The effect of red blood cell transfusion on tissue oxygenation and microcirculation in severe septic patients. Ann Intensive Care. 2011;1:46.

37 Creteur J, Neves AP, Vincent JL. Near-infrared spectroscopy technique to evaluate the effects of red blood cell transfusion on tissue oxygenation. Crit Care. 2009;13 Suppl 5:S11.

38 Weinberg JA, Maclennan PA, Vandromme-Cusick MJ, et al. Microvascular response to red blood cell transfusion in trauma patients. Shock. 2012;37:276–81.

39 Fowler RA, Berenson M. Blood conservation in the intensive care unit. Crit Care Med. 2003;31:S715–S720.

40 Tinmouth AT, McIntyre LA, Fowler RA. Blood conservation strategies to reduce the need for red blood cell transfusion in critically ill patients. CMAJ. 2008;178:49–57.

41 Smoller BR, Kruskall MS, Horowitz GL. Reducing adult phlebotomy blood loss with the use of pediatric-sized blood collection tubes. Am J Clin Pathol. 1989;91:701–3.

42 Sanchez-Giron F, varez-Mora F. Reduction of blood loss from laboratory testing in hospitalized adult patients using small-volume (pediatric) tubes. Arch Pathol Lab Med. 2008;132:1916–19.

43 Mukhopadhyay A, Yip HS, Prabhuswamy D, et al. The use of a blood conservation device to reduce red blood cell transfusion requirements: a before and after study. Crit Care. 2010;14:R7.

44 Rickard CM, Couchman BA, Schmidt SJ, et al. A discard volume of twice the deadspace ensures clinically accurate arterial blood gases and electrolytes and prevents unnecessary blood loss. Crit Care Med. 2003;31:1654–8.

45 Merlani P, Garnerin P, Diby M, et al. Quality improvement report: Linking guideline to regular feedback to increase appropriate requests for clinical tests: blood gas analysis in intensive care. BMJ. 2001;323:620–4.

46 Kumwilaisak K, Noto A, Schmidt UH, et al. Effect of laboratory testing guidelines on the utilization of tests and order entries in a surgical intensive care unit. Crit Care Med. 2008;36:2993–9.

47 Harber CR, Sosnowski KJ, Hegde RM. Highly conservative phlebotomy in adult intensive care–a prospective randomized controlled trial. Anaesth Intensive Care. 2006;34:434–7.

48 Mann MC, Votto J, Kambe J, et al. Management of the severely anemic patient who refuses transfusion: lessons learned during the care of a Jehovah's Witness. Ann Intern Med. 1992;117:1042–8.

49 Russell WC, Greer R, Harper NJ. The effect of neuromuscular blockade on oxygen supply, consumption, and total chest compliance in patients with high oxygen requirements undergoing mechanical ventilation. Anaesth Intensive Care. 2002;30:192–7.

50 Hayes MA, Timmins AC, Yau EH, et al. Elevation of systemic oxygen delivery in the treatment of critically ill patients. N Engl J Med. 1994;330:1717–22.

51 Gattinoni L, Brazzi L, Pelosi P, et al. A trial of goal-oriented hemodynamic therapy in critically ill patients. SvO2 Collaborative Group. N Engl J Med. 1995;333: 1025–32.

52 Lobo SM, Salgado PF, Castillo VG, et al. Effects of maximizing oxygen delivery on morbidity and mortality in high-risk surgical patients. Crit Care Med. 2000; 28:3396–404.

53 McLoughlin PL, Cope TM, Harrison JC. Hyperbaric oxygen therapy in the management of severe acute anaemia in a Jehovah's witness. Anaesthesia. 1999;54:891–5.

54 Lamy ML, Daily EK, Brichant JF, et al. Randomized trial of diaspirin cross-linked hemoglobin solution as an alternative to blood transfusion after cardiac surgery. The DCLHb Cardiac Surgery Trial Collaborative Group. Anesthesiology. 2000;92:646–56.

55 Gannon CJ, Napolitano LM. Severe anemia after gastrointestinal hemorrhage in a Jehovah's Witness: new treatment strategies. Crit Care Med. 2002;30:1893–5.

56 Lanzinger MJ, Niklason LE, Shannon M, et al. Use of hemoglobin raffimer for postoperative life-threatening anemia in a Jehovah's Witness. Can J Anaesth. 2005;52:369–73.

57 Natanson C, Kern SJ, Lurie P, et al. Cell-free hemoglobin-based blood substitutes and risk of myocardial infarction and death: a meta-analysis. JAMA. 2008; 299:2304–12.

58 Elmer J, Alam HB, Wilcox SR. Hemoglobin-based oxygen carriers for hemorrhagic shock. Resuscitation. 2012;83:285–92.

59 Creteur J, Vincent JL. Potential uses of hemoglobin-based oxygen carriers in critical care medicine. Crit Care Clin. 2009;25:311–24, Table.

60 Rogiers P, Zhang H, Leeman M, et al. Erythropoietin response is blunted in critically ill patients. Intensive Care Med. 1997;23:159–62.

61 Corwin HL, Gettinger A, Rodriguez RM, et al. Efficacy of recombinant human erythropoietin in the critically ill patient: a randomized, double-blind, placebo-controlled trial. Crit Care Med. 1999;27:2346–50.

62 Corwin HL, Gettinger A, Pearl RG, et al. Efficacy of recombinant human erythropoietin in critically ill patients: a randomized controlled trial. JAMA. 2002; 288:2827–35.

63 Corwin HL, Gettinger A, Fabian TC, et al. Efficacy and safety of epoetin alfa in critically ill patients. N Engl J Med. 2007;357:965–76.

64 Napolitano LM, Fabian TC, Kelly KM, et al. Improved survival of critically ill trauma patients treated with recombinant human erythropoietin. J Trauma. 2008; 65:285–97.

65 Retter A, Wyncoll D, Pearse R, et al. Guidelines on the management of anaemia and red cell transfusion in adult critically ill patients. Br J Haematol. 2013;160:445–64.

66 Pieracci FM, Henderson P, Rodney JR, et al. Randomized, double-blind, placebo-controlled trial of effects of enteral iron supplementation on anemia and risk of infection during surgical critical illness. Surg Infect (Larchmt). 2009;10:9–19.

CHAPTER 10

The changing transfusion practice of neonatal and pediatric surgery

Pamela J. Kling[1] and Nicolas Jabbour[2]

[1]University of Wisconsin, Madison School of Medicine and Public Health, Madison, WI, USA
[2]Service de Chirurgie et Transplantation Abdominale, Cliniques Universitaires Saint-Luc, Bruxelles, Belgium

Introduction

About two-thirds of all erythrocyte transfusions have traditionally been administered in the perioperative period [1]. In 1988, an NIH Consensus Development Panel reported it inappropriate to utilize single perioperative transfusion criteria of hemoglobin (Hb) less than 100 g/L and recommended ongoing study of transfusion criteria [1]. A practice parameter developed by the Task Force of the College of American Pathologists agreed a single Hb value was arbitrary and inappropriate [2]. Although without prospective data, experts recommend a Hb transfusion threshold of 80 g/L in surgical patients without risk factors for tissue ischemia, and 100 g/L in those at risk for ischemia [3]. In current clinical, and specifically surgical practice, very few randomized clinical trials examining transfusion triggers are found [4, 5]. In pediatric surgery patients, even less information is understood about transfusion. In pediatric patients, severe anemia is seen in prematurity and in several disease processes. Against this background, we will provide an overview of the special considerations relevant to transfusions in the pediatric population and describe the application of strategies to curtail need for transfusions in children undergoing surgery.

Transfusion considerations specific to the pediatric population

Other than in premature infants, most of our understanding of transfusion requirements and outcomes in children has been extrapolated from the

---

Transfusion-Free Medicine and Surgery, Second Edition. Edited by Nicolas Jabbour.
© 2014 John Wiley & Sons, Ltd. Published 2014 by John Wiley & Sons, Ltd.

Table 10.1 Limitations of treating anemia in neonates compared to adults.

	Neonates	Adults
Circulating blood volume	40–320 mL	≥3500 mL
Hematocrit on Admission	36–46%	36–46%
Phlebotomy loss first 24 hours in ICU	3–10 mL	12–28 mL
First 24 hr phlebotomy in ICU as% blood volume	0.9–25%	≤0.8%
Weekly phlebotomy in ICU as% blood volume	6–50%	≤2.5%

adult literature. While common ground does exist between these two populations of patients, children present with some unique problems related to anemia. Children, for example, have proportionately smaller circulating blood volumes compared to phlebotomy loss (Table 10.1).

Transfusion in infants is associated with some potential drawbacks unique to children, such as a possible role in promoting retinopathy of prematurity or promoting necrotizing enterocolitis [6–9]. Additional microbial infectious complications may be more serious in children with long life spans, because clinical manifestations may occur many years after transfusion. Lastly, several interventions, including the use of artificial oxygen carriers, or 'blood substitutes,' are inadequately studied in pediatric patients. For these reasons, a comprehensive knowledge of the problem of anemia and steps that can effectively restrict transfusion requirements is necessary. In adult ICU patients, restrictive transfusion practices (at low Hb thresholds) lead to improved survival [10], leading investigators to design randomized, prospective studies in both NICUs and PICUs examining transfusion triggers (*as described below*). However, interpreting these prospective studies in the subset of pediatric surgical patients is problematic, because study designs sometimes allowed transfusion decisions to be made at the discretion of the surgeons, outside of the acuity or postnatal age guidelines in the larger studies.

Strategies to limit need or transfusion

Use of recombinant human erythropoietin

In the pediatric population, anemia can be caused by a variety of reasons, including phlebotomy blood loss, but the most common is prematurity. A combination of the need to support rapid growth in the neonatal period and the shorter half-life of neonatal red blood cells (RBCs) in comparison to adult cells places an enormous demand on the neonatal marrow. Plasma erythropoietin (EPO) levels are lower in the neonate compared to older children with comparable degrees of anemia, and the rise in EPO levels is relatively flat with falling Hb levels [11]. Using rHuEPO for anemia of prematurity has a sound physiological basis. Studies have shown reductions in packed RBC transfusions [12–15], but few studies have shown complete elimination of transfusions [16]. Numerous studies have examined optimization of response to rHuEPO by altering the timing of therapy and nutritional support during rHuEPO [15–17]. In a stepwise fashion, published work has refined dosing, dosing interval, nutritional support and has found that early dosing before 8 days of life may be associated with severe retinopathy of prematurity [18], but has shown rHuEPO to be otherwise safe, without identifiable adverse effects.

Although few randomized trials have been performed, using rHuEPO has been extended to the perioperative period in an effort to limit transfusions. Table 10.2 summarizes the evidence for efficacy of rHuEPO in pediatric patients, showing which indications are supported by controlled, retrospective, or descriptive reports. Descriptive reports suggest that rHuEPO may facilitate autologous donation of blood in children undergoing caniosynostosis and orthopedic repairs [19, 20]. rHuEPO may be effective for autologous donation in children weighing as little as 6–0 kg [20]. Adolescents may safely donate more autologous blood in a single setting (up to 20% of their blood volume), decreasing costs [19].

Table 10.2 Evidence for efficacy of rhEPO in decreasing erythrocyte transfusions in pediatric patients.

Indication	U/kg/wk	Randomized/ Controlled Trials	Retrospective/ Descriptive Reports
Anemia of Prematurity	300–1500	++	±
Renal Failure	50–150	++	±
Oncologic Disease	450–1200	±	±
Autologous Marrow Transplant	900–1400	±	±
Allogenic Marrow Transplant	1050–1400	±	±
Cardiac Surgery (pre & post)	300–1200	+	±
Pre-op Autologous Transfusion	200–900	*	±
Pre-op to raise Hct	200–300	±	+
Post-op	450–900	±	*
Burn Patients	50–350	*	±
PICU Patients	900–1500	*	±

Key for studies: ++ indicates multiple randomized/controlled trials supporting efficacy at decreasing transfusions, + indicates one randomized/controlled trial supporting efficacy, ± under randomized/controlled trials indicates equal number supporting and refuting efficacy, ± under retrospective/descriptive studies indicates data supporting rhEPO efficacy, * indicates no study found in that category.

Because collection and storage of preoperative autologous blood donation increases the elective surgical expense, preoperative rhEpo therapy to increase preoperative hematocrit has also been studied [21, 22]. In a retrospective review of their experience in all adolescent orthopedic surgery, preoperative rhEPO resulted in higher preoperative hematocrit and less allogeneic transfusions (4%), compared to those without (24%) preoperative rhEPO [23]. A study of 20 neonates undergoing general surgical procedures, randomized to placebo (n = 10) or rHuEPO (n = 10) for 2 weeks, found rHuEPO stimulated higher reticulocytes than placebo, with stable hematocrit percentages, despite a trend for greater phlebotomy losses in the rHuEPO group [24].

However, the use of rHuEPO in children is associated with some concern. Stimulation by pharmacologic doses of rHuEPO commits iron to erythropoiesis, thereby limiting its availability to nonerythopoietic needs, such as the brain. However, at least one study refutes this, finding serum EPO levels correlated with better neurodevelopment [25]. The theoretical risk that the combined administration of rHuEPO and iron can lead to oxidative injury and may increase retinopathy of prematurity may be true if rHuEPO is given in the first week of life [18], although transfusions may also be linked to retinopathy of prematurity [26]. Use of alternative erythropoietic stimulating agents may also be beneficial in infants and children, but are only now being studied. There remains a lack of consensus on the use of rHuEPO in the pediatric surgical population, although there is increasing use in the critically ill, perioperative child.

Autotransfusion strategies

Acute normovolemic hemodilution (ANH) procedures have been reported in children. ANH removes whole blood from the patient immediately before the surgical procedure and collects it in anticoagulant [27–32]. Depending on patient size, between 1 and 4 units of blood can be collected. During donation, circulating blood volume is maintained with acellular fluid (hetastarch or crystalloid) [29], and compensatory mechanisms, including increased preload, decreased afterload, and increased heart rate help improve cardiac output and maintain perfusion. Although most studies evaluating ANH are performed in adults, one controlled study of adolescent spine surgery showed that 79% of the non-hemodilution patients received transfusions, while 37% received transfusions in the ANH group [33]. An expert panel of the NIH recommends its use [31], while a Consensus Conference on Autologous Transfusion does not recommend its implementation [34]. Many studies utilizing AHN are suboptimal, utilizing historical controls or not defining transfusion criteria. A meta-analysis of 24 prospective, randomized trials of ANH in adults found less exposure to blood and exposure to a smaller number of units, but this finding did not hold up with inclusion of trials with strict transfusion criteria [35]. However, this meta-analysis excluded any studies treating children younger than 18 years. In children, plateletphoresis and plasmaphoresis techniques may enhance the collection of clotting factors in AHN techniques, but these methods have not been systematically studied [36]. Modification of ANH techniques by utilizing a hetastarch and balanced salt/lactate solution or a fluorocarbon emulsion shows promise for optimizing AHN techniques in adults [37, 38].

The application of ANH in the pediatric population has been tempered due to several legitimate concerns. The ability of children to tolerate dilutional coagulopathy from ANH is more limited, especially in neonates due to low baseline levels of clotting factors [39]. In our study on the application of ANH to multiple Jehovah's Witness children [40, 41], all patients developed dilutional coagulopathy as evidenced by laboratory tests. However, whether this finding is a biochemical aberrancy or has clinical relevance is unclear. In one study that included pediatric patients undergoing cardiac surgery for cyanotic heart disease [42], extreme ANH was associated with markedly abnormal laboratory clotting parameters, but not increased clinical bleeding. Another concern with ANH, especially in infants, is the high fraction of HbF resulting in leftward shift of the oxyhemoglobin curve, at least theoretically impairing end organ oxygen delivery. Lastly, while most studies on ANH in children have examined global physiological effects, specific organ function abnormalities have not been individually evaluated. A recent randomized study found similar neurological examinations and mental developmental index scores in infants undergoing cardiopulmonary bypass (CPB) at lower vs. higher Hct (21.5% vs. 27.8%); the lower Hct group had lower psychomotor developmental index scores [43]. Hence, although ANH is a promising strategy for limiting transfusion in children, evidence supporting routine use of ANH is still lacking.

Other autotransfusion strategies such as autologous blood donation have also been evaluated in children. Autologous blood donation results in decreased donor blood use during spinal fusion in children and adolescents [44]. However, in very small children, the technique of autologous donation can be technically challenging and cumbersome. In premature and term neonates with prenatally diagnosed surgical anomalies, collecting cord blood for perioperative autologous transfusion has a moderately low infection rate (<9%), and when not infected provided 50–75% of the PRBCs needed during the stay [45, 46].

Application of hemostatic agents

Blood loss is the most frequent indication for transfusion and hence strategies to limit blood loss are bound to significantly impact transfusion requirements. Following the advent of blood component fractionation, the use of acellular plasma, platelets or plasma coagulation factors such as cryoprecipitate to facilitate clotting has been widely accepted. Recently, several new nonplasma compounds have been introduced for facilitating coagulation. Antifibrinolytic agents, such as aminocaproic acid or tranexamic acid and aprotinin, are currently in widespread clinical use. Aminocaproic acid binds to plasminogen and prevents its breakdown to plasmin by tissue plasminogen activator, thereby stabilizing the clot. Similarly, aprotinin is a serine protease inhibitor that directly inhibits plasmin. Both agents have shown reductions in blood loss in many types of surgical patients [47] and should be studied more carefully in children. Desmopressin, a synthetic analog of the antidiuretic hormone, increases the release of von Willebrand factor from its storage sites on endothelial cells and enhances platelet function, thereby facilitating hemostasis. Conjugated estrogens have been used in children with uremia-related hemorrhage to induce clotting.

Recombinant activated factor VII (rFVIIa) is a synthetic protein derived from transfected hamster kidney cells that is increasingly gaining popularity amongst clinicians to treat reticent coagulopathy. Although its use has been approved only for hemophiliacs with antibodies against factors VIII and IX, several off-label indications are being reported. It has been used successfully in adult trauma patients, hemorrhage associated with liver failure, spontaneous intracranial hemorrhage, and for congenital factor VII deficiency. Recently, case reports have documented its safe and effective application in neonates with liver failure undergoing liver biopsy [48]. Given that rFVIIa acts by binding to activated platelets, its hemostatic effect is largely isolated to the site of active bleeding and is hence a very attractive therapeutic compound. Pilot studies have also evaluated the use of factor XIII in adult CPB and bone marrow transplant patients, though it is not currently approved for clinical use.

Perioperative approaches

Attention to perioperative factors and improved surgical technique can significantly decrease surgical blood losses [49–51]. Strategies for blood conservation include calculation of precise transfusion requirements, preoperative review of specific transfusion criteria for each patient, rehearsal of the operative procedure, shortening operative time and delaying the timing of transfusion as long as possible [50]. Development of specific instruments that minimize surgical blood loss is ongoing [51, 52], but is well behind that in adult surgery. Endoscopic, as compared to open, procedures have shown potential to decrease blood loss in craniofacial surgery [53].

Controlled studies show that hypotensive anesthesia and cell-saving procedures are safe and decrease blood loss during pediatric orthopedic procedures [54], although there is a paucity of controlled studies in other pediatric surgical populations. The use of intraoperative cell salvage (ICS) in the pediatric population was hampered until recently by the lack of appropriate size devices. The introduction of small bowl sizes of cell-saver devices has increased the feasibility of ICS in very small children. Moderate to deep hypothermia can increase the amount of dissolved oxygen and decrease tissue oxygen demands during surgery, especially when hemodilution is being utilized. The use of hyperoxic ventilation strategy in one study offered an increased safety margin allowing for an extreme level of hemodilution to 3.0 g/dl [55].

Monitoring devices within central lines that perform in-line point-of-care blood testing can minimize blood loss pre-, intra- and postoperatively [56, 57]. These devices have shown reliable results in small premature infants, with a decreased blood volume drawn (e.g. whole blood electrolytes and blood gas from 250 ml per test to <25 ml). Studies have yet to show decreased transfusion requirements in perioperative children with these in-line devices.

Physician awareness

A large body of evidence has now confirmed the safety of lower Hb levels even in critically ill children. There may be advantages to lower Hb thresholds. Children undergoing RBC transfusion may take more resources, have longer ICU stay, more days in oxygen and with mechanical ventilation, and more days with vasoactive agent infusions than those not transfused [58]. Results such as these put traditional transfusion cutoff points and arbitrary single-point triggers under question. Physician awareness can thus increase the support for conservative transfusion practices and limit unnecessary transfusions.

The single most important contributing factor to the transfusion practice in any setting is the physician force. Several studies have documented marked variations in physician practice patterns resulting in dramatically different transfusion thresholds [59]. Transfusion medicine is commonly inadequately covered in training [60]. However, more senior physicians may have poorer knowledge of evidence-based transfusion medicine than residents, a finding problematic because the strongest impetus for timing of transfusion by physicians-in-training was the influence of attending physician [61]. Published literature confirms the importance of focused physician education and practice audit as a transfusion-limiting strategy [62]. The most successful methods utilize a combination of education, real-time feedback, administrative control and pharmacological support. Educational programs alter physician transfusion practices [63]. Further, studies have shown that hospitals tend to develop transfusion strategies that are ingrained within the institution and differ little between physicians at that center [64]. Hence, the institution of hospital-wide administrative tools has been evaluated and appears to improve adherence to transfusion guidelines [65]. Additionally, studies show that blood loss, expressed per kilogram body weight is directly associated with RBC transfusions in both PICU and NICU patients [14, 66], so efforts to employ microsampling for blood draws, to eliminate scheduled labs, and to restrict ordering to necessary labs would decrease transfusions in surgical patients.

Applications of transfusion-limiting strategies to specific surgical situations

Neonatal surgery

The most common surgical emergency observed in premature infants is necrotizing enterocolitis (NEC) [67]. In NEC, anemia is common secondary to bleeding associated with thrombocytopenia and disseminated intravascular coagulation (DIC), as well as hemolytic anemia and iatrogenic blood loss [68–71]. In NEC, bleeding may occur as intraluminal, intraperitoneal, intracranial and/or intrapulmonary hemorrhage [71]. Infants with NEC are commonly administered platelet concentrates, coagulation factors, and erythrocytes [71, 72]. The incidence of thrombocytopenia is 65–90% in NEC and 55–80% in any neonatal infection [71–73]. In severe infections and shock, the host defense system disturbs the equilibrium of the coagulation and fibrinolytic systems [74]. DIC, which occurs in 40% of premature infants with NEC and 17% of infants with sepsis, is generally treated with coagulation factors [71]. Although blood loss from DIC and thrombocytopenia is so common in NEC or neonatal infections, a trial of rhEPO in NEC has not been performed.

Premature neonates commonly undergo surgical procedures and pediatric surgeons have long been pioneers in techniques to minimize blood loss and transfusions. Because allogeneic transfusions are commonly given to premature neonates, the potential of autologous cord blood collection at delivery has been investigated, but is limited in practice, due to technical, financial and infection concerns [75, 76]. Adequate volumes of autologous cord blood can be collected at delivery and stored for later transfusion [77–79], and in premature and term neonates with prenatally diagnosed surgical anomalies, collecting cord blood for perioperative autologous transfusion has a low infection rate (<9%) and provides 50–75% of the blood needed [45, 46]. A better alternative may be delaying clamping of the umbilical cord at delivery to increase blood volume and hematocrit percentages in premature and term neonates [80–82]. The practice of delayed clamping or milking of cords in premature and term infants is increasing in frequency in the US and it is likely beneficial for prenatally diagnosed surgical newborns.

Cardiac surgery

Most cardiac surgery procedures performed in neonatal and pediatric patients are those treating congenital heart defects. These children are commonly transfused perioperatively. In one study, the strongest predictor of transfusion in children undergoing open heart surgery was the patient's age [49]. Children undergoing cardiac surgery at <1 year of age received a mean transfusion number of 6, compared to 2 in those >1 year of age [49]. Procedures to decrease blood exposure have been sought, including reducing duration or eliminating time spent on the circuit [83]. Less invasive transcatheter cardiac procedures could eliminate, decrease or delay surgical cardiac procedures in neonates [84]. In addition to the classic balloon atrial septostomy, valvulotomies, balloon dilation of vessels (including coarctation of the aorta), stenting of vessels, coil embolization of vessels (including the patent ductus arteriosis), and biopsies have all been performed by catheter procedures in neonates [84]. Although not yet shown to reduce blood loss, video-assisted thorascopic ligation of the patent ductus arteriosis in premature infants as small as 500 g has resulted in less surgical trauma and faster recovery times [83]. Video-assisted thorascopic techniques have been utilized to divide vascular rings, treat chylothoraces, and plicate the diaphragm in neonates [83].

Techniques used for transfusion avoidance in cardiac surgery include preoperative and postoperative rhEPO therapy, bloodless priming of the CPB circuit, decreasing circuit volume to as low as 95 mL, using smaller pumps, hypothermic, hypotensive anesthesia, monitoring cerebral perfusion with NIRS, returning all blood immediately following bypass, and transfusing with cell-savers [85–87]. Case reports of transfusion avoidance with cardiac surgery in Jehovah's Witnesses, including a 5.3 kg, 14-week-old with cor triatriatum [85], 3.55 kg neonate with tetralogy of Fallot [88], 2.96 kg neonate with hypoplastic aortic arch [87].

A noncontrolled series of 14 cardiac cases in Jehovah's Witnesses ≥6 years of age reported bloodless congenital heart repairs, with lowest hematocrit 15% during perfusion and 16% postoperative [89]. In another report of Jehovah's Witnesses, only 4 of 48 children ≤20 kg undergoing cardiac surgery received perioperative transfusion [90], with a similar ICU outcome to historical controls whose CPB circuits were primed with blood [90]. A prospective controlled study of pre- and postoperative rhEPO therapy was performed in children undergoing CPB surgery (mean age 5.5 years) [86], with transfusion avoided in all those receiving high dose rhEPO, in 91% of moderate dose rhEPO and 69% of those controls (oral iron only) [86]. A recent study described 23 neonates of 4–17 days (1.7–4.2 kg) that underwent bloodless priming of the CPB circuit for transposition of the great vessels, with transfusion threshold of Hb 7 g/dL, showed avoidance of intraoperative transfusion in 17, and 6 needed no transfusion at all [91]. No difference in outcome between those transfused and not transfused was observed, with preoperative Hct being the greatest predictor of transfusion. Another series described miniaturization of circuit eliminating intraoperative blood in 6/13 neonatal CPB cases, including one child at 1.7 kg [92]. Even those with blood-primed circuits report less blood and bicarbonate use in miniaturized circuits [93].

Utilization of blood salvaged from the extracorporeal membrane circuit after cardiac surgery may contribute a significant autologous transfusion volume to the pediatric patient postoperatively (50–150 mL of blood with a Hct of 52.7 ± 9.7%) [94]. Additionally, use of an autotransfusion technique to replace post-operative blood loss through mediastinal drains in pediatric cardiac surgery patients decreases postoperative blood transfusions [95].

Orthopedic surgery

Much work has been done to minimize blood loss in pediatric orthopedic procedures and several retrospective descriptive reports were found [54]. One matched, controlled study was found that showed hypotensive anesthesia decreased blood loss and transfusion administration in spinal fusion procedures, compared to control [96]. A well-designed study using closely matched historical controls showed that cell saving procedures and autologous transfusion may also decrease blood loss and transfusion requirements [97]. In neuromuscular scoliosis, preoperative rHuEPO (n = 35) to 26 non rHuEPO patients showed increased pre- and postoperative Hct percentages, but did not decrease transfusions [98]. In idiopathic scoliosis, preoperative rHuEPO decreased donor transfusions from 23.5% to 3.9% [98]. Although needing prospective study, techniques to minimize blood loss, used in combination with pre- and/or postoperative rhEPO therapy should work better than either strategy alone [54].

Craniosynostosis surgery

Open craniosynostosis surgical procedures are associated with massive surgical blood losses, with reports describing preoperative rHuEPO and blood-conservation techniques including hypervolemic hemodilution, ANH and controlled hypotension being reported. Because most open craniosynostosis repairs occur in children ≤ 1 year of age, transfusion rates are commonly 100% [99]. By careful attention to surgical blood loss, estimated red cell mass, and transfusion criteria, precise control of transfusion volumes can be achieved [100]. One descriptive craniosynostosis repair report utilizing preoperative rhEPO therapy, preoperative autologous blood donation, ANH and intraoperative blood salvage achieved a 15% allogeneic transfusion rate [20]. We performed a retrospective chart review of patients undergoing craniosynostosis repair by the same plastic surgeon at the Children's Hospital of Los Angeles between January 2002 and January 2003. A subgroup of patients (10/19) had consented to preoperative rHuEPO for 4 weeks. In addition, hemodilution techniques were used in eight of ten rHuEPO patients and no controls, while controlled hypotension was used in nine of ten and six of nine patients, respectively. rHuEPO increased preoperative RBC mass by 28%, lowered transfusion rate (4/10 vs. 9/9) and total volume transfused (154 mL vs. 421 mL, p < 0.03). Discharge Hct percentages were not significantly different between the groups. Another recent series described endoscopically treated sagittal craniosynostosis procedures (n = 47) with 29 mL mean blood loss, 6.4% transfusion rate and shorter hospital stay (1.2 days), compared to 42 open surgeries, with mean 218 mL blood loss, with all receiving transfusion and hospital stay of 3.9 days [53].

Hepatic surgery

Blood loss during hepatic procedures can be extremely high. In an early report of blood transfusion in liver transplantation, a median of 11 transfusions was given to 49 pediatric liver transplants [101]. Attention to detail can limit blood loss in liver transplants to 37–75 mL, instead of mean blood losses in the 130–165 mL range [102]. In liver surgeries, hepatic inflow occlusion techniques are commonly employed to minimize blood loss. In hepatic inflow occlusion, the hepatic artery, portal vein and hepatic vein of the affected segment are ligated before the hepatic parenchyma is resected [103, 104]. Although no controlled studies have been performed, blood loss with liver tumor resection in children can be minimized with hypotensive, ANH anesthesia, with autotransfusion via cell saver [27]. Only three of eight children undergoing liver resections received any allogenic blood and those transfused received low (100–125 ml) volumes. Further, ultrasonically activated harmonic scalpels may improve hemostasis [105], but this has not undergone systematic study.

We have recently published our experience with bloodless live-donor liver transplantation (LDLT) in two Jehovah's Witness children, 6 months and 3 years of age [40]. Both children had end-stage liver disease secondary to biliary atresia. The first had undergone a Kasai procedure followed by rapidly deteriorating liver function and gastrointestinal (GI) bleeding. The second patient had previously received a live-donor liver at another institution that was lost to chronic rejection. Using rHuEPO preoperatively, Hct percentages were augmented to 37.1% and 31.5%, facilitating the removal of 170 cc and 250 cc of blood at the beginning of surgery for ANH. ICS recovered 90 cc and 40 cc of the blood loss. Intraoperative coagulopathy was managed by the use of aprotinin, desmopressin and rFVIIa. Despite an average operative duration of 9.25 h and estimated blood loss of 92 cc, the immediate postoperative Hct was 29% in both children. They recovered uneventfully, had an uncomplicated postoperative course and are well at $2\frac{1}{2}$-year follow-up.

Burn surgery

Transfusions are common in burn patients. Pediatric patients (mean age 6.4 ± 1.2 years) with burns covering greater than 60% total body surface area commonly receive and tolerate massive (4.1 ± 1.7 units) transfusion of whole blood for near-total burn excision procedures [106]. Use of rhEPO may decrease transfusion numbers in this population. Thermal injury is associated with lower serum EPO levels, such that rhEPO should be effective at stimulating erythropoiesis [107]. Several case reports describe prevention of erythrocyte transfusions with rhEPO therapy in burn patients [108, 109], including pediatric burn patients [110, 111]. Additional strategies to decrease blood loss in burn patients include injection of adrenaline at donor site and excised wound, utilization of tourniquets for limb procedures [112]. With these conservative techniques, transfusions can be decreased from 3.3 ± 3.1 units per case to 0.1 ± 0.3 units per case.

Trauma surgery

Based on the American Association for the Surgery of Trauma's Organ Injury Scaling System, strategies to decrease the number of acute surgeries in trauma patients has been investigated [113]. As surgical blood losses are commonly massive, identification of the best surgical candidates can eliminate transfusions. A retrospective review of hemodynamically stable patients with blunt hepatic injury, including children, showed that a non-operative strategy including intense observation resulted in less surgery, fewer abdominal infections, decreased hospital stays and fewer transfusions [114]. A pediatric series showed that of 27 patients, 22 qualified for nonoperative management of hepatic injury, while 5 received operative care [115]. Only 4.5% of the non- operative group received transfusions as opposed to 60% of the operative group. Nonoperative management of ruptured spleen secondary to blunt trauma has also been studied in children. In a Turkish study, 56 of 84 children were assigned a nonoperative initial strategy and 57% of these ultimately required transfusion, while 100% of the operative group were transfused [116]. An additional retrospective analysis of nonoperative management of ruptured spleen showed that 78 of 173 adult and pediatric patients met prospective criteria (lower severity score) and were monitored [117]. Only 2 of 78 required surgery with the surgical patients averaging 13 transfusions each and 3/4 of the nonoperative patients avoiding transfusions.

Anemia of prematurity

Premature neonates are among the most frequently transfused group of hospitalized patients [118]. As in adults, Hb and Hct are imprecise measures of tissue oxygenation in neonates, but are commonly utilized to determine timing of erythrocyte transfusion in neonates [119]. In 1989, premature infants with birthweight <1500 g received 8–10 transfusions during initial hospitalization, while currently 2 transfusions per infant are reported [68, 120, 121]. A lowering of the Hb or Hct values that trigger transfusions in premature infants has been observed [122]. Lower patient acuity scores, lower phlebotomy losses, and delayed cord clamping at delivery, or milking of the cord are linked to reduced transfusions [12, 68, 69, 80, 82, 123]. Advances in perinatal care have resulted in improved stability of premature neonates and are therefore associated with fewer transfusion numbers [121], but clinical transfusion practices vary widely [69, 75, 124]. The 1995 US Multicenter rhEPO trial by Shannon et al. is noteworthy for both its use of rhEPO and its adherence to conservative consensus transfusion guidelines [125], including those undergoing surgery. After slight revision [2, 14, 126], many centers have adopted these restrictive transfusion guidelines (see Tables 10.3 and 10.4). However, restrictive vs. liberal transfusions have also been directly addressed in controlled trials and summarized in a Cochrane review of five studies of low (restrictive) vs. high (liberal) Hb thresholds for transfusions in

Table 10.3 Neonatal RBC transfusion guidelines [14, 16, 126].

1 Transfuse if hematocrit ≤20% or hemoglobin <70 g/L and reticulocyte count ≤100 000/mm^3 (or ≤4%).
2 Transfuse if hematocrit ≤25% or hemoglobin <8 g/L and any of below present.
  (a) Increased severity of AB episodes
    ≥ 10 episodes in 24 hrs or
    ≥ 2 episodes requiring bag and mask over previous 24 hrs
  (b) Sustained tachycardia of ≥ 180 beats/minute for 24 hr or Sustained tachypnea of ≥ 80 breaths/minute for 24 hr by averaging monitor data.
  (c) Cessation of previously adequate weight gain (≥ 10g/d) over previous 4d.
  (d) Mild Respiratory Disease: Infants on 1/8 to 1/4 l O$_2$/min nasal cannula or 0.25 to s FIO$_2$ by hood, NPCPAP or ventilator.
3 Transfuse if hematocrit ≤30% or hemoglobin <100 g/L with moderate respiratory distress on > 1/4 l O$_2$/min nasal cannula or >0.35 FIO$_2$ on hood, NPCPAP or ventilator.
4 Transfuse if hematocrit ≤35% or hemoglobin <120 g/L in infants with "severe" respiratory disease requiring mechanical ventilation and FiO$_2$ ≥ 50.%
5 Acute blood loss with shock: blood replacement to reestablish adequate blood volume and hematocrit of 40%.
6 Transfuse if hematocrit ≤30% and undergoing surgery [12].

*FiO$_2$ indicates fraction of inspired oxygen, NCPAP indicates nasal continuous positive airway pressure.

Table 10.4 Alternative neonatal RBC transfusion guidelines [149].

Transfuse to maintain the blood HCT per each clinical situation:
  >40% (35 to 45%*) for severe cardiopulmonary disease
  >30% for moderate cardiopulmonary disease
  >30% for major surgery
  >25% (20 to 25%*) for symptomatic anemia
  >20% for asymptomatic anemia

*Reflects practices that vary among neonatologists. Thus, any value within range is acceptable for local practices.

premature infants and found no difference in short and medium-term outcomes [127]. Two studies, Bell et al. and Kirpalani et al., both showed no difference in initial morbidity, mortality, or primary neurodevelopmental outcomes, except that *post hoc* analysis in one found a trend for increased intraventricular hemorrhage or periventricular in the restrictive group [127–129]. However, follow-up studies of those children suggest a slight advantage in neurodevelopment in the restrictive transfusion criteria [130–133]. Additionally, the study from Bell et al. showed no acute physiological benefit to the liberal transfusion [60]. Another advantage to restrictive transfusion may be lower incidence of chronic lung disease, associated with lower RBC volumes [134].

More than 50 studies treating anemia in premature infants with rhEPO have been reported, with meta-analysis of controlled clinical trials [135], concluding that rhEPO reduced erythrocyte transfusion by 11.0 mL/kg per neonate. Cochrane Reviews conclude that rHuEPO in premature infants reduces any transfusion, transfusion number per infant and total blood given [17, 18, 136] without increased morbidity, mortality or other clinical outcome, except a potential risk for increased retinopathy of prematurity if given in the first week of life. Although not yet standard of care for all premature infants, rhEPO therapy is used, especially in infants whose parents are practicing Jehovah's Witnesses [137, 138].

Anemia in the PICU

Studies have examined transfusions in PICU and postsurgical PICU patients. In a prospective observational study of 30 PICUs in North America, after adjusting for severity of illness, transfused PICU patients had longer mechanical ventilation, longer PICU stays, increased mortality, greater nosocomial infections, and greater evidence of cardiorespiratory dysfunction [66]. Avoidance of erythrocyte transfusion in intensive care units may be beneficial. In adult intensive care unit patients, mortality rates during hospitalization were lower in a restrictive transfusion strategy group [10]. In the postsurgical subset of the multicenter TRIPICU study, randomization of restrictive transfusions to liberal transfusions showed no differences in new or progressive multi-organ dysfunction syndrome, or 28 day mortality in PICU patients, but was beneficial in promoting a shorter mean stay in the restrictive (7.7 days) vs. liberal group (11.6 days) [139]. Use of rhEPO has received only limited study in PICUs, but transfusions were avoided by using rhEPO and close observation in Jehovah's Witness children experiencing massive gastrointestinal hemorrhage [2].

Anemia of oncologic disease

rhEPO has been used to treat anemia in children with hematopoietic malignancy [140–142]. Prospective, controlled rhEPO trials in patients with solid tumors showed higher hemoglobin levels and either a significant decrease or a trend towards lower transfusion requirements with treatment [141, 143]. Reports of rhEPO use in bone marrow or peripheral stem cell transplant resulted in avoidance of blood products in Jehovah's Witness adults [144, 145]. A prospective study of rhEPO in pediatric and adult bone marrow transplantation, rhEPO accelerates erythrocyte recovery and may decrease transfusion requirements after allogeneic transplant, but not autologous bone marrow transplant [146–148].

Conclusion

Transfusion therapy has a unique application in children, both in terms of the narrow safety margin of anemia in this population and the need to tailor therapy with long-term outcomes in mind. Despite these differences, prospective studies that can translate into guidelines for the management of anemia in children are lacking, and much of our current understanding is extrapolation from studies performed on adults. However, evidence supports the application to the pediatric population of several approaches that have been shown to curtail blood loss and limit transfusion requirements in adults. Ongoing investigations at furthering our knowledge of the hematopoietic machinery and coagulation cascades will certainly strengthen efforts aimed at solidifying the practice of transfusion management in children.

Acknowledgements

PJK would like to acknowledge funding by the NIH RO1HD057064, Thrasher Research Fund, Meriter Foundation and the Wisconsin Partnership Collaborative Health Sciences Program Grant.

References

1 NIH Consensus Development Panel. Perioperative red blood cell transfusion. JAMA. 1988;260:2700–3.
2 Simon TL, Alverson DC, AuBuchon J, Cooper ES, DeChristopher PJ, Glenn GC, Gould SA, Harrison CR, Milam JD, Moise KJ, Rodwig FR, Sherman LA, et al. Practice parameter for the use of red blood cell transfusions. Arch Pathol Lab Med. 1998;122:130–8.
3 Goodnough LT, Brecher ME, Kanter MH, AuBuchon JP. Transfusion Medicine. New Engl J Med. 1999;340:438–48,525–33.
4 Carson JL, Chen AY. In search of the transfusion trigger. Clin Orthopaedics. 1998;357:30–5.
5 Wilkinson KL, Brunskill SJ, Doree C, Hopewell S, Stanworth S, Murphy MF, Hyde C. The clinical effects of red blood cell transfusions: an overview of the randomized controlled trials evidence base. Transfusion Med Rev. 2011;25:145–55 e2.
6 Brooks SE, Marcus DM, Gillis D, Pirie E, Johnson MH, Bhatis J. The effect of blood transfusion protocol on retinopathy of prematurity: a prospective, randomized study. Pediatrics. 1999;104:514–8.
7 Agwu JC, Narchi H. In a preterm infant, does blood transfusion increase the risk of necrotizing enterocolitis? Arch Dis Child. 2005;90:102–3.
8 Singh R, Visintainer PF, Frantz ID, 3rd, Shah BL, Meyer KM, Favila SA, Thomas MS, Kent DM. Association of necrotizing enterocolitis with anemia and packed red blood cell transfusions in preterm infants. J Perinatol. 2011;31:176–82.

9 Paul DA, Mackley A, Novitsky A, Zhao Y, Brooks A, Locke RG. Increased odds of necrotizing enterocolitis after transfusion of red blood cells in premature infants. Pediatrics. 2011;127(4):635–41.

10 Hebert P, Wells G, Blajchman M, Marshall J, Martin C, Pagliarello G, Tweeddale M, Schweitzer I, Yetisir E. A multicenter, randomized, controlled clinical trial of transfusion requirements in critical care. The New England Journal of Medicine. 1999;340:409–68.

11 Brown MS, Phibbs RH, Garcia JF, Dallman PR. Postnatal changes in erythropoietin levels in untransfused premature infants. J Pediatr. 1983;103:612–17.

12 Shannon KM, Keith JM, Mentzer WC, Ehrenkranz RA, Brown MS, Widness JA, Gleason CA, Bifano EM, Millard DD, Davis CB, Stevenson DK, Alverson DC, et al. Recombinant human erythropoietin stimulates erythropoiesis and reduces erythrocyte transfusions in very low birth weight preterm infants. Pediatrics. 1995;95:1–10.

13 Maier RF, Obladen M, Mueller-Hansen I, Kattner E, Merz U, Arlettaz R, Gro-neck P, Hammer H, Koessel H, Verellen G, Stock G-J, Lacaze-Masmonteil T, et al. Early treatment with erythropoietin beta ameliorates anemia and reduces transfu-sion requirements in infants with birth weights below 1000 g. J Pediatr. 2002;141: 8–15.

14 Ohls RK, Ehrenkranz RA, Wright LL, Lemons JA, Korones SB, Stoll BJ, Stark AR, Shankaran S, Donovan EF, Close NC, Das A. The effects of early ery-thropoietin therapy on the transfusion requirements of preterm infants below 1250 grams birthweight: A multicenter, randomized controlled trial. Pediatrics. 2001;108:934–42.

15 Haiden N, Schwindt J, Cardona F, Berger A, Klebermass K, Wald M, Kohlhauser-Vollmuth C, Jilma B, Pollak A. Effects of a combined therapy of erythropoietin, iron, folate, and vitamin B12 on the transfusion requirements of extremely low birth weight infants. Pediatrics. 2006;118(5):2004–13.

16 Bishara N, Ohls RK. Current controversies in the management of the anemia of prematurity. Semin Perinatol. 2009;33(1):29–34.

17 Aher SM, Ohlsson A. Early versus late erythropoietin for preventing red blood cell transfusion in preterm and/or low birth weight infants. The Cochrane Col-laboration; 2010 [CD004865].

18 Ohlsson A, Aher S. Early erythropoietin for preventing red blood cell transfusion in preterm and/or low birth weight infants. The Cochrane Collaboration; 2010 [CD004863].

19 Erb T, Moller R, Christen P, Signer E, Frei FJ. Increased withdrawl volume per deposit for pre-opeartive autologous blood donation in adolescents. Vox Sangui-nis. 2000;78:231–4.

20 Velardi F, Chirico AD, Rocco CD, Fundaro C, Genovese O, Rendeli C, Menichella G, Serafini R, Piastra M, Viola L, Pietrini D, Pusateri A, et al. "No allogeneic blood transfusion" protocol for the surgical correction of craniosynostoses. Child's Ner-vous System. 1998;14:732–9.

21 Rothstein P, Roye D, Verdisco L, Stern L. Preoperative use of erythropoietin in an adolescent Jehovah's Witness. Anesthesiology. 1990;73:568–70.

22 Polley JW, Berkowitz RA, McDonald TB, Cohen M, Figeroa A, Penney DW. Craniomaxillofacial surgery in the Jehovah's Witness patient. Plastic and Reconstructive Surgery. 1994;93:1258–63.

23 Roye DP. Recombinant human erythropoietin and blood management in pediatric spine surgery. Orthopedics. 1999;22:s158–s60.

24 Bierer R, Roohi M, Peceny C, Ohls RK. Erythropoietin increases reticulocyte counts and maintains hematocrit in neonates requiring surgery. J Pediatr Surg. 2009;44:1540–5.

25 Bierer R, Peceny MC, Hartenberger CH, Ohls RK. Erythropoietin concentrations and neurodevelopmental outcome in preterm infants. Pediatrics. 2006;118(3):e635–40.

26 Dani C, Reali MF, Bertini G, Martelli E, Pezzati M, Rubaltelli FF. The role of blood transfusions and iron intake on retinopathy of prematurity. Early Human Develop. 2001;62:57–63.

27 Schaller RT, Schaller J, Furman EB. The advantages of hemodiluation anesthesia for major liver resection in children. J Pediatr Surg. 1984;19:705–10.

28 Schaller RT, Schaller J, Morgan A, Furman EB. Hemodilution anesthesia: A valuable aid to major cancer surgery. Am J Surg. 1983;146:79–84.

29 Stehling L, Zauder HL. Acute normovolemic hemodilution. Transfusion. 1991;31:857–68.

30 Roye DP, Rothstein M, Rickert JB, Verdisco L, Farcy J-P. The use of preoperative erythropoietin in scoliosis surgery. Spine. 1992;17:S204–S5.

31 NIH National Consensus Development Panel. Transfusion alert: use of autologous blood. Transfusion. 1995;35:703–11.

32 Goodnough LT, Monk TG, Brecher ME. Acute normovolemic hemodilution should replace preoperative autologous blood donation before elective surgery. Transfusion. 1998;38:473–6.

33 Copley LAB, Richards BS, Safavi FZ, Newton PO. Hemodilution as a method to reduce transfusion requirements in adolescent spine fusion surgery. Spine. 1999;24:219–24.

34 Consensus Conference on Autologous Transfusion. Final consensus statement. Transfusion. 1996;36:667.

35 Bryson GL. Does acute normovolemic hemodilution reduce perioperative allogeneic transfusion? A meta-analysis. Anesth Analg. 1997;86:9–15.

36 Safwat AM, Reitan JA, Benson D. Management of Jehovah's Witness patients for scoliosis surgery: the use of platelet and plasmapheresis. J Clin Anesthesia. 1997;9:510–13.

37 Gan TJ, Bennett-Guerrero E, Phillips-Bute B, Wakeling H, Moskowitz DM, Olufolabi Y, Konstadt SN, C Bradford C, Glass PSA, Machin SJ, Mythen MG. Hextend®, a physiologically balanced plasma expander for large volume use in major surgery: A randomized Phase III clinical trial. Anesth Analg. 1999;88: 992–8.

38 Spahn DR, van Brempt R, Theilmeier G, Reibold J-P, Welte M, Heinzerling H, Birck KM, Keipert PE, Messmer K. Perflubron emulsion delays blood transfusions in orthopedic surgery. Anesthesiology. 1999;91:1195–208.

39 Sloan SR. Neonatal transfusion review. Paediatr Anaesth. 2011;21:25–30.

40 Jabbour N, Gagandeep S, Mateo R, Sher L, Genyk Y, Selby R. Transfusion free surgery: single institution experience of 27 consecutive liver transplants in Jehovah's Witnesses. J Am Coll Surg. 2005;201:412–17.

41 Farlo J. Management of hemostasis during exrerme normovolemic hemodilution in pediaric Jehovah's Witenss patietns undergoin high-risk surgical procedures. Anesthesiology. 2003;99:A1425.

42 Milam JD, Austin SF, Nihill MR, Keats AS, Cooley DA. Use of sufficient hemodilution to prevent coagulopathies following surgical correction of cyanotic heart disease. J Thorac Cardiovasc Surg. 1985;89(4):623–9.

43 Jonas RA, Wypij D, Roth SJ, Bellinger DC, Visconti KJ, du Plessis AJ, Goodkin H, Laussen PC, Farrell DM, Bartlett J, McGrath E, Rappaport LJ, et al. The influence of hemodilution on outcome after hypothermic cardiopulmonary bypass: results of a randomized trial in infants. J Thorac Cardiovasc Surg. 2003;126: 1765–74.

44 Murray DJ, Forbes RB, Titone MB, Weinstein SL. Transfusion management in pediatric and adolescent scoliosis surgery. Efficacy of autologous blood. Spine. 1997;22:2735–40.

45 Imura K, Kawahar H, Kitayama Y, Yoneda A, Yagi M, Suehara N. Usefulness of cord-blood harvesting for autologous transfusion in surgical newborns with antenatal diagnosis of congenital anomalies. J Pediatr Surg. 2001;36: 851–4.

46 von Lindern JS, Brand A. The use of blood products in perinatal medicine. Semin Fetal Neonatal Med. 2008;13:272–81.

47 Dunn CJ, Goa KL. Tranexamic acid: A review of its use in surgery and other indications. Drugs. 1999;57:1005–32.

48 Sendensky A, Gutzwiller JP, Schneider-Frost J, Wuillemin WA, Graeni R, Beglinger C. Recombinant activated factor VII (NovoSeven) stops severe intra-abdominal bleeding after liver needle biopsy without surgery. Blood Coagul Fibrinolysis. 2004;15:701–2.

49 Williams GD, Bratton SL, Ramamoorthy C. Factors associated with blood loss and blood product transfusions: a multivariate analysis in children after open-heart surgery. Anesth Analg. 1999;89:57–64.

50 Nelson CL, Fontenot HJ. Ten strategies to reduce blood loss in orthopedic surgery. Am J Surg. 1995;170:64S–8S.

51 Stauffer UG. The Shaw haemostatic scalpel in paediatric surgery: clinical report on 3000 operations. Progress in Pediatric Surgery. 1990;25:40–7.

52 Majeski J. Advances in general and vascular surgical care of Jehovah's Witnesses. International Surgery. 2000;85:357–265.

53 Shah MN, Kane AA, Petersen JD, Woo AS, Naidoo SD, Smyth MD. Endoscopically assisted versus open repair of sagittal craniosynostosis: the St. Louis Children's Hospital experience. J Neurosurg Pediatr. 2011;8:165–70.

54 Tate DE, Friedman RJ. Blood conservation in Spinal Surgery. Spine. 1992;17:1450–6.

55 Fontana JL, Welborn L, Mongan PD, Sturm P, Martin G, Bunger R. Oxygen consumption and cardiovascular function in children during profound intraoperative normovolemic hemodilution. Anesth Analg. 1995;80:219–25.

56 Widness JA, Kulhavy JC, Johnson KJ, Cress GA, Kromer IJ, Acarregui MJ, Feld RD. Clinical performance of an in-line point-of-care monitor in neonates. Pediatrics. 2000;106:497–504.

57 Moya MP, Clark RH, Nicks J, Tanaka DT. The effects of bedside blood gas monitoring on blood loss and ventilator management. Biol Neonate. 2001;80: 257–61.

58 Goodman AM, Pollack MM, Patel KM, Luban NL. Pediatric red blood cell transfusions increase resource use. J Pediatr. 2003;142:123–7.

59 Soumerai SB, Salem-Schatz S, Avorn J, Casteris CS, Ross-Degnan D, Popovsky MA. A controlled trial of educational outreach to improve blood transfusion practice. Jama. 1993;270:961–6.

60 Fredrickson LK, Bell EF, Cress GA, Johnson KJ, Zimmerman MB, Mahoney LT, Widness JA, Strauss RG. Acute physiological effects of packed red blood cell transfusion in preterm infants with different degrees of anaemia. Arch Dis Child Fetal Neonatal Ed. 2011;96:F249–53.

61 Salem-Schatz SR, Avorn J, Soumerai SB. Influence of clinical knowledge, organizational context, and practice style on transfusion decision making. Implications for practice change strategies. JAMA. 1990;264:476–83.

62 Toy P. The transfusion audit as an educational tool. Transfus Sci. 1998;19(1):91–6.

63 Morrison JC, Sumrall DD, Chevalier SP, Robinson SV, Morrison FS, Wiser WL. The effect of provider education on blood utilization practices. Am J Obstet Gynecol. 1993;169:1240–5.

64 Surgenor DM, Churchill WH, Wallace EL, Rizzo RJ, McGurk S, Goodnough LT, Kao KJ, Koerner TA, Olson JD, Woodson RD. The specific hospital significantly affects red cell and component transfusion practice in coronary artery bypass graft surgery: a study of five hospitals. Transfusion. 1998;38:122–34.

65 Baer VL, Henry E, Lambert DK, Stoddard RA, Wiedmeier SE, Eggert LD, Ilstrup S, Christensen RD. Implementing a program to improve compliance with neonatal intensive care unit transfusion guidelines was accompanied by a reduction in transfusion rate: a pre-post analysis within a multihospital health care system. Transfusion. 2011;51:264–9.

66 Bateman ST, Lacroix J, Boven K, Forbes P, Barton R, Thomas NJ, Jacobs B, Markovitz B, Goldstein B, Hanson JH, Li HA, Randolph AG. Anemia, blood loss, and blood transfusions in North American children in the intensive care unit. Am J Respir Crit Care Med. 2008;178:26–33.

67 Ballance WA, Dahms BD, Shenker N, Kliegman RM. Pathology of neonatal necrotizing enterocolitis: A ten-year experience. J Pediatr. 1990;177:S6–S13.

68 Kling PJ, Sullivan TM, Leftwich ME, Roe DJ. Score for neonatal acute physiology predicts erythrocyte transfusions in premature infants. Arch Dis Pediatr Adolesc Med. 1997;151:27–31.

69 Ringer SA, Richardson DK, Sacher RA, Keszler M, Churchill WH. Variations in transfusion practice in neonatal intensive care. Pediatrics. 1998;101:194–200.

70 Mehta P, Vasa R, Neumann L, Karpatkin M. Thrombocytopenia in the high-risk infant. J Pediatr. 1980;97:791–4.

71 Kling PJ, Hutter JJ. Hematologic abnormalities in severe neonatal necrotizing enterocolitis: 25 years later. J Perinatol. 2003;23:523–30.

72 Sola M, Vecchio A, Rimsza L. Evaluation and treatment of thrombocytopenia in the neonatal intensive care unit. Neonatal Hematology. 2000;27:655–79.

73 Aronis S, Platokouki H, Photopoulos S, Eftychia A, Xanthou M. Indications of Coagulation and/or Fibrinolytic systems activation in healthy and sick very low birth weight neonates. Biol Neonate. 1998;74:337–44.

74 Tapper H, Herwald H. Modulation of hemostatic mechanisms in bacterial infectious diseases. Blood. 2000;96:2329–37.

75 Hume H. Red blood cell transfusions for preterm infants: The role of evidence-based medicine. Sem Perinatol. 1997;21:8–19.

76 Strauss RG, Widness JA. Is there a role for autologous/placental red blood cell transfusions in the anemia of prematurity? Transfusion medicine reviews. 2010;24:125–9.

77 Ballin A, Arbel E, Kenet G, Berar M, Kohelet D, Tanay A, Zakut H, Meytes D. Autologous umbilical cord blood transfusion. Arch Dis Child. 1995;73:F181–3.

78 Beattie R, Stark JM, Wardrop CAJ, Holland BM, Kinmond S. Autologous umbilical cord blood transfusion. Arch Dis Child. 1996;74:F221.

79 Eichler H, Schaible T, Richter E, Zieger W, Voller K, Leveringhaus A, Goldmann SF. Cord blood as a source of autologous RBCs for transfusion to preterm infants. Transfusion. 2000;40:1111–7.

80 Mercer JS, Vohr BR, McGrath MM, Padbury JF, Wallach M, Oh W. Delayed cord clamping in very preterm infants reduces the incidence of intraventricular hemorrhage and late-onset sepsis: a randomized, controlled trial. Pediatrics. 2006;117:1235–42.

81 Hutton EK, Hassan ES. Late vs early clamping of the umbilical cord in full-term neonates: systematic review and meta-analysis of controlled trials. Jama. 2007;297:1241–52.

82 Oh W, Fanaroff AA, Carlo WA, Donovan EF, McDonald SA, Poole WK. Effects of delayed cord clamping in very-low-birth-weight infants. J Perinatol. 2011;31 (Suppl 1):S68–71.

83 Burke RP, Hannan RL. Reducing the trauma of congenital heart surgery. Surg Clin North Am. 2000;80:1593–605.

84 Kreutzer J. Transcatheter intervention in the neonate with congenital heart disease. Clin Perinatol. 2001;28:137–57.

85 Alexi-Meskhishvili V, Ovroutski S, Dahnert I, Fischer T. Correction of cor triatriatum sinistrum in a jehova's witness infant. Eur J Cardio-Thorac Surg. 2000;18:724–6.

86 Shimpo H, Mizumoto T, Onoda K, Yuasa H, Yada I. Erythropoietin in pediatric cardiac surgery. Chest. 1997;111:1565–70.

87 Huebler M, Habazettl H, Boettcher W, Kuppe H, Hetzer R, Redlin M. Transfusion-free complex cardiac surgery: with use of deep hypothermic circulatory arrest in a preterm 2.96-kg Jehovah's witness neonate. Texas Heart Institute J. 2011;38:562–4.

88 Huebler M, Boettcher W, Koster A, Emeis M, Lange P, Hetzer R. Transfusion-free complex cardiac surgery with cardiopulmonary bypass in a 3.55-kg Jehovah's Witness neonate. Ann Thorac Surg. 2005;80:1504–6.

89 Chikada M, Furuse A, Kotsuka Y, Yagyu K. Open-heart surgery in Jehovah's Witness patients. Cardiovascular Surgery. 1996;4:311–4.

90 Ashraf H, Subrmanian S. Bloodless cardiac surgery in children. Saudi Heart Bulletin. 1990;1:15–22.

91 Redlin M, Huebler M, Boettcher W, Kukucka M, Schoenfeld H, Hetzer R, Habazettl H. Minimizing intraoperative hemodilution by use of a very low priming volume cardiopulmonary bypass in neonates with transposition of the great arteries. J Thorac Cardiovasc Surg. 2011;142:875–81.

92 Koster A, Huebler M, Boettcher W, Redlin M, Berger F, Hetzer R. A new miniaturized cardiopulmonary bypass system reduces transfusion requirements during neonatal cardiac surgery: initial experience in 13 consecutive patients. J Thorac Cardiovasc Surg. 2009;137:1565–8.

93 Kotani Y, Honjo O, Nakakura M, Ugaki S, Kawabata T, Kuroko Y, Osaki S, Yoshizumi K, Kasahara S, Ishino K, Sano S. Impact of miniaturization of cardiopulmonary bypass circuit on blood transfusion requirement in neonatal open-heart surgery. ASAIO J. 2007;53:662–5.

94 Calza G, Zannini L, Lerzo F, Nitti P, Mangraviti S, Perutelli P, Porlezza M. Quantitative and qualitative evaluation of blood salvaged after extracorporeal circulation in paediatric heart surgery. Int J Artificial Organs. 2000;23:398–406.

95 Schaff HV, Hauer J, Gardner TJ, Donahoo JS, Watkins L, Gott VL, Brawley RK. Routine use of autotransfusion following cardiac surgery: experience in 700 patients. Ann Thorac Surg. 1978;27:493–9.

96 Malcolm-Smith NA, McMaster MJ. The use of induced hypotension to control bleeding during posterior fusion for scoliosis. J Bone Joint Surg. 1983;65-B:255–8.

97 Kruger LM, Colbert JM. Intraoperative autologous transfusion in children undergoing spinal surgery. J Pediatr Orthoped. 1985;5:330–2.

98 Vitale MG, Privitera DM, Matsumoto H, Gomez JA, Waters LM, Hyman JE, Roye DP, Jr. Efficacy of preoperative erythropoietin administration in pediatric neuromuscular scoliosis patients. Spine. 2007;32:2662–7.

99 Stricker PA, Shaw TL, Desouza DG, Hernandez SV, Bartlett SP, Friedman DF, Sesok-Pizzini DA, Jobes DR. Blood loss, replacement, and associated morbidity in infants and children undergoing craniofacial surgery. Paediatr Anaesth. 2010;20:150–9.

100 Kang JK, Lee SW, Baik MW, Son BC, Hong YK, Jung CK, Ryu KH. Perioperative specific management of blood volume loss in craniosynostosis surgery. Child's Nervous System. 1998;14:297–301.

101 Butler P, Israel L, Nusbacher J, Jenkins DE, Starzl TE. Blood transfusion in liver transplantation. Transfusion. 1985;25:120–3.

102 Ulukaya S, Acar L, Ayanoglu HO. Transfusion requirements during cadaveric and living donor pediatric liver transplantation. Pediatr Transplant. 2005;9:332–7.

103 Kim YI, Ishii T, Aramaki M, Nakashima K, Yoshida T, Kobayashi M. The Pringle maneuver induces only partial ishcemia of the liver. Hepato-Gastroenterology. 1995;42:169–71.

104 Quan D, Wall W. The safety of continuous hepatic inflow occlusion during major liver resection. Liver Transplantation and Surgery. 1996;2:99–104.

105 Gertsch P, Pelloni A, Guerra A, Krpo A. Initial experience with the harmonic scalpel in liver surgery. Hepato-Gastroenterology. 2000;47:763–6.

106 Barret JP, Desai MH, Herndon DN. Massive transfusion of reconstituted whole blood is well tolerated in pediatric burn surgery. J Trauma Injury: Injury Infect Crit Care. 1999;47:526–8.

107 Deitch EA, Sitting KM. A serial study of the erythropoietic response to thermal injury. Ann Surg. 1993;217:293–9.

108 Boshkov LK, Tredget EE, Janowska-Wieczorek A. Recombinant human erythropoietin for a Jehovah's Witness with anemia of thermal injury. Am J Hematol. 1991;37:53–4.

109 Moghtader JC, Edlich RF, Mintz PD, Zachmann GC, Himel HN. The use of recombinant human erythropoietin and cultured epithelial autografts in a Jehovah's Witness with a major thermal injury. Burns. 1994;20:176–7.

110 Deitch EA, Guillory D, Cruz N. Successful use of recombinant human Erythropoietin in a Jehovah's Witness with a thermal injury. J Burn Care Rehabil. 1994;15:42–5.

111 Law EJ, Still JM, Gattis CS. The use of erythropoietin in two burned patients who are Jehovah's Witnesses. Burns. 1991;1991:75–7.

112 Cartotto R, Musgrave MA, Beveridge M, Fish J, Gomez M. Minimizing blood loss in burn surgery. J Trauma. 2000;49:1034–9.

113 Moore E, Shackford SR, Pachter HL, et al. Organ injury scaling: Spleen, liver and kidney. J Trauma. 1989;1989:1664–6.

114 Malhotra AK, Fabian TC, Croce MA, Gavin TJ, Kudsk KA, Minard G, Pritchard SC. Blunt hepatic injury: A paradigm shift from operative to nonoperative management in the 1990's. Ann Surg. 2000;231:804–13.

115 Leone RJ, Hammond JS. Nonoperative management of pediatric blunt hepatic trauma. The American Surgeon. 2001;67:138–42.

116 Kilic N, Gurpinar A, Kiristioglu I, OA, Balkan E, Dogruyol H. Ruptured spleen due to blunt trauma in children: analysis of blood transfusion requirements. Eur J Emerg Med. 1999;6:135–9.

117 Smith JS, Cooney RN, Mucha P. Nonoperative management of the ruptured spleen: A revalidation of criteria. Surgery. 1996;120:745–51.

118 Strauss RG. Controversies in the management of the anemia of prematurity using single-donor red blood cell transfusions and/or recombinant human erythropoietin. Transfusion medicine reviews. 2006;20:34–44.

119 Jones JG, Holland BM, Hudson IRB, Wardrop CAJ. Total circulating red cells versus haematocrit as the primary descriptor of oxygen transport by the blood. Br J Haematol. 1990;1990:288–94.

120 Strauss RG. Transfusion therapy in neonates. Am J Dis Child. 1991;145:904–11.

121 Widness JA, Seward VJ, Kromer IJ, Burmeister LF, Bell EF, Strauss RG. Changing patterns of red blood cell transfusion in very low birth weight infants. J Pediatr. 1996;129:680–7.

122 Maier RF, Sonntag J, Walka MM, Liu G, Metze BC, Obladen M. Changing practices of red blood cell transfusions in infants with birth weights less than 1000g. J Pediatr. 2000;136:220–4.

123 Kinmond S, Aitchison TC, Holland BM, Jones JG, Turner TL, Wardrop CAJ. Umbilical cord clamping and preterm infants: a randomised trial. Brit Med J. 1993;306:172–5.

124 Bednarek FJ, Weisberger S, Richardson DK, Frantz ID, Shah B, Rubin L. Variations in blood transfusions among newborn intensive care units. J Pediatr. 1998;133:601–7.

125 Shannon K. Recombinant erythropoietin in anemia of prematurity: five years later. Pediatrics. 1993;92:614–16.

126 Ohls RK. Erythropoietin to prevent and treat the anemia of prematurity. Curr Opin Pediatr. 1999;11:108–14.

127 Whyte RK. Low versus high haemoglobin concentration threshold for blood transfusion for preventing morbidity and mortality in very low birth weight infants. Cochrane Collaboration. 2011.

128 Bell EF, Strauss RG, Widness JA, Mahoney LT, Mock DM, Seward VJ, Cress GA, Johnson KJ, Kromer IJ, Zimmerman MB. Randomized trial of liberal versus restrictive guidelines for red blood cell transfusion in preterm infants. Pediatrics. 2005;115:1685–91.

129 Kirpalani H, Whyte RK, Andersen C, Asztalos EV, Heddle N, Blajchman MA, Peliowski A, Rios A, LaCorte M, Connelly R, Barrington K, Roberts RS. The Premature Infants in Need of Transfusion (PINT) study: a randomized, controlled trial of a restrictive (low) versus liberal (high) transfusion threshold for extremely low birth weight infants. J Pediatr. 2006;149:301–7.

130 Whyte RK, Kirpalani H, Asztalos EV, Andersen C, Blajchman M, Heddle N, LaCorte M, Robertson CM, Clarke MC, Vincer MJ, Doyle LW, Roberts RS. Neurodevelopmental outcome of extremely low birth weight infants randomly assigned to restrictive or liberal hemoglobin thresholds for blood transfusion. Pediatrics. 2009;123:207–13.

131 Crowley M, Kirpalani H. A rational approach to red blood cell transfusion in the neonatal ICU. Curr Opin Pediatr. 2010;22:151–7.

132 Nopoulos PC, Conrad AL, Bell EF, Strauss RG, Widness JA, Magnotta VA, Zimmerman MB, Georgieff MK, Lindgren SD, Richman LC. Long-term outcome of brain structure in premature infants: effects of liberal vs restricted red blood cell transfusions. Arch Pediatr Adolesc Med. 2011;165(5):443–50.

133 McCoy TE, Conrad AL, Richman LC, Lindgren SD, Nopoulos PC, Bell EF. Neurocognitive profiles of preterm infants randomly assigned to lower or higher hematocrit thresholds for transfusion. Child Neuropsychol. 2011;17:347–67.

134 Chen HL, Tseng HI, Lu CC, Yang SN, Fan HC, Yang RC. Effect of blood transfusions on the outcome of very low body weight preterm infants under two different transfusion criteria. Pediatrics and neonatology. 2009;50:110–16.

135 Vamvakas EC, Strauss RG. Meta-analysis of controlled clinical trials studying the efficacy of rHuEPO in reducing blood transfusions in the anemia of prematurity. Transfusion. 2001;41:406–15.

136 Aher SM, Ohlsson A. Late erythropoietin for preventing red blood cell transfusion in preterm and/or low birth weight infants. The Cochrane Collaboration; 2010 [CD004868].

137 Bausch LC. Blood transfusions and the Jehovah's Witness -- neonatal perspectives. Nebraska Medical J. 1991;76:283–4.

138 Davis P, Herbert M, Davies DP, Verrier Jones ER. Case study. Erythropoietin for anaemia in a preterm Jehovah's Witness. Early Hum Devel. 1992;28:279–83.

139 Rouette J, Trottier H, Ducruet T, Beaunoyer M, Lacroix J, Tucci M. Red blood cell transfusion threshold in postsurgical pediatric intensive care patients: a randomized clinical trial. Ann Surg. 2010;251:421–7.

140 Beck MN, Beck D. Recombinant erythropoietin in acute chemotherapy-induced anemia of children with cancer. Medical and Pediatric Oncology. 1995;25:17–21.

141 Leon P, Jimenez M, Barona P, Sierraseumaga L. Recombinant human erythropoietin for the treatment of anemia in children with solid malignant tumors. Medical and Pediatric Oncology. 1998;30:110–16.

142 Bolonaki I, Stiakaki E, Lydaki E, Dimitriou H, Kambourakis A, Kalmantis T, Kalmanti M. Treatment with recombinant human erythropoietin in children with malignancies. Pediatric Hematol Oncol. 1998;13:111–21.

143 Csaki C, Ferencz T, Schuler D, Borsi JD. Recombinant human erythropoietin in the prevention of chemotherapy-induced anaemia in children with malignant solid tumors. Eur J Cancer. 1998;34:364–7.

144 Ballen KK, Ford PA, Witkus H, Emmons RVB, Levy W, Doyle P, Stewart FM, Quesenberry PJ, Becker PS. Successful autologous bone marrow transplant without use of blood product support. Bone Marrow Transplantation. 2000;26:227–9.

145 Estrin JT, Ford PA, Henry DH, Stradden AP, Mason BA. Erythropoietin permits high-dose chemotherapy with peripheral blood stem-cell transplant for a Jehovah's Witness. Am J Hematol. 1997;55:51–2.

146 Beguin Y, Oris R, Fillet G. Dynamics of erythropoietic recovery following bone marrow transplantation: role of marrow proliferative capacity and erythropoietin production in autologous versus allogenic transplants. Bone Marrow Transplantation. 1993;11:285–92.

147 Locatelli F, Zecca M, Pedrazzoli P, Prete L, Quaglini S, Comoli P, DeStefano P, Beguin Y, Robustelli della Cuna G, Severi F, et al. Use of recombinant human erythropoietin after bone marrow transplantation in pediatic patients with acute leukemia: effect on erythroid repopulation in autologous verus allogeneic transplants. Bone Marrow Transplantation. 1994;13:403–10.

148 Biggs JC, Atkinson SA, Booker V, Concannon A, Dart DW, Dodds A, Downs A, Szer J, Turner J, Worthington R. Prospective randomised double-blind trial of the *in vivo* use of recombinant human erythrpoietin in bone marrow transplantation from HLA-identical sibling donors. Bone Marrow Transplant. 1995;15:129–34.

149 Strauss RG. Anaemia of prematurity: pathophysiology and treatment. Blood reviews. 2010;24:221–5.

CHAPTER 11

Current management of anemia in oncology

Shelly Sharma[1] and Sharad Sharma[2]

[1]Department of Radiation Oncology, St. Jude Children's Research Hospital, Memphis, TN, USA
[2]Department Of Transplant Surgery, UTMB, Galveston, TX, USA

Overview

Anemia in cancer patients is the most common hematological morbidity with the reported prevalence ranging from 30% to 90%. Various studies have shown association of anemia in cancer patients with decreased quality of life and reduced overall survival. Correction of anemia in cancer patients is required not only for improving the physical and functional status of the patient, but in fact this correction is also warranted to improve oxygenation of tumor tissue, which may be exhibited as low sensitivity to radiation and some chemotherapy drugs under hypoxic circumstances. Typically, anemia in these patients is multifactorial. It can be secondary to direct and/or indirect effects of tumor cells and cancer treatment (cancer-related anemia), or related to underlying comorbidities independent of cancer or any combination of these. Path physiologic mechanisms underlying anemia in cancer patients can involve any stage of erythropoiesis. The aim of anemia treatment is to correct any reversible cause if possible and to provide supportive therapy using erythropoiesis-stimulating agents (ESAs) with or without iron supplementation or blood transfusions. Choice of the treatment option depends on individualized risk assessment based on the acuteness and severity of anemia, presence of symptoms, comorbid conditions and phase of treatment. ESAs had been the most frequent agents used to manage anemia in oncology until recently. However, there has been a shift in the paradigm as safety of these agents has been questioned. This may compromise the transfusion-sparing benefit gained by ESAs.

Transfusion-Free Medicine and Surgery, Second Edition. Edited by Nicolas Jabbour.
© 2014 John Wiley & Sons, Ltd. Published 2014 by John Wiley & Sons, Ltd.

In this chapter we will discuss the path physiology of anemia in oncology with the current management guidelines; touching the controversies associated with the use of various options and their implications on the trend of use of transfusions in near future. The discussion will be limited to cancer-related anemia in adult patients with non-myeloid malignancies.

Epidemiology and pattern of treatment

Anemia is defined as a reduction of hemoglobin (Hb) concentration, red blood cell (RBC) count or packed cell volume below normal levels. Definition of normal levels in oncology is as variable as in the general population secondary to inter and intrapopulation variations in the ranges of Hb levels in healthy individuals. Anemia is prevalent in 30 to 90% of cancer patients [1]. Increased awareness of the negative impact of anemia on the local tumor control and survival has led to changes in the patterns of anemia correction in this patient population. Prevalence of anemia varies widely among cancer patient populations depending on the site of tumor, stage of disease, type of the treatment (radiotherapy or chemotherapy or surgery or combination of any of these) and definition of anemia. Anemia is more prevalent among patients with metastatic diseases, bone marrow infiltrating disease and in patients with advanced solid tumors [1]. In the systematic review by Knight et al. [1], prevalence of anemia was 7% in Hodgkin patients when anemia was defined as Hb < 90.0 g/L and was 86% when Hb cut off value was <110 g/L. Similarly, on review of studies considering anemia in patients with colon cancer, anemia was prevalent in 40% of patients with early stage and frequency reached to 80% in patients with advanced disease. The European Cancer Anemia Survey (ECAS) [2], a large multinational prospective survey conducted in Europe between 2001 and 2002, revealed that approximately 40% of patients had Hb < 12.0 g/dL and 75% of patients undergoing chemotherapy developed anemia within 6 months. Risk factors identified for anemia development in this population were baseline Hb level, site of primary tumor, use of platinum containing regimens, female gender, advanced stage and low performance status. Low Hb levels correlated significantly with poor performance status, but anemia was treated only in 40% of patients (ESAs, 17.4%; transfusion, 14.9%; and iron, 6.5%). Contrary to this, the Anemia of Cancer Therapy (ACT) study [3], a retrospective observational study done on 2192 cancer patients, revealed that around 70% of anemic patients were treated. ESAs were used in 62.2%; Blood transfusion in 19.4% and 32.8% received iron supplementation. This discrepancy in the rates of treatment of anemia reflects the increasing awareness of the impact of anemia on cancer prognosis leading to increased enthusiasm for correction of anemia.

Prognostic significance and rationale for correcting anemia in oncology

Anemia is a well-known independent prognostic factor in cancer patients. Pre-treatment anemia has been extensively investigated with fewer reports evaluating anemia during treatment as a prognostic factor. Pre-treatment anemia in this population has been associated with poor local tumor control and reduced overall survival [4]. For example, inferior survival has been reported in anemic patients with lung, ovarian, cervical, laryngeal cancers treated with surgery, chemotherapy or radiation therapy [4–8]. A meta-analysis of 60 studies estimated an overall 65% increase in risk of death in cancer patients who were anemic [9].

In addition, the negative impact of anemia on quality of life (QoL) has also been identified [1]. Anemia results in symptoms like palpitations, fatigue, dyspnea, nausea, depression, heart failure, impairment of cognitive function and dizziness [10]. There is enough evidence in literature suggesting that Hb levels below 12 g/dL are associated with fatigue, decreased quality of life and functional status in cancer patients as compared to higher Hb levels [11–15].

A variety of explanations exists in the literature to justify the negative prognostic impact of anemia. The most accepted theoretical explanation is the association between anemia and hypoxia [1, 12, 15, 16]. Experimental tumor tissue models, in which anemia was induced, led to decreased tumor tissue oxygenation (hypoxia) [17]. The hypoxic tumor tissue may become resistant to radiation therapy because of lack of free oxygen to fix highly reactive free radicals that mediate the indirect hit of radiation on tumor cell DNA [14, 18]. Clinically, this resistance to irradiation is reflected by the observation that poor prognosis in anemic patients if treated with radiotherapy, mainly results from poor local control [12, 18]. Also, all the studies that have analyzed the effect of Hb levels prior to and during radio therapy have revealed that Hb levels during radiotherapy are more important than pre-treatment Hb levels in patients being treated with radiotherapy [8, 12, 19, 20] potentiating the importance of optimal oxygenation of tumor tissue during irradiation. Similar mechanisms are thought to be responsible for resistance to chemotherapy drugs like cyclophosphamide [15, 16].

However, the association of poor outcomes observed in anemic patients treated with surgery alone or with chemotherapeutic drugs not requiring oxygen for their cytotoxic effect indicate the possibility of anemia being a surrogate of aggressiveness of tumor [21]. Inflammatory cytokines like IL-6 secreted by aggressive tumors have not only been implicated for development of anemia but studies have also shown them to increase tumor cell proliferation and increase angiogenesis as in breast and prostate tumors [15, 21, 22]. In addition, hypoxia may promote more aggressive phenotype by selecting for p53 mutations, making tumor cells genetically more unstable and aggressive [16]. Furthermore, impaired tissue oxygenation itself can induce generation of angiogeneic factors that can promote tumor growth or anemia may impact tumor behavior via hypoxia inducible factor 1alpha or it may impair immune function with subsequent increased risk of tumor progression [16, 23, 24].

Pathophysiology of anemia in cancer patients

Anemia in cancer patients is typically multifactorial. It may result from malignant disease itself, or can be caused by specific therapy such as chemotherapy, radiation therapy or surgery or it may result from independent concomitant diseases (Table 11.1) [15, 25]. Multiple causes are in play simultaneously in most of the cases but during the course of the disease and therapy one mechanism may predominate. Anemia could be a direct effect of cancer cells or a paraneoplastic manifestation mediated by inflammatory cytokines and autoantibody produced secondary to immune turmoil in the body following cancer [15, 25, 26].

Interestingly, cancer has been implicated with affecting almost each phase erythropoiesis. Hence, similar to the non-oncologic population, pathophysiologic mechanisms of anemia in cancer can be characterized as following:
1 Decreased RBC production(Hypoproliferative state)
2 Increased RBC destruction (Hyperproliferative state)
3 Blood loss secondary to bleeding or hemorrhage

This categorization can very well form the basis of characterization of anemia in these patients. For instance, a plethora of cytokines secreted as a part of immunological turmoil following malignancy can lead to a hypoproliferative state with decreased RBC production. This is the most common mechanism underlying anemia in cancer patients [25]. These inflammatory cytokines can inhibit red cell production directly or indirectly by activating cytotoxic macrophages or by impairing erythropoietin production. Also, these cytokines may decrease iron availability by iron sequestration into cells leading to decreased RBC production. Besides, tumor cells may directly suppress erythropoiesis by bone marrow

Table 11.1 Multifactorial causation of anemia in cancer patients categorized based on its etiology linked to tumor, cancer treatment or coexisting morbidities independent of cancer. Anemia in patients on or after recent chemotherapy is often known as "chemotherapy induced anemia".

Causes of Anemia in Cancer Patients

Causes of anemia secondary to tumor itself

1 Tumor-related anemia (similar to anemia of chronic disease, mediated by inflammatory cytokines)
2 Acute or chronic blood loss from tumor site
3 Compromised nutritional intake (e.g. esophageal and head and neck cancers compromising oral intake)
4 Bone marrow infiltration by tumor cells
5 Immune mediated hemolysis or pure red cell aplasia secondary to immune response to tumor
6 Activation of coagulation by tumor leading to microangiopathic hemolytic anemia
7 Hypersplenism secondary to tumor infiltration or portal hypertension leading to increased hemolysis

Causes of anemia secondary to cancer treatment

1 Myelosupressive effects of chemotherapy (chemotherapy induced anemia)
2 Nephrotoxic effect of chemotherapy decreasing production of erythropoietin by kidney e.g. platinum-containing agents(chemotherapy induced anemia)
3 Myelosupressive effect of radiotherapy to skeleton with red marrow (e.g. cranium and spine)
4 Blood loss during surgery

Causes of anemia secondary to co-existent morbidities independent of cancer

1 Concurrent medical illness (e.g. renal insufficiency, esophageal varicosis, GI ulcers, chronic inflammatory disease etc.)
2 Concomitant medication (NSARs, Dapsone)
3 Hereditary anemias

infiltration. Additional suppression of RBC production can occur because of nutritional deficiencies secondary to decreased appetite or secondary to myelosupressive effects of chemotherapy and/or radiation therapy. Radiation to spine and/or cranium can result in grade 3 to 4 hematotoxicity [15, 25, 27]. Similarly, chemotherapeutic agents can not only directly impair hematopoiesis by their toxic effect on progenitor cells in marrow, but also a few, such as platinum compounds, can suppress erythropoietin production secondary to their nephrotoxicity [26]. Similarly, there can be increased destruction of RBCs secondary to hemolytic auto-antibodies, microangiopathic destruction following disseminated coagulation or hypersplenism seen in some cancer patients [15, 25]. Hemolytic anemia of this type is common amongst chronic leukemias.

Diagnostic evaluation and risk assessment

The aim of this evaluation is to characterize anemia and look for any under-lying co-morbidity that can be corrected. Considering the broad range of Hb levels among healthy individuals, there isn't any consensus regarding a normal level of Hb in cancer patients as well. However, National Com-prehensive Cancer Network (NCCN) panelists have recommended eval-uation of anemia at Hb levels of 11 g/dl or below in adult cancer patients with solid tumors or chronic lymphoid leukemias [28]. In addition, in a patient with high baseline Hb, a drop of 2 g/dl or more has also been rec-ommended for anemia evaluation [28].

Considering the complexity of these patients' illnesses, integrating information from thorough physical examination and detailed medical histories is essential to reach accurate diagnosis of anemia and plan the treatment strategy. Detailed physical examination may reveal jaundice, splenomegaly, heart murmurs or bleeding revealing the underlying pathogenic process. Similarly, a detailed history should include the duration and severity of symptoms, comorbidities, family history and history of chemotherapeutic drugs and radiation therapy [28].

Following these details various blood indices are used to complete the picture [15, 28]. These include, but are not limited to; Hematocrit or red blood cell (RBC) mass, peripheral blood smear (PBS), complete blood count (CBC), mean corpuscular volume (MCV), reticulocyte count, reticulocyte index (RI), and bone marrow biopsy. Besides, additional tests for common underlying mechanisms and ailments can be used, e.g. serum iron and total iron binding capacity (TIBC), transferrin saturation in absolute iron deficiency; B12 and folate levels for their deficiencies; stool guaiac test and endoscopy for hemorrhage; coombs test, disseminated intravascular coagulation (DIC) panel, haptoglobin and bilirubin levels for hemolysis; GFR and erythropoietin levels for chronic renal disease.

CBC gives a clue if other cytopenia are present and also informs about the mean corpuscular volume (MCV). Hematocrit or RBC mass represents the balance between RBC production and destruction. Added to this, mean corpuscular volume (MCV) helps in morphological characterization of anemia based on the average RBC size (Table 11.2). Reticulocyte count (young immature RBCs) represents the productive capacity of the marrow, thus reticulocyte count corrected against anemia (reticulocyte index; RI) is helpful in understanding if marrow is at fault. Peripheral blood smear provides information about the size, shape and color of the RBCs, thus elaborating the specific changes as seen in autoimmune hemolysis or hemolysis secondary to microangiopathy. Bone marrow

Table 11.2 Hematological indices and their interpretations used to characterize anemia in cancer patients with pertinent examples. Morphological indices are based on the size and volume of RBCs while kinetic indices suggest the underlying mechanism of anemia distinguishing production, destruction and loss of RBCs.

Morphological Indices	*Interpretations*
MCV < 80 fl; microcytic RBC	Iron deficiency, thalassemia, anemia of chronic disease(also seen in cancer) or sideroblastic anemia
MCV > 100 fl; macrocytic RBC	Majority are megaloblastic with B12 or folate deficiency Non megaloblastic anemia secondary to alcoholism, myelodysplatic syndrome or hydroxyurea, diphentoin
Normocytic; MCV 80–100 fl	Hemorrhage, hemolysis, bone marrow failure, anemia of chronic inflammation or renal insufficiency.
Kinetic indices	
Low Reticulocyte index	Indicates decreased RBC product; e.g., iron deficiency, B12/Folate deficiency, Aplastic anemia, bone marrow dysfunction secondary to cancer or chemotherapy/radiotherapy
High Reticulocyte index	Indicates normal or increased RBC production; e.g., in normal marrow following blood loss or hemolysis in the anemic patient

biopsy can give an accurate assessment of cellularity, fibrotic changes and tumor metastases

As an example, in anemia secondary to blood loss or hemolysis, RI will be increased if marrow is competent. To narrow the differential further, peripheral smear can show changes specific to autoimmune or microangiopathic hemolysis. If no such cause is identified then search for bleeding will point to the cause of anemia. However, anemia in oncology is generally accompanied by low reticulocyte count indicative of hypoproliferative state. Red cell morphologic indices and red cell distribution width in such hypoproliferative states can help characterize the anemia (Table 11.2). In this hypoproliferative state an increased MCV can indicate nutritional deficiency of vitamin B12 or folic acid or effects of methotrexate or hydroxyurea. On the other hand, a low MCV would point towards deficiency of iron or anemia of chronic inflammatory state. Bone marrow biopsy can also help in Hypoproliferative anemia. It may reveal absent iron stores or megaloblastic maturation or red cell aplasia or myelopdysplasia or a sideroblastic anemia.

Often anemia in cancer patients resembles anemia of chronic disease, but this is a diagnosis of exclusion only after ruling out other causes. It is characterized by low or normal MCV, low serum iron and iron binding capacity and normal or elevated serum ferritin. Also, functional iron deficiency often arises secondary to continued erythropoietin use (discussed later) [15].

If no cancer independent cause is identified, the cancer-related inflammation or myelosupressive chemotherapy/radiotherapy should be considered as a cause of anemia in the cancer patient. Once this is established, the next step is to do individualized risk assessment of anemia to decide which intervention is required. The factors that need to be considered for **risk assessment** are [28]:

1 Individual patient characteristics
2 Degree and severity of anemia
3 Presence and severity of comorbidities
4 Clinical judgment of the physician also addressing the phase of treatment and the anticipated risk of further deterioration of anemia with therapy.

As an example, recent intensive chemotherapy or radiation with progressive decline in hemoglobin (Hb) may place the patient in the high risk group necessitating immediate correction with PRBC transfusion. Similarly, in an acute setting, asymptomatic anemic patients without significant comorbidities can be followed up with observation while asymptomatic patients with significant comorbidities (e.g. cardiovascular, pulmonary or cerebrovascular diseases) or symptomatic patients may be considered for transfusion [28]. Other important factors that need attention while evaluating the risk is the phase of treatment, e.g. in chemotherapy-induced anemia; the nadir Hb levels, time to the nadir levels and whether the Hb values is pre or post nadir will affect the choice of intervention [29].

Treatment options

The aim is to correct reversible causes of anemia if any and to provide supportive correction with the following options.

1 Erythropoiesis stimulating agents (ESAs)
2 Peripheral Red Blood Cell Transfusion (PRBCT)
3 Iron supplementation with ESA

Each option has its own risks and benefits, as discussed in detail below and summarized in Table 11.3.

Erythropoiesis stimulating agents (ESAs)

Erythropoietin is a cytokine, stimulating the production of RBCs, is secreted mainly by the kidneys and to a lesser extent by the liver during postnatal life. ESAs are synthetic recombinant human erythropoietin that can enhance erythropoiesis in patients with low RBC mass. Epoetin alpha and darbepoietin alpha are the two such synthetic types presently available in the US [30]. Avoidance of transfusion has been their most important benefit in this population. Also, ESAs were shown to improve cancer-related fatigue and QoL in this population further raising their popularity. However, their safety has been questioned recently with increasing reports on their potential detrimental effects on survival leading to significant revisions of national and international recommendations for their use [28, 31].

Physiologic basis for ESA use in oncology

The biologic effects of erythropoietin on the target cells are conferred by interaction of erythropoietin with its receptor [32, 33]. Studies have revealed that erythropoietin receptors are found in increased numbers only in the later phases of erythropoietic development, with near absence on mature RBCs [25]. Erythropoietin thus affects the later stages of erythroid proliferation and maturation. Its production is up regulated by hypoxia thereby correcting RBC mass quickly. However, in cancer patients, erythropoietin level is inappropriately low for the degree of hypoxia because of blunted response to tissue hypoxia leading to erythropoietin deficient state [15, 34]. In addition, various inflammatory cytokines produced in cancer patients, like interleukin-1, tumor necrosis factor or transforming growth factor-beta, have been implicated as negative regulators suppressing erythropoietin production [25]. Also, these cytokines suppress RBC production, independent of erythropoietin, by impairing the proper use of iron by erythropoietic cells, discussed in detail later and forms the basis for iron supplementation with ESAs. Therefore, theoretically use of ESAs can mitigate the blunted erythropoietin response in cancer patients.

Benefits of ESAs

1. Avoidance of transfusion

ESAs efficiently increase Hb levels in cancer patients and decrease the requirement for blood transfusion. Transfusion risk was evaluated in more than 10 meta-analyses and reduction in transfusion risk in anemic patients on ESAs has been fairly consistent (RR range 0.58–0.67) in favor of ESA arm [35–37]. A randomized placebo-controlled study in patients receiving chemotherapy with anemia revealed a significant decrease in transfusion requirement in patients using epoetin alpha arm compared with placebo (24.7% versus 39.5%, p = 0.0057) [38]. A Cochrane review of 42 randomized controlled clinical trials including a total of 6510 patients also revealed a significant decrease in relative risk of transfusion in the patients who received erythropoietin (RR = 0.64; 95% CI, 0.60–0.68) [39].

2. Improved quality of life (QoL)

ESAs improve fatigue and energy rating scores in patients with chemotherapy induced anemia [40–42]. Unlike transfusion that raises Hb levels temporarily but instantaneously, ESAs raise Hb levels after a lag of around two weeks. However, repeated administration of ESAs is capable of maintaining the required Hb level. Increases in Hb levels have been associated with improved QoL as well [40–42]. In a systemic literature review of randomized controlled trials; 40 studies including 21 378 patients published during 1980 and July 2005; where patients received ESAs and QoL data was collected, patients receiving ESAs experienced a significant improvement in QoL; the mean difference in Functional Assessment of Cancer Therapy-Fatigue score (FACT-F score) for ESAs versus controls was 0.23 (95% CI, 0.10–0.36; P = 0.001) [40, 43]. Data from two open-label, community-based trials of epoetin alpha therapy that enrolled 4382 anemic cancer patients undergoing chemotherapy were used to evaluate the relationship between hemoglobin changes and QOL changes [44]. Their data revealed a positive and nonlinear relationship between change in hemoglobin level and change in QOL with greatest gain in QOL occurring when hemoglobin changed from 11 to 12 gm/dl with little increase when Hb level rises further to 14 gm/dl, and the gain leveled off in spite of further improvement of Hb levels [44]. Investigators suggest that there exists an optimal Hb level according to the size of blood volume, and oxygen transport increases until a Hb level is reached beyond which oxygen transport falls because of hyper viscosity [16]. Interestingly, this is reflected in the QoL and Hb level relationship in these patients as well.

Risks of ESAs

In 2007, the U.S. food and Drug administration issued a black box warning for recombinant ESA, warning of greater mortality, serious cardiovascular and thromboembolic events (TE), and tumor progression [30].

1. Decreased overall survival rates and tumor progression

The black box warnings by the FDA were based on increased mortality observed in patients receiving ESAs than the controls in eight randomized trials including patients treated with radiotherapy for head and neck cancer (erythropoietin to treat anemia in head and neck patients, ENHANCE study), patients treated with chemotherapy or radiotherapy for breast cancer patients with breast cancer (breast cancer erythropoietin survival trial, BEST study), and in anemic patients not receiving chemotherapy (EPO-CAN-20 non-small cell lung cancer [NSCLC] study and Amgen

103 study) [35, 42, 45, 48]. First meta-analysis of these studies refuted these findings, showing benefit for ESA patients (adjusted HR 0.84, 95% CI 0.67–0.99) [49], but later updated results of this meta-analysis showed the opposite [50]. In an independent individual patient data based meta-analysis including both published and unpublished data, risk of death during study period was increased in ESA patients; HR 1.17 (95% CI 1.06–1.30) but the detrimental effects of ESAs on overall survival were smaller; HR 1.06 (95% CI 1.00–1.12) [51]. The debate of the ESA effect on survival is still ongoing and literature has contradicting results from various systemic reviews and meta-analysis [35]. Several pharmacovigilance trials reported no decrease in survival with ESA use. In light of the emerging concept of optimal range of Hb [12, 16], higher than recommended Hb levels achieved in various RCTs leading to increased thromboembolic events accounting for mortality have been disputed as well [12, 32]. On the other hand, concerns have been raised regarding tumor progression by ESAs secondary to erythropoietin receptor stimulation on tumor cells but lack of specificity of antibodies used for these immunological assays has been questioned [32]. Until these controversies are settled in the coming years it is difficult to refute the possibility of increased mortality associated with ESA use in cancer patients. Therefore, in clinical practice the increased risk of death with ESA use needs to be balanced against the benefits of treatment with ESAs [28, 31].

2. Thromboembolic complications

Increased thromboembolic risks have been associated with ESA use. ESAs have the potential to increase thrombotic events secondary to their effect of increasing RBS mass, increased platelet number or reactivity, endothelial activation, reduction in plasma volume, and other mechanisms [16, 35]. Also, in general, cancer patients are at increased risk of thrombovascular events (TVEs) because of a hypercoaguable state secondary to inflammatory cytokines released in malignancy itself [16]. The majority of the randomized controlled trials comparing ESA with no ESA in cancer patients, though not designed or powered to detect this difference, have reported increased risk of TVEs in patients receiving ESAs [35]. In addition, this association has been potentiated by various meta-analyses; increased risk of thrombotic events with ESA use has been reported by Bennett et al. (RR = 1.57; 955 CI, 1.31–1.87), Tonelli et al. (RR = 1.69; 95% CI, 1.27–1.72), Glaspy et al. (OR = 1.48; 95% CI, 1.28–1.72) [36, 37, 52, 53]. In two IPD-based meta-analyses restricted to specific ESAs, first evaluating Epoetin β in seven trials including 2112 patients and second on darbepoietin in 12 trials including 2297 patients, RR for TVEs was increased for patients on ESAs (RR = 1.62; 95% CI, 1.13–2.31 and RR = 1.57; 95% CI, 1.10–2.26) [36, 54]. Therefore in light of current evidence oncologists need to be aware of increased risk of thromboembolic events in anemic patients on ESA.

3. Anti-erythropoietin antibodies induced pure red cell aplasia (PRCA)

PRCA is a rare occurrence, characterized by anti-erythropoietin antibodies, low reticulocyte count, loss of erythroblasts in marrow and resistance to ESA therapy. It has been reported mostly in patients with chronic renal disease on ESA and its occurrence in cancer patients is still unclear [55]. After its initial reports in 1998 the incidence reached its peak in 2001; up to 2004, 191 cases had been reported [56]. It was primarily associated with use of Eprex, a recombinant erythropoietin used outside the US. The association was implicated to the subcutaneous route, uncoated rubber stoppers and formulations without human albumin [55]. Interventions aimed at these associations led to decrease in incidence by 90% [55]. PRCA led to a class label change for all ESAs. Based on these observations, ESA withdrawal is recommended in cancer patients developing sudden loss of response to ESA accompanied by severe anemia and decreased reticulo-cyte count and should be evaluated for anti-erythropoietin antibodies [28].

4. Other

Seizures have been reported in patients receiving ESAs for chronic renal failure but their incidence and risk in the oncology population is still unknown [30]. However, Hb level monitoring is recommended to decrease the risk of such events in cancer patients [28].

Iron supplementation with ESA

Currently, iron administration is recommended as a supplement to ESA therapy only [28]. Its role as a monotherapy for cancer-related anemia is still being evaluated in different clinical trials. Different oral and I/V formulations of iron are available however only intravenous (I/V) iron supplementation has been found to accentuate Hb response in anemic cancer patients receiving ESA [57]. The basis of this supplementation roots from the reasoning that continued use of erythropoietin can cause functional iron deficiency. It is hypothesized that, similar to patients with chronic renal failure, the rapid erythropoiesis induced by ESA leads to slower release of iron as it causes iron mobilization from reticuloen-dothelial cells to bone marrow [15]. Also, hepcidin, a molecule known to block the release of iron by reticuloendothelial cells to its transporter transferrin, is up-regulated by inflammatory cytokines released during malignancy or after ESA administration [57, 58]. Hence, baseline and periodic monitoring of iron, C reactive protein, TFS and ferritin levels are recommended [28, 31], with ESA use to rule out this functional iron deficiency. Also, absolute iron deficiency (TSAT < 15%, serum ferritin < 30 ng/ml), identified prior to ESA use, may respond to oral or I/V iron. However, I/V or oral iron as monotherapy in cancer-related anemia are still being evaluated in various clinical trials.

Peripheral red blood cell (PRBC) transfusion

Peripheral red blood cell (PRBC) is the whole blood fraction of choice for treating anemia. PRBC fraction is separated from the whole blood using centrifugation or aphaeresis. Further processing includes processes such as anticoagulation, addition of preservatives, leukoreductions, irradiation, freezing and washing. Since, PRBC transfusion is administration of RBCs from a healthy individual (donor)to a patient (recipient) [16]; therefore this process does involve a "tissue transplant", having its specific implications in the oncology population. Besides the possibility of a plethora of transfusion reactions (ref), similar to that encountered in the non-oncologic population, its immunosuppressive and pro-inflammatory effects have implications on survival and tumor progression in cancer patients as well. Transfusion is rarely indicated in oncology for Hb level above 10 g/dl. The transfusion practice varies in oncology but it is often restrictive [59, 60]. The need for PRBC transfusion is not judged based on some "trigger" threshold Hb [28], but is judged based on an individualized approach as per the aforementioned risk assessment criteria. However, an increase in transfusion usage for anemia correction may be observed following the restrictions on ESA use in cancer patients being treated with curative intent [61].

Benefits
1. Rapid correction of anemia
Rapid correction of anemia being its major advantage, this is a modality of preference in acute settings and in phases of therapy that need immediate correction of anemia. One unit of PRBC is estimated to raise Hb level by 1 g/dl and Hematocrit by 3% in a normal sized adult with no active bleeding [62].

2. Improved survival in a subset
Improved survival has been observed in selective populations receiving transfusion for maintaining Hb in the optimal range during radiation as

discussed later [19, 20, 60, 63]. However, investigators believe that anemia, hypoxia, and transfusion have complex interaction that may vary in different cancer subtypes and needs further research [64].

Risks

1. Immunosupression and cancer progression

Interestingly patients receiving blood transfusion prior to organ transplantation have long been reported to have better graft and patient survival [65, 66]. This led to the hypothesis that host immune surveillance against tumor cells may get compromised secondary to this immunosupression following transfusion translating into increased tumor recurrence. This was potentiated by various prospective and retrospective cancer colon studies [65]. Various animal and clinical studies potentiated this observation though a causal relationship could not be established yet. Allogenic leukocytes were implicated for this effect but trials with leukodepletion in colorectal cancer and other cancers showed no benefit in terms of recurrence rates though improved survival was reported [67, 68].

Though the mechanism of transfusion-induced immunomodulation are still to being elucidated but potential mediators mentioned in literature include decreased natural killer cells [69], interleukin2 production, pro-cancer cytokine accumulation in stored blood, activation of suppressor t lymphocytes with decreased helper/suppressor ratio, and decreased macrophage antigen presentation [70, 71]. This immunosupression is also responsible for increased post-surgical infections. The complex effect of PRBC transfusion on cancer prognosis will be discussed later.

2. Infectious and non-infectious complications

Though blood transfusion is increasingly safe following specific donor screening essays and other interventions, the plethora of complications associated with it historically, worldwide travel enabling non-endemic pathogens, and the ever existing vulnerability to as yet unknown potentially lethal viruses and other pathogens warrants its cautious use [16, 72]. Other hazards, such as human error resulting in the inadvertent transfusion of incompatible blood, acute and delayed transfusion reactions, transfusion-related acute lung injury (TRALI), transfusion-associated graft-versus-host disease (TA-GVHD) are still prevalent and need consideration in this setting as well [72–77].

3. Arterial and venous thromboembolism

In a retrospective study of 70542 investigating the associations between transfusions and venous thromboembolism, arterial thromboembolism, and mortality in hospitalized cancer patients using the discharge database, reported increased venous and arterial thromboembolism in addition to increased risk of hospital mortality associated with transfusions in these patients [78].

4. Iron overload

This condition is generally observed in patients requiring repeated transfusions over years to manage their anemia as in patients with myelodysplatic syndrome(MDS) [79], and is less expected with transfusions used for chemotherapy-induced anemia (period generally less than a year) or perioperative transfusions.

5. Limited supply

Finally, limited supply of PRBC, a finite source, needs consideration as well.

6. Blood transfusion and cancer prognosis; an ongoing controversy

The effect of transfusions on cancer prognosis has long been debated and it appears that transfusions used in different settings in oncology have different implications. Literature reports poorer survivals with perioperative transfusions while some positive associations were observed when used in anemic patients on radiation. However, the impact of transfusions on survival in advanced cancer for symptomatic palliation is still elusive.

Peri-operative allogenic blood transfusion association with poorer prognosis in terms of tumor recurrence and increased mortality is often reported, but its independent effect on prognosis is still eluded by various confounding factors [66, 80, 82]. Largely because most of these studies had been retrospective with variable endpoints. So, there exists a possibility that circumstances necessitating blood transfusion, rather than transfusion itself, underlie such outcomes. Also, it is ethically impossible to randomize preoperatively patients into those who will and who will not receive transfusions. A meta-analysis including 12127 patients with colon cancer treated with curative resection support the hypothesis that peri-operative transfusions have a detrimental effect on the recurrence of curable colorectal cancers [82]. Similarly, in a meta-analysis of patients undergoing resection for gastric cancer, preoperative transfusion was a statistically significant negative influence on 5-year survival and overall survival rate (58.2% vs 79.9% [P = 0.00], 58.2% vs 76.8% [P = 0.00]) [83]. Different hypothesis exist in literature explaining the underlying mechanisms for transfusion-induced tumor progression; immunosuppressive effect mediated by leukocytes or soluble bioactive molecules in products producing

Table 11.3 Risks and benefits associated with various treatment options for anemia in cancer patients.

ESA

Benefits	Risks
1 Avoidance of PRBC transfusion 2 Improved QoL	1 Shortened survival 2 Tumor progression 3 Thromboembolic events 4 Pure red cell aplasia

PRBC transfusion

Benefits	Risks
1 Almost immediate correction of anemia 2 Rapid symptomatic improvement	1 Transfusion reactions 2 Infectious complications 3 Immunosupression 4 Limited supply 5 Compromised survival in certain cases

Iron Supplementation

Benefits	Risks
1 Improved response in Hb levels when used with ESA for functional iron deficiency	1 Use as monotherapy for cancer-related anemia is still being evaluated

immune turmoil during the peri-operative period thus enabling the escape of less cohesive malignant cells from the attack of already decreased natural killer cells [16]. Others have proposed the release of active lipids from aged RBCs, promoting tumor cell proliferation [82]. Though the causal relationship cannot be established clearly because of inherent limitations mentioned early, but almost none have reported any positive correlation with survival in perioperative setting therefore investigators have suggested restrictive strategies for transfusion in this setting.

However, transfusion used in a subset of anemic patients on radiation reveals some benefits. A study in 56 consecutive patients with unresectable esophageal cancer treated with chemo radiation revealed increase in overall survival (hazard ratio = 0.26; 95% CI 0.09–0.75, p = 0.01) [60]. In addition, benefits in terms of increased local control and disease free survival were also observed in patients with cervix cancer treated with definitive radiotherapy and transfusions used to maintain the Hb level around 12 g/dl [19, 20, 63].

Transfusion use in advanced cancer setting evaluated in the Cochrane review by Preston et al. [84], revealed high 14 day mortality rate; however, the fact that only 12 studies identified with a total of 653 patients were conducted limited the power to distinguish potential harms of blood transfusion at end of life from inappropriate transfusion in patients dying from advanced cancer. The authors concluded that higher quality studies are still required to identify the subgroup that will be benefitted the most in this setting by transfusion.

Trend of increased transfusions because of decreased ESA use

As discussed earlier, the current recommendations restricting use of ESAs in cancer patients being treated with curative intent may increase their use in the near future [85]. In a modeling simulation employed to evaluate the excess number of RBC units that would be required with limited ESA treatment as per current recommendations, revealed limiting ESA use would impose considerable pressure on the available blood supply margin given the small margin between usable blood and transfusion demand [61]. Approximately 202 000 additional units of PRBCs would be required if ESA use was reduced by 75% [23].

Current recommendations

An individualized approach for risk vs. benefit assessment [28, 31], is recommended while opting for the treatment option of anemia. ESAs in patients with solid tumors are only recommended to be used for chemotherapy-induced anemia and to be discontinued on completion of chemotherapy course. Also, in the light of aforementioned concerns, FDA has mandated risk evaluation and mitigation strategy (REMS) for hospitals and physicians prescribing ESA therapy [30]. Though ESAs' association with tumor progression and mortality is still disputed, but based on present negative clinical data, their use in patients being treated with curative intent is strongly discouraged. However, for patients undergoing palliative treatment ESAs can be used preferentially over transfusion [28]. Also in light of an emerging concept of existence of optimal Hb levels, FDA mandates individualized titration of ESA dosing to maintain Hb levels within 10–12 g/dl. Use of ESA in proximity of PRBC transfusion is not recommended because of probable additive thrombotic effect. Iron therapy is only indicated for absolute or functional iron deficiency.

Evolving concepts

The possibility of the negative impact of ESAs on survival being secondary to higher than optimal HB levels achieved in various RCTs is being investigated in current trials. Ongoing Phase III trials (NCT00338286 and NCT00858364) are evaluating the impact of use of ESAs according to label guidance on tumor progression in patients with metastatic cancer on standard chemotherapy. Also, trials (NCT01168505 and NCTO1145638) are underway to evaluate the impact of iron on preventing and treating chemotherapy-induced anemia. Besides, hemoglobin-based oxygen carriers and perflourocarbons are being studied as oxygen carriers that can supplement hemoglobin in humans.

Conclusion

ESAs had been the most frequent agents used for anemia management in oncology practice until recently, but the latest studies showing association of ESAs with decreased survival have brought a change in the paradigm leading to revised guidelines for their use. ESAs' use outside the treatment period of cancer-related chemotherapy has been discouraged. Blood transfusions are generally offered when immediate boost of Hb is required. Results of studies evaluating the effect of transfusion on survival in cancer patients have been conflicting; some raising the possibility of increased mortality and decreased time to tumor progression in patients receiving transfusions. However, the contemporary phase of limiting the use of ESAs may substantially lean towards increased use of transfusions in these patients. In light of recognized limited supply of blood in the US, and potential side effects associated with transfusions, future trials are required to evaluate the role of IV iron and other preventive and prophylactic measures to curtail transfusion needs.

References

1 Knight K, Wade S, Balducci L. Prevalence and outcomes of anemia in cancer: a systematic review of the literature. Am J Med. 2004 Apr 5;116 (Suppl 7A):11S–26S.

2 Ludwig H, Van Belle S, Barrett-Lee P, Birgegard G, Bokemeyer C, Gascon P, et al. The European Cancer Anaemia Survey (ECAS): a large, multinational, prospective survey defining the prevalence, incidence, and treatment of anaemia in cancer patients. Eur J Cancer. 2004 Oct;40(15):2293–306.

3 Ludwig H, Aapro M, Bokemeyer C, Macdonald K, Soubeyran P, Turner M, et al. Treatment patterns and outcomes in the management of anaemia in cancer patients in Europe: findings from the Anaemia Cancer Treatment (ACT) study. Eur J Cancer. 2009 Jun;45(9):1603–15.

4 Grant DG, Hussain A, Hurman D. Pre-treatment anaemia alters outcome in early squamous cell carcinoma of the larynx treated by radical radiotherapy. J Laryngol Otol. 1999 Sep;113(9):829–33.

5 Munstedt K, Kovacic M, Zygmunt M, Von Georgi R. Impact of hemoglobin levels before and during chemotherapy on survival of patients with ovarian cancer. Int J Oncol. 2003 Sep;23(3):837–43.

6 Wigren T, Oksanen H, Kellokumpu-Lehtinen P. A practical prognostic index for inoperable non-small-cell lung cancer. J Cancer Res Clin Oncol. 1997;123(5): 259–66.

7 Watine J, Bouarioua N. Anemia as an independent prognostic factor for survival in patients with cancer. Cancer. 2002 May 15;94(10):2793–6; author reply 6–7.

8 Dunst J, Kuhnt T, Strauss HG, Krause U, Pelz T, Koelbl H, et al. Anemia in cervical cancers: impact on survival, patterns of relapse, and association with hypoxia and angiogenesis. Int J Radiat Oncol Biol Phys. 2003 Jul 1;56(3):778–87.

9 Caro JJ, Salas M, Ward A, Goss G. Anemia as an independent prognostic factor for survival in patients with cancer: a systemic, quantitative review. Cancer. 2001 Jun 15;91(12):2214–21.

10 Ludwig H, Strasser K. Symptomatology of anemia. Semin Oncol. 2001 Apr;28 (2 Suppl 8):7–14.

11 Cella D. The effects of anemia and anemia treatment on the quality of life of people with cancer. Oncology (Williston Park). 2002 Sep;16(9 Suppl 10):125–32.

12 Dunst J. Management of anemia in patients undergoing curative radiotherapy. Erythropoietin, transfusions, or better nothing? Strahlenther Onkol. 2004 Nov;180(11):671–81.

13 Gabrilove JL, Cleeland CS, Livingston RB, Sarokhan B, Winer E, Einhorn LH. Clinical evaluation of once-weekly dosing of epoetin alfa in chemotherapy patients: improvements in hemoglobin and quality of life are similar to three-times-weekly dosing. J Clin Oncol. 2001 Jun 1;19(11):2875–82.

14 Glimelius B, Linne T, Hoffman K, Larsson L, Svensson JH, Nasman P, et al. Epoetin beta in the treatment of anemia in patients with advanced gastrointestinal cancer. J Clin Oncol. 1998 Feb;16(2):434–40.

15 Spivak JL. The anaemia of cancer: death by a thousand cuts. Nat Rev Cancer. 2005 Jul;5(7):543–55.

16 Spivak JL, Gascon P, Ludwig H. Anemia management in oncology and hematology. Oncologist. 2009;14 Suppl 1:43–56.

17 Kelleher DK, Baussmann E, Friedrich E, Vaupel P. The effect of erythropoietin on tumor oxygenation in normal and anemic rats. Adv Exp Med Biol. 1994;345: 517–24.

18 Rofstad EK, Sundfor K, Lyng H, Trope CG. Hypoxia-induced treatment failure in advanced squamous cell carcinoma of the uterine cervix is primarily due to hypoxia-induced radiation resistance rather than hypoxia-induced metastasis. Br J Cancer. 2000 Aug;83(3):354–9.

19 Grogan M, Thomas GM, Melamed I, Wong FL, Pearcey RG, Joseph PK, et al. The importance of hemoglobin levels during radiotherapy for carcinoma of the cervix. Cancer. 1999 Oct 15;86(8):1528–36.

20 Bush RS. The significance of anemia in clinical radiation therapy. Int J Radiat Oncol Biol Phys. 1986 Nov;12(11):2047–50.

21 Yovino S, Kwok Y, Krasna M, Bangalore M, Suntharalingam M. An association between preoperative anemia and decreased survival in early-stage non-small-cell lung cancer patients treated with surgery alone. Int J Radiat Oncol Biol Phys. 2005 Aug 1;62(5):1438–43.

22 Yamaji H, Iizasa T, Koh E, Suzuki M, Otsuji M, Chang H, et al. Correlation between interleukin 6 production and tumor proliferation in non-small cell lung cancer. Cancer Immunol Immunother. 2004 Sep;53(9):786–92.

23 Aebersold DM, Burri P, Beer KT, Laissue J, Djonov V, Greiner RH, et al. Expression of hypoxia-inducible factor-1alpha: a novel predictive and prognostic parameter in the radiotherapy of oropharyngeal cancer. Cancer Res. 2001 Apr 1;61(7): 2911–6.

24 Vaupel P. Hypoxia and aggressive tumor phenotype: implications for therapy and prognosis. Oncologist. 2008;13 Suppl 3:21–6.

25 Moliterno AR, Spivak JL. Anemia of cancer. Hematol Oncol Clin North Am. 1996 Apr;10(2):345–63.

26 Schwartz RN. Anemia in patients with cancer: incidence, causes, impact, management, and use of treatment guidelines and protocols. Am J Health Syst Pharm. 2007 Feb 1;64(3 Suppl 2):S5–13; quiz S28–30.

27 Jefferies S, Rajan B, Ashley S, Traish D, Brada M. Haematological toxicity of cranio-spinal irradiation. Radiother Oncol. 1998 Jul;48(1):23–7.

28 National Comprehensive Cancer Network: NCCN Clinical Practice Guidelines in Oncology:Cancer and Chemotherapy-induced anemia. http://www.nccnorg/ professionals/physician_gls/f_guidelinesasp#supportive. accessed May 27, 2011.

29 Wilson J, Yao GL, Raftery J, Bohlius J, Brunskill S, Sandercock J, et al. A systematic review and economic evaluation of epoetin alpha, epoetin beta and darbepoetin alpha in anaemia associated with cancer, especially that attributable to cancer treatment. Health Technol Assess. 2007 Apr;11(13):1–202, iii–iv.

30 Food and Drug Administration. FDA information on ESAs. 2010. http://www .fdagov/drugs/drugsafety/postmarketdrugsafetyinformationforpatientsand providers/ucm109375htm. Accessed May 27, 2012.

31 Schrijvers D, De Samblanx H, Roila F. Erythropoiesis-stimulating agents in the treatment of anaemia in cancer patients: ESMO Clinical Practice Guidelines for use. Ann Oncol. 2010 May;21 (Suppl 5):v244–7.

32 Aapro M, Jelkmann W, Constantinescu SN, Leyland-Jones B. Effects of erythropoietin receptors and erythropoiesis-stimulating agents on disease progression in cancer. Br J Cancer. 2012 Mar 27;106(7):1249–58.

33 Osterborg A, Aapro M, Cornes P, Haselbeck A, Hayward CR, Jelkmann W. Preclinical studies of erythropoietin receptor expression in tumour cells: impact on clinical use of erythropoietic proteins to correct cancer-related anaemia. Eur J Cancer. 2007 Feb;43(3):510–9.

34 Spivak JL. The blood in systemic disorders. Lancet. 2000 May 13;355(9216):1707–12.

35 Bohlius J, Tonia T, Schwarzer G. Twist and shout: one decade of meta-analyses of erythropoiesis-stimulating agents in cancer patients. Acta Haematol. 2011;125(1–2):55–67.

36 Ludwig H, Crawford J, Osterborg A, Vansteenkiste J, Henry DH, Fleishman A, et al. Pooled analysis of individual patient-level data from all randomized, double-blind, placebo-controlled trials of darbepoetin alfa in the treatment of patients with chemotherapy-induced anemia. J Clin Oncol. 2009 Jun 10;27(17):2838–47.

37 Tonelli M, Hemmelgarn B, Reiman T, Manns B, Reaume MN, Lloyd A, et al. Benefits and harms of erythropoiesis-stimulating agents for anemia related to cancer: a meta-analysis. CMAJ. 2009 May 26;180(11):E62–71.

38 Littlewood TJ. Management options for cancer therapy-related anaemia. Drug Saf. 2002;25(7):525–35.

39 Bohlius J, Wilson J, Seidenfeld J, Piper M, Schwarzer G, Sandercock J, et al. Erythropoietin or darbepoetin for patients with cancer. Cochrane Database Syst Rev. 2006(3):CD003407.

40 Vadhan-Raj S, Mirtsching B, Charu V, Terry D, Rossi G, Tomita D, et al. Assessment of hematologic effects and fatigue in cancer patients with chemotherapy-induced anemia given darbepoetin alfa every two weeks. J Support Oncol. 2003 Jul–Aug; 1(2):131–8.

41 Jones M, Schenkel B, Just J, Fallowfield L. Epoetin alfa improves quality of life in patients with cancer: results of metaanalysis. Cancer. 2004 Oct 15;101(8): 1720–32.

42 Littlewood TJ, Bajetta E, Nortier JW, Vercammen E, Rapoport B. Effects of epoetin alfa on hematologic parameters and quality of life in cancer patients receiving non-platinum chemotherapy: results of a randomized, double-blind, placebo-controlled trial. J Clin Oncol. 2001 Jun 1;19(11):2865–74.

43 Ross SD, Allen IE, Henry DH, Seaman C, Sercus B, Goodnough LT. Clinical benefits and risks associated with epoetin and darbepoetin in patients with chemotherapy-induced anemia: a systematic review of the literature. Clin Ther. 2006 Jun;28(6):801–31.

44 Crawford J, Cella D, Cleeland CS, Cremieux PY, Demetri GD, Sarokhan BJ, et al. Relationship between changes in hemoglobin level and quality of life during chemotherapy in anemic cancer patients receiving epoetin alfa therapy. Cancer. 2002 Aug 15;95(4):888–95.

45 Henke M, Laszig R, Rube C, Schafer U, Haase KD, Schilcher B, et al. Erythropoietin to treat head and neck cancer patients with anaemia undergoing radiotherapy: randomised, double-blind, placebo-controlled trial. Lancet. 2003 Oct 18; 362(9392):1255–60.

46 Leyland-Jones B. Breast cancer trial with erythropoietin terminated unexpectedly. Lancet Oncol. 2003 Aug;4(8):459–60.

47 Wright JR, Ung YC, Julian JA, Pritchard KI, Whelan TJ, Smith C, et al. Randomized, double-blind, placebo-controlled trial of erythropoietin in non-small-cell lung cancer with disease-related anemia. J Clin Oncol. 2007 Mar 20;25(9):1027–32.

48 Smith RE, Jr., Aapro MS, Ludwig H, Pinter T, Smakal M, Ciuleanu TE, et al. Darbepoetin alpha for the treatment of anemia in patients with active cancer not receiving

chemotherapy or radiotherapy: results of a phase III, multicenter, randomized, double-blind, placebo-controlled study. J Clin Oncol. 2008 Mar 1;26(7):1040–50.

49 Bohlius J, Langensiepen S, Schwarzer G, Seidenfeld J, Piper M, Bennett C, et al. Recombinant human erythropoietin and overall survival in cancer patients: results of a comprehensive meta-analysis. J Natl Cancer Inst. 2005 Apr 6;97(7):489–98.

50 Bohlius J, Weingart O, Trelle S, Engert A. Cancer-related anemia and recombinant human erythropoietin--an updated overview. Nat Clin Pract Oncol. 2006 Mar;3(3):152–64.

51 Bohlius J, Schmidlin K, Brillant C, Schwarzer G, Trelle S, Seidenfeld J, et al. Erythropoietin or Darbepoetin for patients with cancer--meta-analysis based on individual patient data. Cochrane Database Syst Rev. 2009(3):CD007303.

52 Bennett CL, Silver SM, Djulbegovic B, Samaras AT, Blau CA, Gleason KJ, et al. Venous thromboembolism and mortality associated with recombinant erythropoietin and darbepoetin administration for the treatment of cancer-associated anemia. JAMA. 2008 Feb 27;299(8):914–24.

53 Glaspy J, Crawford J, Vansteenkiste J, Henry D, Rao S, Bowers P, et al. Erythropoiesis-stimulating agents in oncology: a study-level meta-analysis of survival and other safety outcomes. Br J Cancer. 2010 Jan 19;102(2):301–15.

54 Aapro M, Scherhag A, Burger HU. Effect of treatment with epoetin-beta on survival, tumour progression and thromboembolic events in patients with cancer: an updated meta-analysis of 12 randomised controlled studies including 2301 patients. Br J Cancer. 2008 Jul 8;99(1):14–22.

55 McKoy JM, Stonecash RE, Cournoyer D, Rossert J, Nissenson AR, Raisch DW, et al. Epoetin-associated pure red cell aplasia: past, present, and future considerations. Transfusion. 2008 Aug;48(8):1754–62.

56 Bennett CL, Luminari S, Nissenson AR, Tallman MS, Klinge SA, McWilliams N, et al. Pure red-cell aplasia and epoetin therapy. N Engl J Med. 2004 Sep 30; 351(14):1403–8.

57 Weiss G, Goodnough LT. Anemia of chronic disease. N Engl J Med. 2005 Mar 10;352(10):1011–23.

58 Henry DH. Supplemental Iron: A Key to Optimizing the Response of Cancer-Related Anemia to rHuEPO? Oncologist. 1998;3(4):275–8.

59 Hill SR, Carless PA, Henry DA, Carson JL, Hebert PC, McClelland DB, et al. Transfusion thresholds and other strategies for guiding allogeneic red blood cell transfusion. Cochrane Database Syst Rev. 2002(2):CD002042.

60 Kader AS, Lim JT, Berthelet E, Petersen R, Ludgate D, Truong PT. Prognostic significance of blood transfusions in patients with esophageal cancer treated with combined chemoradiotherapy. Am J Clin Oncol. 2007 Oct;30(5):492–7.

61 Vekeman F, Bookhart BK, White J, McKenzie RS, Duh MS, Piech CT, et al. Impact of limiting erythropoiesis-stimulating agent use for chemotherapy-induced anemia on the United States blood supply margin. Transfusion. 2009 May;49(5):895–902.

62 Wiesen AR, Hospenthal DR, Byrd JC, Glass KL, Howard RS, Diehl LF. Equilibration of hemoglobin concentration after transfusion in medical inpatients not actively bleeding. Ann Intern Med. 1994 Aug 15;121(4):278–30.

63 Kapp KS, Poschauko J, Geyer E, Berghold A, Oechs AC, Petru E, et al. Evaluation of the effect of routine packed red blood cell transfusion in anemic cervix cancer

patients treated with radical radiotherapy. Int J Radiat Oncol Biol Phys. 2002 Sep 1;54(1):58–66.

64 Fyles AW, Milosevic M, Pintilie M, Syed A, Hill RP. Anemia, hypoxia and transfusion in patients with cervix cancer: a review. Radiother Oncol. 2000 Oct;57(1):13–19.

65 Vamvakas EC, Blajchman MA. Transfusion-related immunomodulation (TRIM): an update. Blood Rev. 2007 Nov;21(6):327–48.

66 Vamvakas EC, Blajchman MA. Deleterious clinical effects of transfusion-associated immunomodulation: fact or fiction? Blood. 2001 Mar 1;97(5):1180–95.

67 van de Watering LM, Brand A, Houbiers JG, Klein Kranenbarg WM, Hermans J, van de Velde C. Perioperative blood transfusions, with or without allogeneic leucocytes, relate to survival, not to cancer recurrence. Br J Surg. 2001 Feb;88(2):267–72.

68 Houbiers JG, Brand A, van de Watering LM, Hermans J, Verwey PJ, Bijnen AB, et al. Randomised controlled trial comparing transfusion of leucocyte-depleted or buffy-coat-depleted blood in surgery for colorectal cancer. Lancet. 1994 Aug 27;344(8922):573–8.

69 Gascon P, Zoumbos NC, Young NS. Immunologic abnormalities in patients receiving multiple blood transfusions. Ann Intern Med. 1984 Feb;100(2):173–7.

70 Weitz J, D'Angelica M, Gonen M, Klimstra D, Coit DG, Brennan MF, et al. Interaction of splenectomy and perioperative blood transfusions on prognosis of patients with proximal gastric and gastroesophageal junction cancer. J Clin Oncol. 2003 Dec 15;21(24):4597–603.

71 Benson DD, Beck AW, Burdine MS, Brekken R, Silliman CC, Barnett CC, Jr. Accumulation of pro-cancer cytokines in the plasma fraction of stored packed red cells. J Gastrointest Surg. 2012 Mar;16(3):460–8.

72 Alter HJ, Klein HG. The hazards of blood transfusion in historical perspective. Blood. 2008 Oct 1;112(7):2617–26.

73 Walther-Wenke G, Schmidt M. Impact of Bacterial Contamination on Blood Supply. Transfus Med Hemother. 2011;38(4):229–30.

74 Wallis JP. Progress in TRALI. Transfus Med. 2008 Oct;18(5):273–5.

75 Brand A. Immunological aspects of blood transfusions. Blood Rev. 2000 Sep; 14(3):130–44.

76 Vamvakas EC, Blajchman MA. Transfusion-related mortality: the ongoing risks of allogeneic blood transfusion and the available strategies for their prevention. Blood. 2009 Apr 9;113(15):3406–17.

77 Vamvakas EC, Blajchman MA. Blood still kills: six strategies to further reduce allogeneic blood transfusion-related mortality. Transfus Med Rev. 2010 Apr; 24(2):77–124.

78 Khorana AA, Francis CW, Blumberg N, Culakova E, Refaai MA, Lyman GH. Blood transfusions, thrombosis, and mortality in hospitalized patients with cancer. Arch Intern Med. 2008 Nov 24;168(21):2377–81.

79 Jabbour E, Kantarjian HM, Koller C, Taher A. Red blood cell transfusions and iron overload in the treatment of patients with myelodysplastic syndromes. Cancer. 2008 Mar 1;112(5):1089–95.

80 Blumberg N, Heal JM. Noncausal relationship between cancer recurrence and perioperative blood transfusions. Ann Surg. 1995 Dec;222(6):757–8.

81 Heiss MM, Mempel W, Delanoff C, Jauch KW, Gabka C, Mempel M, et al. Blood transfusion-modulated tumor recurrence: first results of a randomized study of autologous versus allogeneic blood transfusion in colorectal cancer surgery. J Clin Oncol. 1994 Sep;12(9):1859–67.

82 Amato A, Pescatori M. Perioperative blood transfusions for the recurrence of colorectal cancer. Cochrane Database Syst Rev. 2006(1):CD005033.

83 Kim SH, Lee SI, Noh SM. Prognostic significance of preoperative blood transfusion in stomach cancer. J Gastric Cancer. 2010 Dec;10(4):196–205.

84 Preston NJ, Hurlow A, Brine J, Bennett MI. Blood transfusions for anaemia in patients with advanced cancer. Cochrane Database Syst Rev. 2012;2:CD009007.

85 Henry DH, Langer CJ, McKenzie RS, Piech CT, Senbetta M, Schulman KL, et al. Hematologic outcomes and blood utilization in cancer patients with chemotherapy-induced anemia (CIA) pre- and post-national coverage determination (NCD): results from a multicenter chart review. Support Care Cancer. 2011 Dec 11.

CHAPTER 12

Artificial blood

Aryeh Shander, Mazyar Javidroozi, and Seth Perelman

Department of Anesthesiology and Critical Care Medicine, Englewood Hospital and Medical Center, Englewood, NJ, USA

Background

As one of the most prominent tissues of the body, blood plays several vital functions. In addition to being the largest buffer, it provides a medium to transport gases, nutrients, waste products, and biochemical signals throughout the body, supports the osmotic and electrochemical balance in the body, provides volume and viscosity to maintain organ and tissue perfusion, and serves as the cornerstone of the coagulation and immune system. To perform these and other known and yet-to-be-discovered functions, blood relies on various components such as red blood cells (RBCs), white blood cells (WBCs), platelets, and a myriad of plasma factors. Needless to say, recreating all these tasks *de novo* in a synthetic product – to make an omni-functional "artificial blood" capable of completely replacing human blood – is a very difficult challenge and not likely to be achievable in near future.

Alternatively, products intended to replace one or a few functions of blood have been under investigation and some have been in clinical use for years. In many ways, various crystalloid and colloid fluids widely in use in clinical practice can be a viewed as "blood substitutes" due to their hemodynamic and circulatory role, impairment of which can quickly lead to circulatory collapse and death. Transportation of oxygen is the other critical function of blood under active investigation, giving rise to "artificial oxygen carriers" (AOCs). It is this aspect that is most commonly considered today when discussing artificial blood. While our focus in this chapter will be on these products, it should be remembered that such products are not, by any means, true substitutes for blood, and they often provide temporary replacement for a few of the many vital blood functions.

Transfusion-Free Medicine and Surgery, Second Edition. Edited by Nicolas Jabbour.
© 2014 John Wiley & Sons, Ltd. Published 2014 by John Wiley & Sons, Ltd.

Basics of blood oxygen transportation

Oxygen is carried in the blood mainly in two forms: chemically-bound to the iron in the heme group of hemoglobin (Hb) molecules within the RBCs, and physically dissolved in plasma. Each Hb molecule can carry up to four oxygen molecules, yielding a maximum oxygen binding capacity of 1.34 mL/g of Hb under normal physiologic conditions. Hb is a large molecule and its complex tetrameric structure allows its affinity for oxygen to be regulated at various levels. Binding of the oxygen molecule to a Hb subunit results in conformational changes that would affect the other subunits in the tetramer and increase their affinity for oxygen. This "cooperative binding" of oxygen to Hb creates the classic sigmoidal Hb-oxygen dissociation curve (Figure 12.1). Additionally, various external factors can affect the affinity of Hb for oxygen. For example, decreased pH (due to increased level of carbon dioxide [Bohr effect], a condition that is prevalent at tissue sites) and increased 2,3-diphosphoglycerate (2,3-DPG) would reduce the affinity of Hb for oxygen and facilitate the release of oxygen from Hb molecules (Figure 12.1). Affinity of Hb for oxygen is often quantified by P_{50}, which is the partial pressure of the oxygen (PO_2) that results in 50% Hb oxygen saturation (SO_2 50%) (Figure 12.1). Normal adult human Hb (Hb-A) has a P_{50} of approximately 26 mmHg. Altogether, these factors dynamically regulate the affinity of Hb for oxygen and optimize oxygen uptake in the lungs and oxygen release in the tissues where it is needed [1–3]. Total Hb-bound oxygen of blood (in liters) can be calculated based on the equation below using Hb concentration in g/L and SO_2 expressed as a value between 0 and 1.0 [1, 4]:

$$Hb - bound\ oxygen = Hb\ concentration \times Hb\ oxygen\ saturation\ (SO_2) \times 0.00134$$

The other component of oxygen carried by blood, the plasma-dissolved oxygen, obeys the much simpler rule of Henry's law, which states that at any given temperature, the amount of a gas dissolved in a liquid is directly (and linearly) proportional to the partial pressure of the gas in equilibrium with the liquid, i.e. the higher the partial pressure of the gas, the higher the dissolved amount of gas will be [1, 4]:

$$Plasma - dissolved\ oxygen = PO_2 \times Henry's\ law\ constant$$

Under normal physiologic conditions and temperature of 37 °C, each liter of plasma is capable of dissolving about 0.00003 L oxygen per each

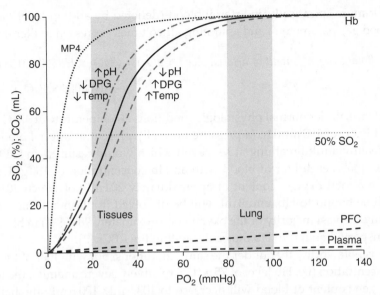

Figure 12.1 Relation between partial pressure of oxygen (PO_2) and oxygen saturation/content of Hb molecules, plasma, and two artificial oxygen carriers, in a 150 mL sample with 75 g total Hb content at 37 °C. For PFC sample, it was assumed that it completely replaced the plasma (75 mL). These numbers were selected in order to keep the numeric values of the Hb oxygen content (CO_2, mL) and Hb-oxygen saturation (SO_2, %) the same. The solid black line represents normal Hb in RBCs (as well as some of the HBOCs, although individual differences exist). The dashed gray lines represent the shift to left or right in Hb-oxygen dissociation curve as a result of changes in pH, 2,3-DPG or temperature. The dotted black line represents MP4, an HBOC with particularly high affinity for oxygen (low P_{50}), which is expected to release its oxygen content at very low oxygen levels (e.g. ischemic sites). Dashed black lines represent the oxygen dissolved in plasma or PFC. As can be seen, despite higher capacity of PFCs to dissolve oxygen compared with plasma, higher PO_2 levels are still needed to allow adequate oxygen delivery using PFCs. The horizontal dotted line represents the 50% SO_2. For each Hb-oxygen dissociation curves, the PO_2 that results in 50% SO_2 is the P_{50}. It should be noted that given the higher molecular weight of MP4, the oxygen content of an MP4 solution at any given SO2 will be lower than the oxygen content of a native Hb solution at similar concentration, and hence the CO_2 values on the vertical axis of the graph do not apply to MP4. Data to plot the graphs were obtained from Winslow RM [25] and Farmer M et al. [26].

1 mmHg PO_2 [1, 2] (Figure 12.1). Combining these two components would give us the total oxygen content of blood:

$$Total\ oxygen\ content\ of\ blood = Hb - bound\ oxygen + Plasma$$
$$- dissolved\ oxygen$$

Or more specifically, in arterial blood (denoted by adding letter "a" to blood gas parameters) and assuming all volumes expressed in liter units:

$$\textit{Total oxygen content of arterial blood } (CaO_2) = (SaO_2 \times Hb \times 0.00134)$$
$$+ (0.00003 \times PaO_2)$$

Hence, under normal physiologic conditions at temperature of 37 °C and at a PaO_2 of 100 mmHg (a pressure normally present in arterial blood of a healthy adult breathing at sea level) which would result in an SaO_2 of near 100%, each liter of blood with an Hb concentration of 150 g/L will have a total oxygen content of approximately 204 mL, of which 201 mL will be bound to Hb, and 3 mL will be dissolved in plasma. Hence, normally the vast majority of the oxygen (approximately 98–99%) in blood is transported bound to Hb molecules within the RBCs [2].

It is noteworthy that under the same conditions, but with half of the Hb concentration (i.e. Hb level of 75 g/L, a relatively severe anemia), the total oxygen content of blood will decrease to 103.5 mL: 100.5 mL, the halved Hb-bound component plus 3 mL, the dissolved component which stays relatively unchanged despite reduced Hb. Alternatively, at any given Hb level, the total oxygen content of each liter of blood can increase by 3 mL for every 100 mmHg increase in the PO_2. Unlike the Hb-bound oxygen that is quickly saturated as PO_2 approaches ~100 mmHg, the plasma-dissolved oxygen increases linearly with the increasing PO_2 and it does not reach a plateau (Figure 12.1). In severe anemia, all available Hb molecules are often fully saturated with oxygen (SaO_2 100%, a common finding in arterial blood gas [ABG] analysis of severely anemic patients that is often misinterpreted to incorrectly assume that the patient has normal oxygen delivery), but the total Hb-bound oxygen content of blood is reduced because of the reduced total Hb amount. Here, increased PaO_2 can increase the oxygen dissolved in plasma, independent of the Hb level. The resulting increase in total oxygen content of blood can be potentially life-saving if the oxygen demand of the tissues in a severely anemic patient is met and this approach is sometimes used in clinical practice when 100%fiO$_2$ and/or hyperbaric oxygen therapy is administered [5].

Defining the need for artificial oxygen carriers

When the oxygen content of the blood cannot meet the tissues' requirements, other approaches to quickly increase the blood's capacity to transport oxygen are needed. Blood transfusions (allogeneic or autologous) are the most commonly considered short-term solution in this situation and they are discussed in detail in the other chapters. There are, however, several issues of risks, costs, availability, and patient's preference/acceptance involved with use of allogeneic blood transfusions, which would make them less preferable, or occasionally even unacceptable or unavailable [6]. Artificial oxygen carriers can be an option in these cases.

Notwithstanding years of research and development, currently there is no artificial oxygen carrier approved in the United States by the Food and Drug Administration (FDA) that is available for clinical use. The regulatory status of these products globally is similar (with a few exceptions discussed below) but this could change anytime and readers are advised to seek the latest information on their availability. Regardless, and given the promising potential of these therapeutics, this is still a field of active research and several products are under various stages of investigation and development.

Artificial oxygen carriers are particularly promising given a number of potential characteristics of these products. While the reputation of allogeneic blood transfusions have been historically marred by their infectious risks [7], artificial oxygen carriers can be developed and produced to be free of most or all of the infectious risks of allogeneic blood (particularly true for synthetic products and those not derived from human/animal sources). Another feature that can be built in these products by design is the lack of requirement for blood grouping and cross matching, which could facilitate the timely infusion of the product and minimize the risk of transfusion errors. Artificial oxygen carriers can be designed to have an extended shelf-life and be stored either cooled or at room temperature. Another related advantage is the potential for virtually unlimited (and stable) availability of the products, an issue that occasionally emerges and affects the use of allogeneic blood, with some suggesting more shortages and related challenges still ahead [8]. Finally, allogeneic blood is inherently a complex product with a plethora of different components (cells, proteins, and others) that are constantly changing, even when blood is processed and stored. These components, many of which are not well described, are together considered a "black box." Numerous components and aspects of allogeneic blood (leukocytes, residual plasma, and storage duration, to name a few) have been scrutinized for their potential harmful effects adding to the quandary of the safety and efficacy of allogeneic blood [9, 10]. Given the theoretical possibility for controlled design and production, it may be feasible to develop artificial oxygen carriers with precisely defined and controlled characteristics that are optimized to achieve the goal of oxygen delivery without the other unwanted consequences [2, 11–13].

Artificial oxygen carriers achieve their oxygen transportation function by increasing the Hb-bound and/or plasma-dissolved oxygen content of blood. The products of the former group often provide additional Hb molecules that uptake more oxygen, while the latter group of artificial oxygen carriers provide fluids that can dissolve more oxygen at any given PO_2. The expected net result in either case is increased total oxygen content in the blood, beyond what is normally achieved by the patient's own Hb level, or the PaO_2 in equilibrium with blood perfusing the lungs. We will discuss the artificial oxygen carriers according to these two functional categories.

Hb-based oxygen carriers

As the name implies, Hb-based oxygen carriers (HBOCs) rely on the physiologic capability of Hb molecules to deliver oxygen. With the exception of pathological conditions resulting in hemolysis, Hb molecules are not free in plasma and are normally contained in the cytoplasm of RBCs circulating in the blood. In addition to providing an extra level of containment to keep the Hb molecules in the blood and prevent them from extravasating, the affinity of Hb for oxygen can also be tightly regulated by the factors present in the cytoplasm of RBCs (e.g. 2,3-DPG as mentioned earlier). These two aspects are often disrupted or missing in free HBOCs and as will be described, this is an area of concern.

Hb used to make HBOCs can be procured from various sources such as expired allogeneic blood units, animal blood, and more recently thanks to advances in biotechnology, *in vitro* synthesis (recombinant Hb) [14]. In addition to the various sources, the Hb molecules often undergo extensive processing and modifications to purify and modulate their pharmacodynamic and pharmacokinetic profiles, toxicity potential, and oxygen-dissociation curves. The first products in this category that underwent clinical experimentation in the 40s were free Hb solutions in saline. The initial trials provided the proof-of-concept that these solutions were capable of transporting oxygen, but also indicated the associated risks and complications, namely renal toxicity [15], which was attributed to impurities such as residual stromal phospholipids in the preparations [16]. Later developments to improve the safety of free Hb solutions led to the development of stroma-free Hb solutions [17]. However, further evaluation of these products indicated that the free Hb was susceptible to dissociation into dimers. This resulted in reduced half-life due to quick clearance by glomerular filtration, direct renal toxicity and abnormally high affinity for oxygen molecules (i.e. low P_{50} levels) with inability to release oxygen at tissue sites where needed [16]. Subsequently, other approaches such as polymerization, cross-linking, conjugation with other molecules, and other chemical modifications were considered and investigated with varying success. More recently, intriguing strategies to more closely replicate the Hb molecules contained in the RBC by encapsulating them in vesicles or other nano-particles have been devised and are still under investigation [16].

Characteristics of some of the most-studied HBOCs are summarized and compared with those of typical packed RBC units in Table 12.1 [16, 18–25]. HemAssist (Baxter, Deerfield, IL) also known as diaspirin cross-linked Hb

Table 12.1 Characteristics of some of the most-studied HBOCs compared with typical stored packed RBC units.

Product	HemAssist (Baxter, Deerfield, IL)	Hemopure (Biopure, Cambridge, MA)	PolyHeme (Northfield, Evanston, IL)	Hemolink (Hemosol, Toronto, Canada)	Hemospan (Sangart, San Diego, CA)	Stored Packed RBC
Hb modifications	Cross-linked	Polymerized	Cross-linked and polymerized	Cross-linked and polymerized	PEG-conjugated Hb	None (Hb in RBCs)
Hb source	Human	Bovine	Human	Human	Human	Human
Average Hb weight (kDa)	64–70	87–500	150–250	32–600	95	64
Hb Tetramers (%)	96–98	<5	<1	34–42	<1	100
Hb concentration (g/L)	100	120–140	100	100	42	130
P_{50} (mmHg)	30–32	38–40	26–32	27–51	5	26
Oncotic pressure (mmHg)	42	25	20–25	26	50	25
Viscosity (cp)	1.2	1.3	1.9–2.2	1–2	2.5	5–10
Methemoglobon (%)	<5	<10	<8	<15	<0.5	<1
Half-life in circulation (h)	6–12	18–24	24	12–24	24	744
Shelf life (yr)	>1	>2	>1	>2	>2	0.1
Storage temperature (°C)	<5	2–30	4	4	-20	4
Highest development stage reached in the US (Subject to change)	Phase III trial	Phase III trial	Phase III trial	Phase III trial	Phase III trial	–

(DCLHb) was developed using Hb extracted from outdated human allogeneic blood units and contains approximately 100 g/L cross-linked Hb [20]. The product was heat-treated to inactivate viruses that could be present in the donated blood [26]. In a US multicenter, single-blind, randomized trial on 112 patients with traumatic hemorrhagic shock, infusion of up to 1 liter of HemAssist during initial resuscitation attempts was associated with significantly higher mortality rates at 48 hours and 28 days compared with saline infusion, resulting in premature termination of the trial [27]. In another study in Europe, 121 trauma patients with severe hemorrhagic shock were randomized to receive up to 1 liter HemAssist or standard treatment. While the use of HemAssist was associated with decreased use of other blood products, it did not affect the occurrence of organ failure or 5- and 28-day mortality rates; the trial was also prematurely-terminated due to safety concerns and no benefits observed over the standard treatment [28]. Since publication of the initial reports, the data from these trials have been pooled and re-analyzed by the investigators and they have concluded that use of HemAssist was not associated with blood pressure variation or poor perfusion, suggesting that increased mortality observed in the patients randomized to HemAssist in these trials was not directly related to the vasoconstrictive effects of the product [27, 29]. Nonetheless and based on disappointing data from clinical studies, the manufacturer has suspended the development of HemAssist.

Hemopure (Biopure, Cambridge, MA) also known as HBOC-201 is a polymerized purified bovine Hb with a concentration of approximately 120–140 g/L. In addition to purification methods intended to remove most pathogens, the product is procured from tightly controlled and managed herds with known origins as a measure to protect against the potential risk of transmitting bovine spongiform encephalopathy (BSE). In a phase-III randomized single-blind trial, 688 stabilized orthopedic surgery patients were randomized to receive Hemopure or packed RBC at first transfusion decision. The study showed that although Hemopure was highly effective in eliminating the subsequent need for allogeneic blood transfusions, it was also associated with increased risk of serious adverse events. However, the observed increased rate of unfavorable outcomes could also have been partially explained by the older average age of patients in the Hemopure arm and other imbalances in volume overload and under-treatment [30]. In a follow-up reanalysis of the data, investigators reaffirmed that peak systolic blood pressure responses were more common in patients randomized to Hemopure compared with those randomized to RBC transfusion, but this was largely limited to older patients and the difference in outcomes between the groups narrowed substantially when patients younger than 50 years old with hypotension and stable trauma were included. This reanalysis was suggestive of subgroups that may benefit from this product, particularly when blood transfusion is not available [31]. Given concerns over the safety of Hemopure, further randomized trials were abandoned in the United States. Nonetheless, per-patient approval to use Hemopure on compassionate care basis for patients with life-threatening anemia who could not be transfused has been granted in the United States and elsewhere. In a report of 54 compassionate care cases, the duration and severity of life-threatening anemia was found to be a significant predictor of mortality, and early administration of Hemopure was suggested to be associated with better survival in these patients [32]. Other case reports of patients with critically low Hb levels who were considered to be at imminent risk of death and could not be transfused have been promising [33, 34], suggesting that HBOCs can be life-saving "oxygen bridges" in such cases to stabilize patients at extremely low Hb levels [35, 36]. Hemopure was the first HBOC to gain regulatory approval for human clinical use in South Africa in 2001 and Russia in 2011, and a related product, Oxyglobin (HBOC-301) was the first HBOC approved in the United States and European Union for veterinary use, with promising results from ongoing studies [37–39].

PolyHeme (Northfield, Evanston, IL) is based on cross-linked and polymerized human Hb sourced from outdated allogeneic RBC units with an Hb level of $100\,g/L$ [20]. In a phase-III multicenter trial in the United States, 714 trauma patients with hemorrhagic shock (systolic blood pressure $\leq90\,mmHg$) were randomized to field resuscitation with PolyHeme or crystalloid. Upon arrival to the trauma center, patients randomized to PolyHeme continued to receive the HBOC for the first 12 hours after the trauma, while the control patients were allowed to receive allogeneic blood transfusion. Use of allogeneic blood products in the first 12 hours was lower in patients randomized to PolyHeme while the 30-day mortality rates were not statistically significantly different between the study arms (13.4% in PolyHeme and 9.6% in control arms on intention-to-treat basis; 11.1% in PolyHeme and 9.3% in control arms on as-treated basis). The risks of adverse events and serious adverse events (particularly myocardial infarction) were moderately higher in the PolyHeme arm. The investigators concluded that given the comparable outcomes and despite increased adverse events, PolyHeme can have a favorable benefit-to-risk ratio in patients who need blood transfusion when blood transfusion is unavailable [40]. Further analysis of the data from the randomized controlled trial indicated that PolyHeme was able to sustain survival following trauma for a longer period compared with the control treatment [41]. Some have voiced concerns on the ethical issues of the design of this trial, namely given the waiver of the informed consent despite potential risks and the fact that the patients randomized to PolyHeme continued to receive it after hospital admission even though blood transfusion was available [42–44].

Hemolink (Hemosol, Toronto, Canada) also known as Hb raffimer is based on O-raffinose cross-linked and polymerized Hb molecules obtained from outdated allogeneic blood units, but the product also contains a substantial proportion of free Hb tetramers. In a phase-III multi-center, double-blind trial, 299 patients undergoing primary coronary artery bypass grafting (CABG) surgery were randomized to receive 750 mL of Hemolink or 10% pentastarch after removal of 500–1500 mL autologous blood at the start of cardiopulmonary bypass (CPB) – a methodology reminiscent of the blood conservation technique known as acute normovolemic hemodilution (ANH) discussed elsewhere in the book, although normovolemia was not necessarily maintained in this study [45]. The frequency and total number of allogeneic RBC transfusions were significantly lower in the patients randomized to Hemolink. Although all patients enrolled in the study experienced at least one adverse event, the total number of adverse events was higher in patients who received Hemolink, with the incidence of hypertension, hyperbilirubinemia, elevated amylase and urological complications particularly high in the Hemolink arm [45].

Hemospan (Sangart, San Diego, CA) also known as MP4 or MP4OX (the oxygenated form) is a polyethylene glycol (PEG)-modified HBOC derived from human blood units. Conjugation of Hb with PEG molecules results in increased effective size of the molecules, prolonged half-life in circulation, and increased affinity for oxygen, as indicated by the much lower P_{50} of Hemospan compared with other HBOCs (Table 12.1; Figure 12.1) [46]. This feature may make Hemospan particularly effective in delivering oxygen to ischemic tissues with particularly low oxygen levels. Two recent phase-III, multi-center, double-blind randomized controlled trials evaluated the safety and efficacy of MP4OX in prevention [47] and treatment [48] of hypotension in patients undergoing primary hip arthroplasty under spinal anesthesia. In the first trial, 367 patients were randomized to receive MP4OX or a hydroxyethyl starch solution at induction of anesthesia as well as when having a predefined hypotension episode. Patients randomized to MP4OX experienced significantly lower hypotensive episodes (66.1% versus 90.2% in hydroxyethylstarch group), but they also had higher occurrence of adverse events (72.7% versus 61.4%) and transient enzyme elevations in blood. The incidence of serious adverse events and the composite morbidity and ischemia outcome was similar in study arms [47]. In the other study, 474 patients were randomized to receive MP4OX or a hydroxyethyl starch solution when reaching a predefined hypotensive trigger. Of all the randomized patients, 405 reached the hypotensive trigger and received the study or control drug. Total duration of hypotensive episodes was significantly lower in patients randomized to MP4OX (52 ± 71 minutes versus 138 ± 120 minutes in the hydroxyethyl starch group), but again, patients who received MP4OX experienced more adverse events (namely, nausea, bradycardia, hypertension and oliguria) despite comparable incidence of serious adverse events [48]. Overall, the investigators concluded that the safety profile of the product was not favorable enough to recommend its use in routine low-risk surgical patients. A phase-IIb multi-center (world-wide, non-US), double-blind, randomized controlled study to evaluate the safety and efficacy of MP4OX compared with saline in traumatic patients with lactic acidosis due to hemorrhagic shock (TRA-205 trial; ClinicalTrials.gov Identifier NCT01262196) began enrolling patients in June 2011 but results were not available at time of this writing.

The data from the trials on HBOCs are generally indicative of some efficacy, in addition to increased risk of various adverse events and unfavorable outcomes. As briefly alluded to at the beginning of this section, presence of Hb molecules outside of the RBCs by itself can have several unwanted consequences. Despite effective oxygen transportation, increased incidence of a number of adverse events such as hypertension, myocardial infarction, cerebral vascular accidents, gastrointestinal complications, acute renal failure and increased risk of death have been observed in patients treated with HBOCs [19]. A 2008 meta-analysis of 16 trials on various HBOCs concluded that regardless of the products or indications studied, use of HBOCs was associated with increased risk of death (relative risk of 1.30) and myocardial infarction (relative risk of 2.71) compared with the controls, which included a mixed pool of allogeneic blood transfusion as well as various crystalloids and colloid fluids [49]. While such heterogeneities and other potential methodological issues may undermine the validity of some of the conclusions drawn by this study, there is little doubt of the risks associated with current HBOCs [50].

HBOC-related hypertension (systemic and pulmonary) is due to the vasoactivity of these products which results in vasoconstriction and increased systemic vascular resistance [19]. Several factors including over-supplying of oxygen molecules, proximity of HBOC molecules to endothelium, extravasation of the HBOC to interstitial space and scavenging nitric oxide (NO) are likely to be involved [25, 51]. Depletion of NO as well as oxidative stress are likely to be involved in other HBOC-associated complications such as cardiac toxicity as well [19]. The reactive heme group in HBOCs and its participation in various oxidative reactions has been put forward as another main culprit in the toxicity associated with use of these products [18].

With more insights gained on the underlying mechanisms of complications related to HBOCs, more opportunities to prevent or alleviate these complications will also emerge. For example, zero-linked polymerization processes have been developed that allow production of much larger Hb polymers and the increased size and other modifications may avoid some of the issues affecting HBOCs discussed here [52]. Another actively researched field is encapsulation of Hb molecules in various nano-particles (e.g. Hb-vesicles) to more closely resemble the physiologic conditions present in the RBCs. While these products are still largely at pre-clinical level of developments, available evidence is suggestive of potentials for improved function and reduced toxicity [53, 54].

Clinical use of HBOCs has some fundamental differences compared with allogeneic blood transfusion. Cross-matching is usually not needed. Given the intravascular short half-life of the products, periodic infusion of additional doses may be needed following the initial dose and the total dose given should be tracked and kept under the recommended maximum total dose of each product. Presence of cell-free Hb in plasma following infusion of HBOCs means that traditional laboratory blood parameters such as hematocrit will not be useful in measuring and monitoring the amount of HBOCs in blood and clinical signs and symptoms should be monitored to guide treatment. Photometric measurement of free Hb in plasma has been shown to be accurate to measure the level of various HBOCs [30, 55]. Presence of free Hb in plasma may also interfere with some other laboratory measurements performed on blood samples obtained from patients treated with HBOCs (e.g. albumin, total protein, cholesterol, and several enzymes) as well as tests that rely on optical properties of blood or plasma such as pulse oximetry and some coagulation tests. HBOCs are more susceptible to oxidation of iron in their heme group from Fe^{2+} to Fe^{3+}, giving rise to formation of methemoglobin which is unable to transport oxygen. Hence, methemoglobinemia in patients treated with HBOCs should be considered and treated [30].

Perfluorocarbons

As discussed earlier, 1–2% of the total oxygen carried by blood under physiologic conditions is dissolved in plasma in accordance with Henry's law. Perfluorocarbons (PFCs) are biologically- and chemically-inert compounds that are capable of dissolving substantially more amounts of oxygen compared with plasma and other similar aqueous solutions at any given PO_2. For comparison, while each liter of plasma is capable of dissolving about 3 mL oxygen at a PO_2 of 100 mmHg at 37 °C, the same volume of PFCs can dissolve 50–70 mL oxygen (depending on the PFC formulations) under the same conditions (Figure 12.1) [56].

PFCs are water-insoluble, and to be clinically functional they are often emulsified. The difference between various PFC emulsions is due to the specific chemical structures of the PFC molecules, emulsifiers used, and physical properties of the emulsion particles. Although PFC molecules are biologically inert, the same does not necessarily apply to other chemicals present in these products (e.g. surfactants added for emulsification). Since the amount of oxygen transported by PFCs is directly proportional to PO_2, supplemental oxygen and increased FiO_2 are usually required to maximize the effectiveness of these products (Figure 12.1) [56].

Fluosol-DA (Green Cross, Osaka, Japan) was a first-generation PFC emulsion that made history in the 1980s by becoming the first and only artificial oxygen carrier ever approved by the FDA for clinical use in the United States. However, its clinical use faced several shortcomings including limited effectiveness and short half-life as well as logistical problems, resulting in its removal from the market [24, 57]. Oxygent (Alliance Pharmaceutical, San Diego, CA) is a second-generation PFC emulsion, with a substantially higher concentration of the PFC to improve its efficacy, with improved safety profile and simpler storage and preparation requirements. In a phase-III single-blind study in Europe, 492 non-anemic patents undergoing high-blood-loss non-cardiac surgeries were randomized to ANH with Oxygent plus additional doses of Oxygent given, or treatment with allogeneic blood transfusions at predefined transfusion triggers. Patients randomized to Oxygent had fewer transfusions overall, but they had more serious adverse events [58]. Another phase-III randomized study in the United States using Oxygent in patients undergoing CPB was prematurely terminated over concerns on possibly higher risk of cerebrovascular events in patients treated with Oxygent [24, 56].

Similar to HBOC infusions, treatment of patients using PFCs involves specific considerations. As discussed, supplemental oxygen is usually required to allow sufficient oxygen delivery (Figure 12.1). Rather than relying on hematocrit, an alternative measure – the so-called "fluorocrit," i.e. the percentage of whole blood taken up by PFC identifiable crudely by the white or cloudy layer in centrifuged blood sample – must be used [59]. Additionally, the physical effects of PFC emulsions in blood (the plasma volume they replace and their specific oxygen content at various PO_2 levels) must be considered in calculating the total oxygen content of blood [56].

Conclusion

Despite enormous potential, artificial oxygen carrier research has been impeded by several obstacles. Many of the products investigated in clinical studies have been found effective in reducing allogeneic blood transfusion in various settings, but this has often been achieved at the cost of increased adverse events, including higher risk of morbidity and mortality. On the other hand, several case series attest to the clinical usefulness of artificial oxygen carriers in specific cases, mostly patients with extremely low Hb levels (as low as 20–30 g/L) who could not be transfused for various reasons [32–34, 60]. The condition of these patients (critical anemia with no transfusion permissible) is often in sharp contrast with patients studied in randomized controlled trials performed on artificial oxygen carriers (e.g. elective surgical cases with mild to moderate anemia), suggesting that by better defining target groups, the benefits of artificial oxygen carriers might outweigh their risks in special subgroups of patients. While products with better safety profiles are needed as substitutes for allogeneic blood transfusions, a case can still be made for currently available artificial oxygen carriers as "oxygen bridges" to help patients survive critically-low Hb levels when blood transfusions are not available or not acceptable. It is hoped that ongoing research in this field with the help of the lessons learned from past and current products, will change the landscape, and make safer products available for routine clinical use to replace allogeneic blood transfusions in the near future.

References

1 Madjdpour C, Dettori N, Frascarolo P, Burki M, Boll M, Fisch A, et al. Molecular weight of hydroxyethyl starch: is there an effect on blood coagulation and pharmacokinetics? Br J Anaesth. 2005 May;94(5):569–76.
2 Kocian R, Spahn DR. Haemoglobin, oxygen carriers and perioperative organ perfusion. Best Pract Res Clin Anaesthesiol. 2008 Mar;22(1):63–80.

3 Berg JM, Tymoczko JL, Stryer L. Hemoglobin: Portrait of a Protein in Action. Biochemistry. 7th ed. New York: W. H. Freeman & Co Ltd.; 2011.

4 Istaphanous GK, Wheeler DS, Lisco SJ, Shander A. Red blood cell transfusion in critically ill children: a narrative review. Pediatr Crit Care Med. 2011 Mar;12(2):174–83.

5 Van Meter KW. A systematic review of the application of hyperbaric oxygen in the treatment of severe anemia: an evidence-based approach. Undersea Hyperb Med. 2005 Jan;32(1):61–83.

6 Shander A, Goodnough LT. Why an alternative to blood transfusion? Crit Care Clin. 2009 Apr;25(2):261–77.

7 Buddeberg F, Schimmer BB, Spahn DR. Transfusion-transmissible infections and transfusion-related immunomodulation. Best Pract Res Clin Anaesthesiol. 2008 Sep;22(3):503–17.

8 Drackley A, Newbold KB, Paez A, Heddle N. Forecasting Ontario's blood supply and demand. Transfusion. 2012 Feb;52(2):366–74.

9 Shander A, Javidroozi M, Ozawa S, Hare GM. What is really dangerous: anaemia or transfusion? Br J Anaesth. 2011 Dec;107 Suppl 1:i41–i59.

10 Shander A, Fink A, Javidroozi M, Erhard J, Farmer SL, Corwin H, et al. Appropriateness of allogeneic red blood cell transfusion: the international consensus conference on transfusion outcomes. Transfus Med Rev. 2011 Jul;25(3):232–46.

11 Shander A, Goodnough LT. Why an alternative to blood transfusion? Crit Care Clin. 2009 Apr;25(2):261–77, Table.

12 Goodnough LT, Shander A. Blood management. Arch Pathol Lab Med. 2007 May;131(5):695–701.

13 Goodnough LT, Shander A. Evolution in alternatives to blood transfusion. Hematol J. 2003;4(2):87–91.

14 Fronticelli C, Koehler RC, Brinigar WS. Recombinant hemoglobins as artificial oxygen carriers. Artif Cells Blood Substit Immobil Biotechnol. 2007;35(1):45–52.

15 AMBERSON WR, JENNINGS JJ, RHODE CM. Clinical experience with hemoglobin-saline solutions. J Appl Physiol. 1949 Jan;1(7):469–89.

16 Inayat MS, Bernard AC, Gallicchio VS, Garvy BA, Elford HL, Oakley OR. Oxygen carriers: a selected review. Transfus Apher Sci. 2006 Feb;34(1):25–32.

17 Rabiner SF, Helbert JR, Lopas H, Friedman LH. Evaluation of a stroma-free hemoglobin solution for use as a plasma expander. J Exp Med. 1967 Dec 1;126(6):1127–42.

18 Alayash AI. Setbacks in blood substitutes research and development: a biochemical perspective. Clin Lab Med. 2010 Jun;30(2):381–9.

19 Buehler PW, D'Agnillo F, Schaer DJ. Hemoglobin-based oxygen carriers: From mechanisms of toxicity and clearance to rational drug design. Trends Mol Med. 2010 Oct;16(10):447–57.

20 Chen JY, Scerbo M, Kramer G. A review of blood substitutes: examining the history, clinical trial results, and ethics of hemoglobin-based oxygen carriers. Clinics (Sao Paulo). 2009;64(8):803–13.

21 Eastman AL, Minei JP. Comparison of Hemoglobin-based oxygen carriers to stored human red blood cells. Crit Care Clin. 2009 Apr;25(2):303–10, Table.

22 Silverman TA, Weiskopf RB. Hemoglobin-based oxygen carriers: current status and future directions. Anesthesiology. 2009 Nov;111(5):946–63.

23 Napolitano LM. Hemoglobin-based oxygen carriers: first, second or third generation? Human or bovine? Where are we now? Crit Care Clin. 2009 Apr;25(2):279–301, Table.

24 Ness PM, Cushing MM. Oxygen therapeutics: pursuit of an alternative to the donor red blood cell. Arch Pathol Lab Med. 2007 May;131(5):734–41.

25 Winslow RM. Cell-free oxygen carriers: scientific foundations, clinical development, and new directions. Biochim Biophys Acta. 2008 Oct;1784(10):1382–6.

26 Farmer M, Ebeling A, Marshall T, Hauck W, Sun CS, White E, et al. Validation of virus inactivation by heat treatment in the manufacture of diaspirin crosslinked hemoglobin. Biomater Artif Cells Immobilization Biotechnol. 1992;20(2–4): 429–33.

27 Sloan EP, Koenigsberg M, Gens D, Cipolle M, Runge J, Mallory MN, et al. Diaspirin cross-linked hemoglobin (DCLHb) in the treatment of severe traumatic hemorrhagic shock: a randomized controlled efficacy trial. JAMA. 1999 Nov 17;282(19):1857–64.

28 Kerner T, Ahlers O, Veit S, Riou B, Saunders M, Pison U. DCL-Hb for trauma patients with severe hemorrhagic shock: the European "On-Scene" multicenter study. Intensive Care Med. 2003 Mar;29(3):378–85.

29 Sloan EP, Koenigsberg MD, Philbin NB, Gao W. Diaspirin cross-linked hemoglobin infusion did not influence base deficit and lactic acid levels in two clinical trials of traumatic hemorrhagic shock patient resuscitation. J Trauma. 2010 May;68(5):1158–71.

30 Jahr JS, Mackenzie C, Pearce LB, Pitman A, Greenburg AG. HBOC-201 as an alternative to blood transfusion: efficacy and safety evaluation in a multicenter phase III trial in elective orthopedic surgery. J Trauma. 2008 Jun;64(6):1484–97.

31 Freilich D, Pearce LB, Pitman A, Greenburg G, Berzins M, Bebris L, et al. HBOC-201 vasoactivity in a phase III clinical trial in orthopedic surgery subjects--extrapolation of potential risk for acute trauma trials. J Trauma. 2009 Feb;66(2):365–76.

32 Mackenzie CF, Moon-Massat PF, Shander A, Javidroozi M, Greenburg AG. When blood is not an option: factors affecting survival after the use of a hemoglobin-based oxygen carrier in 54 patients with life-threatening anemia. Anesth Analg. 2010 Mar 1;110(3):685–93.

33 Fitzgerald MC, Chan JY, Ross AW, Liew SM, Butt WW, Baguley D, et al. A synthetic haemoglobin-based oxygen carrier and the reversal of cardiac hypoxia secondary to severe anaemia following trauma. Med J Aust. 2011 May 2;194(9):471–3.

34 Donahue LL, Shapira I, Shander A, Kolitz J, Allen S, Greenburg G. Management of acute anemia in a Jehovah's Witness patient with acute lymphoblastic leukemia with polymerized bovine hemoglobin-based oxygen carrier: a case report and review of literature. Transfusion. 2010 Jul;50(7):1561–7.

35 Levy JH. The use of haemoglobin glutamer-250 (HBOC-201) as an oxygen bridge in patients with acute anaemia associated with surgical blood loss. Expert Opin Biol Ther. 2003 Jun;3(3):509–17.

36 Philbin N, Handrigan M, Rice J, McNickle K, McGwin G, Williams R, et al. Resuscitation following severe, controlled hemorrhage associated with a 24 h delay to

surgical intervention in swine using a hemoglobin based oxygen carrier as an oxygen bridge to definitive care. Resuscitation. 2007 Aug;74(2):332–43.

37 Rempf C, Standl T, Schenke K, Chammas K, Gottschalk A, Burmeister MA, et al. Administration of bovine polymerized haemoglobin before and during coronary occlusion reduces infarct size in rabbits. Br J Anaesth. 2009 Oct;103(4):496–504.

38 Rice J, Philbin N, Light R, Arnaud F, Steinbach T, McGwin G, et al. The effects of decreasing low-molecular weight hemoglobin components of hemoglobin-based oxygen carriers in swine with hemorrhagic shock. J Trauma. 2008 May;64(5):1240–57.

39 Wehausen CE, Kirby R, Rudloff E. Evaluation of the effects of bovine hemoglobin glutamer-200 on systolic arterial blood pressure in hypotensive cats: 44 cases (1997-2008). J Am Vet Med Assoc. 2011 Apr 1;238(7):909–14.

40 Moore EE, Moore FA, Fabian TC, Bernard AC, Fulda GJ, Hoyt DB, et al. Human polymerized hemoglobin for the treatment of hemorrhagic shock when blood is unavailable: the USA multicenter trial. J Am Coll Surg. 2009 Jan;208(1):1–13.

41 Bernard AC, Moore EE, Moore FA, Hides GA, Guthrie BJ, Omert LA, et al. Postinjury resuscitation with human polymerized hemoglobin prolongs early survival: a post hoc analysis. J Trauma. 2011 May;70(5 Suppl):S34–S37.

42 Kipnis K, King NM, Nelson RM. An open letter to institutional review boards considering Northfield Laboratories' PolyHeme(R) trial. Am J Bioeth. 2010 Oct;10(10):5–8.

43 Kipnis K, King NM, Nelson RM. Trials and errors: barriers to oversight of research conducted under the emergency research consent waiver. IRB. 2006 Mar;28(2):16–19.

44 Grassley C. Americans should not be on a game show in U.S. emergency rooms and ambulances. Am J Bioeth. 2010 Oct;10(10):9–10.

45 Greenburg AG, Kim HW. Use of an oxygen therapeutic as an adjunct to intraoperative autologous donation to reduce transfusion requirements in patients undergoing coronary artery bypass graft surgery. J Am Coll Surg. 2004 Mar;198(3):373–83.

46 Vandegriff KD, Winslow RM. Hemospan: design principles for a new class of oxygen therapeutic. Artif Organs. 2009 Feb;33(2):133–8.

47 Olofsson CI, Gorecki AZ, Dirksen R, Kofranek I, Majewski JA, Mazurkiewicz T, et al. Evaluation of MP4OX for prevention of perioperative hypotension in patients undergoing primary hip arthroplasty with spinal anesthesia: a randomized, double-blind, multicenter study. Anesthesiology. 2011 May;114(5):1048–63.

48 van der LP, Gazdzik TS, Jahoda D, Heylen RJ, Skowronski JC, Pellar D, et al. A double-blind, randomized, multicenter study of MP4OX for treatment of perioperative hypotension in patients undergoing primary hip arthroplasty under spinal anesthesia. Anesth Analg. 2011 Apr;112(4):759–73.

49 Natanson C, Kern SJ, Lurie P, Banks SM, Wolfe SM. Cell-free hemoglobin-based blood substitutes and risk of myocardial infarction and death: a meta-analysis. JAMA. 2008 May 21;299(19):2304–12.

50 Shander A, Javidroozi M, Thompson G. Hemoglobin-based blood substitutes and risk of myocardial infarction and death. JAMA. 2008 Sep 17;300(11):1296–7.

51 Hai CM. Systems Biology of HBOC-Induced Vasoconstrictio. Curr Drug Discov Technol. 2011 Jul 4.

52 Harrington JP, Wollocko H. Pre-clinical studies using OxyVita hemoglobin, a zero-linked polymeric hemoglobin: a review. J Artif Organs. 2010 Dec;13(4):183–8.

53 Taguchi K, Maruyama T, Otagiri M. Pharmacokinetic properties of hemoglobin vesicles as a substitute for red blood cells. Drug Metab Rev. 2011 Aug;43(3):362–73.

54 Sakai H, Sou K, Horinouchi H, Kobayashi K, Tsuchida E. Hemoglobin-vesicle, a cellular artificial oxygen carrier that fulfils the physiological roles of the red blood cell structure. Adv Exp Med Biol. 2010;662:433–8.

55 Lurie F, Jahr JS, Driessen B. The novel HemoCu plasma/low hemoglobin system accurately measures small concentrations of three different hemoglobin-based oxygen carriers in plasma: hemoglobin glutamer-200 (bovine) (Oxyglobin), hemoglobin glutamer-250 (bovine) (Hemopure), and hemoglobin-Raffimer (Hemolink). Anesth Analg. 2002 Oct;95(4):870–3, table.

56 Spiess BD. Perfluorocarbon emulsions as a promising technology: a review of tissue and vascular gas dynamics. J Appl Physiol. 2009 Apr;106(4):1444–52.

57 Castro CI, Briceno JC. Perfluorocarbon-based oxygen carriers: review of products and trials. Artif Organs. 2010 Aug;34(8):622–34.

58 Spahn DR, Waschke KF, Standl T, Motsch J, Van HL, Welte M, et al. Use of perflubron emulsion to decrease allogeneic blood transfusion in high-blood-loss non-cardiac surgery: results of a European phase 3 study. Anesthesiology. 2002 Dec;97(6):1338–49.

59 Gardeazabal T, Cabrera M, Cabrales P, Intaglietta M, Briceno JC. Oxygen transport during hemodilution with a perfluorocarbon-based oxygen carrier: effect of altitude and hyperoxia. J Appl Physiol. 2008 Aug;105(2):588–94.

60 Greenburg AG, Light WR, Dube GP. Reconstructing hemoglobin-based oxygen carriers. Transfusion. 2010 Dec;50(12):2764–7.

CHAPTER 13

Translational strategies to minimize transfusion requirement in liver surgery and transplantation: Targeting ischemia-reperfusion injury

Reza F. Saidi and S. Kamran Hejazi Kenari

Division of Organ Transplantation, Department of Surgery, Rhode Island Hospital, Alpert Medical School of Brown University, Providence, RI, USA

Introduction

Liver Surgery is the most effective treatment for benign and malignant liver tumors. Liver transplantation is the treatment of choice for patients with end-stage liver disease. However, a great disparity exists between the number of patients on the waiting list and the number of organs available for transplant, resulting in increased waiting list mortality. One strategy to increase the number of organs available is to use those from marginal donors [1]. Hepatic steatosis is considered to be a criterion for marginality, because it is an important risk factor for early posttransplant liver dysfunction [2]. Obesity is considered a major risk factor for many chronic diseases, including diabetes [2], asthma, coronary artery disease, and liver disease. The incidence of obesity among adults is estimated to be as high as 31%, according to the US Centers for Disease Control and Prevention [3]. In addition, obesity has been linked to increased perioperative morbidity after several types of operations, including major abdominal operations [4, 5].

After restoring the blood supply after ischemia, the liver is prone to further injury aggravating the injury already caused by ischemia [6]. This is termed ischemia-reperfusion (I-R) injury. Endothelial and Kupffer cell swelling [7], vasoconstriction [8], leukocyte infiltration [9], and platelet aggregation in sinusoids [10] characterizes I-R injury. The end result is microcirculatory failure. Activation of Kupffer cells and neutrophils

Transfusion-Free Medicine and Surgery, Second Edition. Edited by Nicolas Jabbour.
© 2014 John Wiley & Sons, Ltd. Published 2014 by John Wiley & Sons, Ltd.

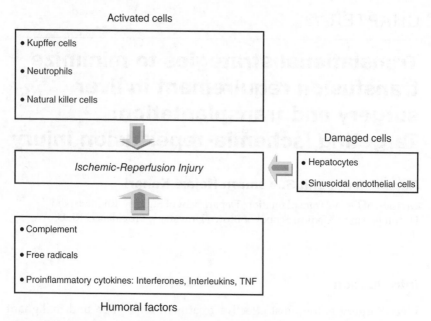

Figure 13.1 Pathophysiology of ischemia-reperfusion injury.

leads to release of inflammatory cytokines [11] and free radicals [12], which further aggravate the liver injury. Tumor necrosis factor (TNF) and interleukins (IL) are the potent cytokines most commonly involved in liver I-R injury (Figure 13.1) [13–15].

A major challenge for the transplant community is to develop strategies to close the gap between the number of patients in need of a transplant and the number of available organs. One way to increase the donor pool is utilization of expanded criteria donors (ECD) or marginal donors (i.e. donors with steatosis, with malignancies, with viral infections, older or elderly donors, donors after cardiac death and others). These marginal livers considered unacceptable for transplantation, are now being transplanted, but the main difficulty is in defining the criteria that can be extended, because these criteria vary between centers and regions. The second way to expand the donor pool is through advances in medical practice, particularly surgical techniques including split liver transplantation (SLT) and living donor liver transplantation (LDLT). Although the organs from marginal donors may not be optimal, the high death rate on the waiting lists produced a stark choice between dying without a liver or proceeding with a liver that was perhaps not ideal [16]. It is known that the marginal grafts exhibit poor tolerance to I/R injury. I/R injury is an important cause of liver damage occurring during surgical procedures including hepatic resections and liver transplantation (LT) [17]. Also, I/R injury is the underlying cause of graft dysfunction in marginal organs [16]. Moreover, I/R negatively affects the process of liver regeneration in surgical conditions including hepatic resections and small-for size LT [17].

Role of ischemia-reperfusion injury in liver surgery and transplantation

As mentioned in this review, I/R negatively affects damage and regeneration in liver surgery and transplantation. A large number of factors and mediators play a part in liver I/R injury [18]. The relationships between the signaling pathways involved are highly complex and it is not yet possible to describe, with absolute certainty, the events that occur between the beginning of reperfusion and the final outcome of either poor function or a non-functional liver which can lead to coagulopathy and bleeding after liver surgery or transplantation. Bleeding and transfusion requirement is associated with mortality and morbidity after liver surgery and transplantation. Bleeding could be multifactorial such as surgical bleeding or coagulopathy. Ischemia-reperfusion (I/R) injury is a major cause of coagulopathy. Strategies to attenuate I/R injury have been shown to decrease the coagulopathy, bleeding, and transfusion requirement after liver surgery and transplantation; therefore, decreasing the mortality and morbidity of the operation.

Cold preservation decreases metabolic activity 10-fold, and increases anaerobic metabolism and lactic acidosis; therefore resulting in mitochondrial energy uncoupling. Depletion of ATP during ischemia causes loss of transcellular electrolyte gradients, influx of free calcium and the subsequent activation of phospholipases, and therefore is the main contributor for cell swelling and lysis. Ischemia creates the basis for the subsequent production of toxic molecules after reperfusion, particularly reactive oxygen intermediates, the basis of the cascade of events that characterize I/R injury. Even with the most effective preservation solutions, cold storage aggravates graft injury at the time of transplantation.

The prolonged times of ischemia negatively affect the post-transplant outcome from ECD livers. Indeed, liver grafts with more than 14 h of cold ischemia have been consistently associated with a two-fold increase in I/R injury resulting in prolonged and complicated postoperative course, biliary stricture, and decreased graft survival. The length of cold preservation has been associated with sinusoidal cell damage and hypercoagulability [16]. The vulnerability of individual grafts to cold ischemia time varies depending on the type of liver. Total ischemic times of less than 12 to 16 h are well tolerated by donor livers without any risk factors, but not by marginal grafts. In liver preservation with University of Wisconsin (UW) solution, the incidence of I/R injury and PNF is quite low if recipients are transplanted with non-marginal grafts. In marginal grafts, however, with such risk factors as steatosis, donor age, donation after cardiac death donor, and reduced size, it is essential that cold ischemia time be minimized [19].

Several hypotheses have been suggested to explain the decreased tolerance of ECD liver to I/R injury. For instance, in the case of steatotic livers, the impairment of the microcirculation is considered a major event of I/R injury [20]. It has been postulated that ECD livers are more susceptible to lipid peroxidation because of either their lower antioxidant defenses or their greater production of reactive oxygen species (ROS) from mitochondria or xanthine/xanthine oxidase (XDH/XOD) system or both [21]. Neutrophils have been involved in the increased vulnerability of steatotic livers to I/R injury, especially in alcoholic steatotic livers. Increased endoplasmic reticulum (ER) stress may be involved in the sensitivity of other marginal grafts to I/R injury, such as steatotic liver grafts and liver grafts from aging donors. Indeed, aging donors have an increased incidence of steatosis, which may favor cold preservation injury [22]. Alterations in the activation of inflammatory transcription factors and expression of cytoprotective proteins, increased intracellular oxidants and decreased mitochondrial function and protein misfolding accumulation, and aggregation also characterize many age-related diseases [23].

In DCD, the heart has stopped when aortic flush commences. During this time, metabolic activity persists in an anoxic environment leading to an increase in intracellular acidosis and accumulation of lactate. Aerobic metabolism converts to an anaerobic state, and ATP stores are rapidly depleted leading to cellular electrolyte imbalances and an increase in harmful inflammatory mediators and proteases ultimately resulting in cell death. In cold preservation at 4 °C, ATP stores are depleted less rapidly [24]. All these aspects make the organs suffer severe ischemic insult. It is necessary to assess the parameters involved in the development of PNF in livers from DCDs in order to improve their viability. The risk of PNF is unacceptably high (>50%) when livers are exposed to >30 minutes of warm ischemia before a short cold ischemia period. In a porcine DCD LT model, the cold preservation of liver grafts is shortened from 20 to 12 to 6 h when warm ischemia time is prolonged from 10 to 20 to 30 minutes. Only liver grafts within these time limits could be safely transplanted [25]. Ma et al. [26], investigated the histological and ultrastructural characteristics of liver grafts during different warm ischemia times in rats and found that the morphological changes are positively related to warm ischemia injury in a time-dependent manner during the reperfusion period. Therefore they consider that a rat liver graft undergoing warm ischemia injury is in the reversible stage when the warm ischemia time is within 30 minutes. A 45-minute warm ischemia time may be a critical point for a rat liver graft to endure warm ischemia injury. When the warm ischemia time is over 60 minutes, the damage is irreversible. In DCDs, PNF is associated with more activated Kupffer cells in recipients, by higher production of tumor necrosis factor (TNF-α) and interleukin-6 (IL-6), with lower alpha-tocopherol and reduced glutathione [25].

Surgical and pharmacological strategies to mimimize I/R injury in liver surgery and transplantation

Effective measures have been taken to improve outcomes when using these marginal livers, include rapid cooling after arrest and minimization of both cold (<8 h) and warm ischemia time. In addition several approaches are being explored to improve the viability of marginal liver grafts, including improvements in donor organ perfusion and preservation methods, additives to preservation solution, pharmacological treatments (modulators of rennin-angiotensin system, modulators of activating pro-survival kinase cascades, adipocytokines derived from liver or adipose tissue, antiapototic strategies, inflammatory cytokines, energy status enhancement, microcirculation amelioration, antioxidant usage), gene therapy, surgical technicals (i.e. ischemic preconditioning), and others.

Static liver preservation

Static cold storage (SCS) is the most commonly used preservation method for all organs. The principles underlying cold preservation are the slowing of metabolism (by cooling) and the reduction of cell swelling due to the composition of preservation solutions. The introduction of the UW solution by Belzer for SCS was a breakthrough and remains the conventional method of preservation [27].

Serine protease and Streptokinase

Pretreatment with serine protease inhibitors has been shown to minimize the damage caused by warm ischemia in experimental models in DCD [28]. Addition of antithrombolytic drugs (Streptokinase) to the perfusion solutions improved the microcirculation of livers after warm ischemia and may thus represent a promising approach to attenuate parenchymal cell injury in liver graft retrieval from DCDs [29]. It is well known that the integrity of liver grafts from DCDs is additionally affected by microvascular alterations, including erythrocyte aggregation and thrombus formation, which might hamper appropriate equilibration of the preservation of grafts microvasculature, precluding cold preservation. In the same line, the elimination of Kupffer cells reduced thromboxane B2 and cytokines and improved sinusoidal microcirculation in DCDs [30].

N-acetylhistidine

Recently, a modified histidine-tryptophan-ketoglutarate (HTK) solution that contains N-acetylhistidine, amino acids and iron chelators (HTK-N) has been developed. Liu et al. [31], demonstrated that HTK-N protect liver grafts with microvesicular steatosis caused by toxic injury from I/R injury better than standard HTK most likely via inhibition of hypoxic injury and oxidative stress and amelioration of the inflammatory reaction occurring upon reperfusion.

Epidermal growth factor (EGF) and Insulin growth actor (IGF-I)

The results, based on isolated perfused liver, indicated that the addition of EGF and IGF-I, separately or in combination to UW reduced hepatic injury and improved function in steatotic and non-steatotic types. EGF increased IGF-I, and both additives up-regulated AKT in both liver types [32].

Pharmacological treatments

Modulators of renin-angiotensin system

Previous researches have observed an important role for the RAS, known for its regulation of blood pressure and fluid homeostasis, in both I/R injury and liver regeneration after partial hepatectomy [33]. In conditions of partial hepatectomy under I/R, Angiotensin receptors (AT1R and AT2R) antagonists for steatotic livers improved regeneration in the remnant liver. AT1R antagonist, through NO inhibition, protected steatotic livers against oxidative stress and damage. The combination of AT1R and AT2R antagonists in steatotic livers showed stronger liver regeneration than either antagonist used separately and also provided the same protection against damage as that afforded by AT1R antagonist alone. These results could be of clinical interest in liver surgery [33, 34]. In LT, Ang-II is an appropriate therapeutic target only in non-steatotic livers. An upregulation of ACE2 in steatotic liver grafts was observed, which was associated with decreased Ang-II and high Ang-(1–7) levels. Ang-(1–7) receptor antagonist reduced necrotic cell death and increased survival mediated by NO inhibition in recipients transplanted with steatotic liver grafts. These results indicate a novel target for therapeutic interventions in LT within the RAS cascade, based on Ang-(1–7), which could be specific for this type of liver [35].

Modulation of inflammatory cytokines and oxidative stress

Livers of mice having a spontaneous mutation in the leptin gene (ob/ob), resulting in global obesity and liver steatosis, are endotoxin sensitive, and do not survive I/R injury. Seventy-five to eighty-three percent of ob/ob mice pre-treated with an anti-LPS mAb prior to initiation of I/R survived after ischemia and 24 h of reperfusion. Furthermore, there was a decrease in ALT and circulating endotoxin levels when treated with an anti-LPS mAb compared with control antibodies.

Corticosteroids have been shown to have a protecting effect on myocardium by diminishing the inflammatory response after cardiopulmonary bypass (CPB), which cause I/R injury [15, 36–38]. Jansen and colleagues [38]. reported that steroid administration before CPB can reduce TNF alpha and IL release, which was associated with a lower postoperative morbidity. Corticosteroids have been used to reduce acute inflammation and to decrease postoperative clinical complications, although the protective mechanisms in the liver are far from being elucidated.

The first reports on the protective effects of steroids on liver ischemia were published in 1975 [39]. Figueroa and Santiago-Delpin found that methylprednisolone (MP) treatment before hepatic occlusion results in increased animal survival and reduced liver damage, as demonstrated by histology when compared with ischemic controls. The hepatic protein synthesis was shown to decrease to the same extent at the end of the ischemic period in rats pretreated with MP as in control animals. However, during the reperfusion period, protein synthesis was restored more quickly and was more complete in animals receiving MP than in control rats. A possible explanation is the protection of the cell membrane by stabilization of the lysosomal membrane or the inhibition of circulating toxic substances liberated from the liver during ischemia. Despite a recent publication showing that MP may enhance hepatic I-R injury in a model of warm liver ischemia [40], corticosteroids have been used for the suppression of inflammatory mechanisms and are used in warm and cold hepatic I/R injury [41].

Saidi et al. [42], showed that on apoptosis and inflammation were markedly influenced by corticosteroids in the lean rats. However, MP made the hepatic I-R worse in the steatotic liver. In the lean rats, MP attenuated the hepatocellular injury as shown by decreases in serum AST levels. Serum IL-6 was also decreased. However, these results were not seen in Zucker rats. It seems that the effects of MP on hepatic I-R are completely different on steatotic liver. The reason for this phenomenon needs further investigation.

In contrast, MP treatment made hepatic I-R injury worse in Zucker rats as shown by increases in serum AST and IL-6 levels and worsening of histopathology grades [42].

Modulation of Kupffer cells and leukocytes

Elimination of Kupffer cells and administration of a protease inhibitor improve graft viability and prevent reperfusion injury in DCD. Franken-berg et al. [43], found that depletion of Kupffer cells with gadolinium chloride (GdCl3) in donor animals prevents PNF of fatty livers after transplantation, and diminishes amino acid release at harvest, but blocks the increased expression of the adhesion molecule ICAM-1 only after transplantation. Moore et al. [44], documented that the interactions between fibronectin, a key extracellular matrix protein, and its integrin receptor $\alpha 4\beta 1$, expressed on leukocytes, specifically up-regulated the expression and activation of metalloproteinase-9 in a well-established steatotic rat liver model of ex vivo ice-cold ischemia followed by LT. The presence of the active form of MMP-9 was accompanied by massive intragraft leukocyte infiltration, high levels of proinflammatory cytokines, such as interleukin-1β and TNF-α, and impaired liver function. Interestingly, MMP-9 activity in steatotic liver grafts was to some extent independent of the expression of its natural inhibitor, the tissue inhibitor of MMP-1. Moreover, the blockade of fibronectin-$\alpha 4\beta 1$ integrin interactions inhibited the expression/activation of MMP-9 in steatotic LT without significantly affecting the expression of metalloproteinase-2 (MMP-2, gelatinase A). These findings reveal a novel aspect of the function of fibronectin-$\alpha 4\beta 1$-integrin interactions, which is of significance in the successful use of marginal steatotic livers in transplantation [44]. Amersi et al. [45], showed the effects of connecting segment-1 (CS1) peptide in a steatotic rat model of ex vivo cold ischemia followed by iso-transplantation. CS1 peptide therapy significantly inhibits the recruitment of T lymphocytes, neutrophil activation/infiltration, and repressed the expression of proinflammatory TNF-α and IFN-γ. Moreover, it resulted in selective inhibition of inducible nitric oxide synthase expression, peroxynitrate formation, and hepatic necrosis. Importantly, CS1 peptide therapy improved function/histological preservation of steatotic liver grafts and extended survival. Also Moore et al. [46], reported that CS1 peptide in steatotic rat LT showed a profound decrease in T-cell and monocyte/macrophage infiltration and significantly reduced levels of cytokine expression such as IL-2 and IFN-γ.

Strategies to minimalize I/R in steotatic liver

Livers with steatotic changes are known to be more susceptible to I-R injury. Several different mechanisms have been proposed to explain this, including mitochondrial dysfunction, predominantly necrotic cell death (as opposed to apoptotic cell death), increased lipid peroxidation, and increased endothelial cell susceptibility. Recently, it was demonstrated that the mechanism of injury pattern after hepatic warm ischemia appears to be different in steatotic livers when compared with lean livers [47, 48].

Livers with steatotic changes are known to be more susceptible to ischemia-reperfusion (I/R) injury [49]. Several mechanisms have been proposed: mitochondrial dysfunction, necrotic (as opposed to apoptotic) cell deaths, increased lipid peroxidation, and increased endothelial cell susceptibility [49].

Strategies to minimize the negative effects of ischemia are now in the forefront of clinical and experimental studies related to liver resection and transplantation. Intermittent clamping (IC) and ischemic preconditioning (IP) have originally been shown to be effective in heart [50] and subsequently liver transplantation [21, 48, 51–55].

IP and IC of the portal triad are the only clinically established protective strategies against liver injury due to prolonged ischemia [56–58].

Steatosis of the liver is common in Western countries, affecting about 25% of donors for liver transplantation and 20% of patients undergoing liver resection [2–5]. Transplantation of livers with severe steatosis (>60%) is associated with a high risk of primary nonfunction; these livers should not be used for organ donation [2]. In contrast, transplantation of livers containing mild steatosis (<30%) yields results similar to those of nonfatty livers [49]. The outcome of livers with moderate steatosis (30% to 60%) vary; the use of these organs depends on the existence of additional risk factors [4]. Similarly, liver resection in patients with steatosis is associated with a risk of postoperative mortality, when compared with patients with nonfatty livers. Although hepatic steatosis is an important risk factor for surgery, little is known about the mechanisms of injury.

Fatty hepatocytes display reduced tolerance against ischemic injury with a predominantly necrotic form of cell death [49]. In addition, the ability of hepatocytes to regenerate after major tissue loss is impaired in the steatotic liver. Few protective strategies are known. IP and IC protect the human liver against prolonged periods of ischemia [54, 55, 57, 58]. These techniques appear to be particularly protective in the steatotic liver.

New insights into the mechanisms of liver failure in steatotic organs are needed to decrease the risk of surgery and increase the pool of organ donors. So far, several studies have demonstrated that IC and IP are better tolerated than continuous clamping. This objective was first described in cardiac surgery and defined as IP [50]. Hereby, the resistance to further sustained ischemic damage was markedly increased after liver resection or cold storage in liver transplantation.

Obese Zucker rats are frequently used as a model for nutritionally induced obesity and the effects of I/R injury. Obese Zucker rats lack cerebral leptin receptors, which results in increased food intake, insulin resistance, and decreased energy expenditure [59–61].

In the steatotic liver subjected to warm ischemia, a predominance of necrosis as the primary form of cell death has been observed [48]. Intracellular mediators of apoptosis were decreased in steatotic livers subjected to ischemia, indicating a failure to activate the apoptotic cascade. A further indication that apoptosis is not the predominant mechanism of injury was the lack of protection when caspase inhibitors were used; unlike in the control liver, treatment with antiapoptotic agents was not as effective in fatty livers [48]. Thus, the question arose whether IP and IC preconditioning may also prevent I/R injury in steatotic livers.

Saidi et al. [62], analyzed the effectiveness of IC and IP compared with CC to prevent IR injury after ischemia in a model of warm liver ischemia in Zucker rats. They found that IP or IC treatment resulted in decreased transaminases. The beneficial effects of IC and IP strategies were additionally underlined by the observation of less hepatocellular damage, as demonstrated by histological examinations. Inflammation were markedly influenced by IC and IP. Serum IL-6 was also decreased. They demonstrated a markedly reduced inflammatory response after IP and IC treatment compared with CC. Staining with hematoxylin and eosin was used to evaluate morphological changes in postischemic liver tissue. In contrast to tissue subjected to continuous inflow occlusion, IC and IP seemed to protect against tissue destruction by preserving liver architecture.

The present experimental results indicated that IP and IC were able to confer protection in steatotic livers. The potential application of IP and IC in clinical practice could improve the tolerance of fatty livers to I/R injury in normothermic conditions, including hepatic resections and transplantation. It could also improve the initial condition of donor livers with low steatosis that are available for transplantation but show reduced post-surgical results. It could also increase the use of donor livers with severe steatosis that are presently discarded for transplantation.

Regulators of lipid metabolism

Manipulation of the chemical composition of hepatic lipids may evolve as a useful strategy to expand the donor pool and improve the outcome after LT [63]. Therefore, normalization of the Ω-6:Ω-3 FA ratio appears to be crucial for protection of the steatotic liver from reperfusion injury. Preoperative dietary omega-3 diet protects macrosteatotic livers against reperfusion injury and might represent a valuable method to expand the live liver donor pool [63]. Clavien et al., treated three live liver donors with moderate degrees of steatosis by oral administration of X-3 FAs. All donors showed a significant reduction of hepatic fatty infiltration within one month. Subsequently, LT was carried out for three candidates with uneventful outcomes for both donors and recipients. A very promising option to prevent post-transplant complications appears to be the use of a pretreatment with X-3 FAs. However, the approach is only feasible in living donation since requires oral administration of X-3 FAs before organ procurement [64]. Cerulenin has been shown by Chavin et al. [65], to reduce body weight and hepatic steatosis in murine model of obesity by inhibiting fatty acid synthase. Indeed when administered prior to I/R it is adequate for protecting steatotic livers subject to LT. Cerulenin inhibited fatty acid metabolism by down-regulating PPARα, as well as mitochondrial uncoupling protein 2 (UCP2), with a concomitant increase in ATP.

Modulators of adenosine

In a model of LT from DCD pigs, Net et al. [66], evaluated the involvement of adenosine and adenosine receptors) during normothermic recirculation (NR). Application of NR after 20 minutes of warm ischemia reversed the lethal injury associated with transplantation of DCD livers, achieving 5-day survival and diminishing glutathione S-transferase (GST), AST, and hyaluronic acid. Adenosine administration prior to warm ischemia simulated the effect of NR. During NR, hepatic adenosine levels increased and xanthine levels decreased [66]. Addition of a selective A2-receptor agonist (CGS 21680) to the preservation solution reduced the biochemical parameters of hepatic damage and promoted an increase in hepatic bile production. This effect, which may represent a promising approach for the use of DCD grafts, seems to be mediated through activation of protein kinase A [67].

Targeting complement system

The complement system of recognition molecules, proteolytic enzymes, effector products and receptors primarily serves host defense. Activation of the complement cascade by three major pathways – classical, lectin and alternative – leads to the deposition of complement component C3 on the surface of the pathogen. This marks the pathogen for removal by the mononuclear phagocyte system or for destruction by the membrane attack complex, which is comprised of complement components C5b, C6, C7, C8, and C9 (referred to as C5b–C9) Pathogenic mechanisms involved in IRI have been extensively investigated. Studies in models of myocardial [68, 69], intestinal [4], renal [5] and hepatic [70–72] IRI have provided evidence for the role of complement in the pathogenesis of IRI [73].

The effect of complement activation during liver IRI is diverse. Several complement components become localized in the ischemic liver [74–77]. Furthermore, plasma levels of activated complement components are increased after liver IRI in pigs and humans [75, 77]. Complement activation products and complement membrane attack complex (MAC) have deleterious effects on the liver and contribute to neutrophil activation, vasoconstriction, impaired microcirculation, increased vascular permeability, and cell lysis [75–77].

Complement activation is an important mediator of IRI after major surgery and transplantation [78]. Activation of the classical complement pathway in this type of tissue damage can occur via antibody-dependent as well as independent mechanisms, which in the latter case may involve the direct binding of C1q to damaged cells and in situ deposited acute phase proteins [76]. To prevent the effects of complement activation, the therapeutic application of complement inhibitor C1-INH, a physiological inhibitor of the serine proteases C1r and C1s of the classical pathway has been preliminary tested in humans [78–80]. The biologic activities of C1 inhibitor may be divided into two broad categories: the regulation of vascular permeability and anti-inflammatory functions. Exogenous administration of C1-INH significantly attenuated liver IRI injury and promoted liver regeneration.

Inhibition of an early step in the classical pathway is of relevance in view of the pro-inflammatory effects of early products of the complement activation cascade, such as C4a [78]. Although in this study the classical pathway of complement was blocked by C1-INH, hepatic IRI injury (i.e. ALT leakage from hepatocytes) was significantly attenuated also in C3−/− mice. This suggests that, although activation of the classical complement pathway is causally involved in harmful complement activation during liver IRI, C1-INH exerts its effects not only via reduction of classical complement activation. C1-INH is also a major inhibitor of the lectin pathway of complement activation, the contact activation system and the intrinsic pathway of coagulation [78]. It is therefore endowed with anti-inflammatory properties. These additional effects of C1-inhibitor probably explain the therapeutic benefit of C1-INH independent of an effect on the classical complement activation. The anti-inflammatory effects of C1 inhibitor appear to result from a variety of activities. These include the regulation of both complement and contact system activation, but also appear to include several activities that are not dependent on protease inhibition [80]. Therefore; further definition of the contribution of the various complement pathways in liver IRI is of major importance for the development of an effective, specific, and safe treatment in liver transplantation.

C1-INH has been found to bind to sinusoidal endothelium or the sinusoidal pole of the liver trabeculae, linked to sinusoidal endothelium, after 8 h of cold storage in UW solution containing C1-inh and 2 h of reperfusion [77]. Deposition of the anti-C3 antibodies on liver cells shows marked heterogeneity, which is likely related to the mainly midzonal expression of I/R injury, but perhaps also to variability in sensitivity to complement activation. We made no attempt to quantify the amount of C3 in hepatocytes after administration of C1-INH or albumin, considering the large variation in those results from assessment of liver sections [80].

The success of liver resection and liver transplantation especially living donor split liver transplantation depends on the liver's ability to regenerate after major tissue loss [1]. Liver has the remarkable ability to regenerate and restore its anatomic and homeostatic integrity in response to partial hepatectomy, toxic exposure, or viral injury [81, 82]. Liver parenchymal cells, including hepatocytes, and nonparenchymal cells such as endothelial, stellate, and Kupffer cells, respond to these stimuli by shedding their quiescent phenotype and synchronously entering the S phase of the cell cycle and proliferation [83].

Previous studies have shown that various parts of the complement system, such as C3 and C5, are essential components in liver regeneration. Mice deficient in these complement proteins were unable to mount a normal regenerative response after liver injury [84, 85]. Our study demonstrated that C1-INH can also promote liver regeneration, in addition to its effect on IRI. The animal which underwent combined IRI and PH showed improve survival after receiving C1-INH. The number of regenerative cells (BrdU and PCNA positive cells) increased in the C1-INH Group (Saidi RF. unpublished data).

Stem cell therapy

Impaired liver regeneration and liver dysfunction have been strongly linked to the extent of hepatic ischemia/reperfusion injury (IRI), an unavoidable consequence of the surgical procedures. Mesenchymal stem cells (MSCs) are a stem cell population within the bone marrow that has been shown to have increasing therapeutic potentials in a wide range of diseases. MSCs are defined as plate-adhering, fibroblast-like cells possessing self-renewal ability with the capacity to differentiate into multiple mesenchymal cell lineages such as osteoblasts, chondrocytes, and adipocytes. MSCs are readily available from a variety of tissues such as bone marrow, umbilical cord blood, trabecular bone, synovial membrane, and adipose tissue. There is some evidence that MSC is playing an important role in tissue repair after IR injury. MSC make up part of the BM stromal microenvironment that provides support to the hematopoietic stem cell and drives the process of hematopoiesis and. Despite their important role within the BM, MSC are rare cells with estimates for MSC frequency ranging from 0.001% to 0.01% of the total nucleated cell population present within the marrow. In addition to the BM, these cells have now been isolated from numerous tissues, including brain, liver, lung, fetal blood, umbilical cord blood, kidney, and even liposuction material, leading one to postulate that MSC are likely to play a critical role in organ homeostasis, perhaps providing supportive factors, such as in the BM, and/or mediating maintenance/repair within their respective tissue. MSC act at different processes required for regeneration of damaged tissue, by releasing growth factors such as vascular endothelial growth factor (VEGF) and hepatocyte growth factor (HGF), MSCs stimulate endogenous tissue repair. Furthermore, MSCs release anti-inflammatory cytokines such as IL-10, IL-6, TGF and nitric oxide (NO). Several animal studies showed the beneficial effect of MSC in I/R injury. Clinical trials using allogenic or autologous MSC in I/R injury are ongoing (www.clinicaltrails.gov) [86–90].

Machine perfusion

Machine liver perfusion has emerged with promising data over the past decade as an alternative preservation method to SCS that can be further categorized based on the temperature employed, and has emerged with promising data over the past decade because it has significant potential in graft preservation and optimization when the use of marginal organs is the objective. Machine perfusion involves pulsatile perfusion of the liver using a machine as opposed to SCS. This can be performed by perfusing the liver with a hypothermic perfusate or with a normothermic perfusate. The safety and efficacy of machine perfusion compared to SCS to decrease liver I/R injury is yet to be assessed in humans by randomized controlled trials [91].

Normothermic machine perfusion (NMP)

The first successful human LT carried out by Starzl et al. [92] were transplanted after liver graft pretreatment by machine perfusion with diluted, hyperbaric oxygenated blood. Most perfusion circuits were assembled from standard cardiopulmonary bypass components. Principle constituents are a centrifugal pump, a membrane oxygenator, and a heat exchanger. Other critical components of the perfusate include nutrition (glucose, insulin, aminoacids), drugs to prevent thrombosis or microcirculatory failure (heparin, prostacyclin) and agents to reduce cellular edema, cholestasis and free radical injury [93]. NMP maintains and mimics normal *in vivo* liver conditions and function during the entire period of preservation, thus avoiding hypothermia and hypoxia and minimizing preservation injury [91]. In contrast to SCS preservation the concept of normothermic preservation is to maintain cellular metabolism. The underlying principle is the combination of continuous circulation of metabolic substrates for ATP regeneration and removal of waste products. Imber et al. [94], found that, after 1 h of warm ischemia, porcine livers that were normothermically perfused had greater bile and factor V production, glucose metabolism, and galactose clearance than SCS. However, Reddy et al. [95], observed no difference in hepatic synthetic function among porcine livers receiving NMP before SCS compared with porcine livers preserved by SCS alone. Schön et al. [96], studied NMP to preserve pig livers for transplantation and to rescue them from warm ischemia in a model of donor after cardiac death. Short (5 h) or prolonged (20 h) NMP preservation is superior to SCS for normal and ischemically damaged livers, respectively [91]. The longest preservation of steatotic livers was the NMP preservation for 48 h in a pig model by Jamisson et al., who employed blood containing additional insulin and vasodilators as perfusate, and observed a mild reduction of steatosis from 28% to 15%. The NMP circuit dually perfuses 1.5 L of autologous heparinized blood at physiological pressures, which allows hepatic blood flow autoregulation. Prostacyclin, taurocholic acid, and essential amino acids are infused continuously. The concept of normothermic recirculation in the context of DCDs was first developed by Garcia-Valdecasas et al. [97], With 4 h of NMP, hepatic damage incurred during 90 minutes of cardiac arrest can be reverted, achieving 100% graft survival after 5 days of postransplant follow-up. Administration of pentoxifylline or arginine to rat and pig respectively may also improve the quality of DCD by reversing ischemic damage [98].

Hypothermic machine perfusion (HMP)

The first and most prominent difference between SCS and (oxygenated) HMP is the restoration of the tissue's energy charge and glycogen content while preventing ATP depletion [91]. Lee et al. [99], reported that HMP for 5 h improves survival and reduces cellular damage of liver tissue that has experienced 30 minutes of warm ischemia in DCD rat livers. Dutkowski et al. [100], showed that 45 minutes of warm in situ ischemia followed by 5 h cold storage followed by 1 h HMP improved DCD rat livers significantly, with a reduction of necrosis and less AST release. This was associated with increased bile flow, ATP preservation and a significant extension of graft survival. Bessems et al. [101], employed HMP preservation with UW-gluconate solution or polysol on DCD rat livers for 24 h. Both alleviated I/R and hepatocellular damage compared to SCS in UW. However, polysol was associated with less cellular edema after preservation and higher flow during reperfusion, bile production and ammonia clearance than UW-gluconate. Extracorporeal membrane oxygenation (ECMO) may be used to reduce warm ischemia time in liver graft obtained from uncontrolled DCDs, thereby increasing graft salvage rates. Rojas et al. [102], evaluated the use of warm blood veno-arterial ECMO reperfusion in preheparinized DCD swine. ECMO was started after 30 or 60 minutes of cardiac arrest and kept running for 120 minutes. In this model, ECMO support restored liver perfusion, oxygenation, and bile production after 1 h of cardiac arrest. Wang et al. [103], reported a liver graft donor who was maintained on ECMO after successful cardiopulmonary resuscitation. The liver was procured using a rapid flush technique 4 h after instituting ECMO. Graft function recovered fully after transplantation. There is a substantial body of research, predominantly in rodents, demonstrating improved preservation by providing oxygen to livers [104]. Nevertheless, clear guidelines towards target values/ranges for oxygen levels regarding the optimal duration of oxygenation during HMP are lacking. HMP can also be applied at the end of the cold storage period, which is attractive for logistical reasons. The disadvantage here is the time-dependent increase in vascular resistance, bearing the risk of damage to the sinusoidal endothelium.

Surgical strategies

Liver is a well vascularized organ with dual blood supply from the hepatic artery and portal vein. Therefore, liver Surgery and transplantation can be associated with significant risk of bleeding. Strategies to prevent blood loss during hepatic resection or transplantation include inflow control (Pringle maneuver) [105] or combined inflow and outflow occlusion

[105–110]. However, all these maneuvers run the risk of hepatic ischemia and irreversible damage occurring about 1 hour after blood supply occlusion. To overcome this problem, intermittent inflow occlusion [111, 112] and ischemic preconditioning [54] has been proposed.

Makuuchi and colleagues [112] described intermittent inflow clamping in 1987. In this technique, a period of inflow occlusion ranging 10 to 30 minutes is followed by a period of 5 to 15 minutes of reperfusion [55, 57, 58, 112]. A number of experimental [55–57] and clinical [111, 112] studies have shown the liver tolerates intermittent clamping better than continuous clamping. However, this maneuver is associated with the risk of bleeding from the liver parenchyma.

Murry and colleagues [113] popularized the concept of ischemic preconditioning by showing that a short period of ischemia prevents myocardial injury from subsequent prolonged periods of ischemia. Ischemic preconditioning consists of a short period of inflow interruption followed by a period of reperfusion, and then followed by a period of a long Pringle maneuver. The protective effects of ischemic preconditioning were subsequently described in the liver as well [114, 115]. One advantage of ischemic preconditioning over intermittent clamping is the absence of blood loss using this technique.

Many protective strategies have been proposed to prevent hepatic I/R injury. IP consists of a brief period of ischemia followed by a short interval of reperfusion before a surgical procedure with prolonged ischemic stress. IC consists of interrupting long ischemic periods with multiple short intervals of reperfusion. Although the benefit of IP and IC in the liver has been suggested in a clinical pilot study [54], knowledge of the molecular mechanisms remains vague. Several mediators have been proposed to play a critical role in the protective pathways including adenosine, nitric oxide, oxidative stress, some heat shock proteins, and tumor necrosis factor-α [7, 8, 11, 14, 59–61]. Furthermore, IP and IC preserved the morphology of the hepatic parenchyma and prevented a rapid increase in general markers of hepatocyte injury, such as the serum transaminase levels [55].

Conclusion

I/R injury is a major cause of mortality and morbidity after liver surgery and transplantation. Strategies to reduce I/R injury could improve post-resection/transplant outcome and help salvage organs that would be discarded otherwise. Multiple methods are currently being investigated to minimize the effects of IR injury to allow the use of ECD organs, including anti-inflammatory approaches to attenuate cytokines, blockade of adhesion molecules, anti-apoptotic strategies, among others. Other strategies with preliminary clinical applications such as IP and other strategies that are still in the experimental stage, including synthetic allografts, and hepatic dialysis, will need to be developed.

Abbreviations

ACE	Angiotensin-converting enzyme
Anti-LPS	Anti-Lipopolysaccharide
ATP	Adenosine Triphosphate
AT1R	Angiotensin 1 receptors
AT2R	Angiotensin 2 receptors
CC	Continuous Clamping
CDC	Centers for Disease Control
CPB	Cardio Pulmonary Bypass
CS1	connecting segment-1
DCD	Donation after Cardiac Death
ECD	Expanded Criteria Donors
ECMO	Extracorporeal Membrane Oxygenation
EGF	Epidermal growth factor
ER	Endoplasmic Reticulum
GdCl3	gadolinium chloride
GSK3β	glycogen synthase kinase-3β
HGF	Hepatocyte Growth Factor
HMP	Hypothermic Machine Perfusion
HTK	Histidine-Tryptophan-Ketoglutarate
HTK-N	HTK solution that contains N-acetylhistidine
IC	Intermittent Clamping
IGF-I	Insulin growth actor
IL-6	Interleukin-6
IP	Ischemic Preconditioning
I/R	Ischemic Reperfusion
IRI	Ischemic Reperfusion Injury
LDLT	Living Donor Liver Transplantation
LT	Liver Transplantation
MAC	Membrane Attack Complex
MP	Methyl Prednisolone
MSCs	Mesenchymal Stem Cells
NMP	Normothermic Machine Perfusion
NO	Nitric Oxide
NR	Normothermic Recirculation

PNF	Primary non-function
RAS	Renin-Angiotensin System
ROS	Reactive Oxygen Species
SCS	Static cold storage
SLT	Split Liver Transplantation
TNF-α	Tumor Necrosis Factor-α
UCP2	uncoupling protein 2
UW	University of Wisconsin
VEGF	Vascular Endothelial Growth Factor
XDH/XOD	xanthine/xanthine oxidase

References

1 Saidi RF. Current status of liver transplantation. Arch Iran Med. 2012;15(12): 772–6.
2 Ploeg RJ, D'Alessandro AM, Knechtle SJ, et al. Risk factors for primary dysfunction after liver transplantation–a multivariate analysis. Transplantation. 1993;55(4):807–13.
3 http://www.cdc.gov/nccdphp/dnpa/obesity/.
4 Lee CT, Dunn RL, Chen BT, Joshi DP, Sheffield J, Montie JE. Impact of body mass index on radical cystectomy. J. Urol. 2004;172(4 Pt 1):1281–5.
5 Tsukada K, Miyazaki T, Kato H, et al. Body fat accumulation and postoperative complications after abdominal surgery. Am Surg. 2004;70(4):347–51.
6 Serracino-Inglott F, Habib NA, Mathie RT. Hepatic ischemia-reperfusion injury. Am. J. Surg. 2001;181(2):160–6.
7 Vollmar B, Glasz J, Leiderer R, Post S, Menger MD. Hepatic microcirculatory perfusion failure is a determinant of liver dysfunction in warm ischemia-reperfusion. Am. J. Pathol. 1994;145(6):1421–31.
8 Marzi I, Takei Y, Rücker M, et al. Endothelin-1 is involved in hepatic sinusoidal vasoconstriction after ischemia and reperfusion. Transpl. Int. 1994;7 (Suppl 1):S503–6.
9 Yadav SS, Howell DN, Gao W, Steeber DA, Harland RC, Clavien PA. L-selectin and ICAM-1 mediate reperfusion injury and neutrophil adhesion in the warm ischemic mouse liver. Am. J. Physiol. 1998;275(6 Pt 1):G1341–52.
10 Cywes R, Packham MA, Tietze L, et al. Role of platelets in hepatic allograft preservation injury in the rat. Hepatology. 1993;18(3):635–47.
11 Colletti LM, Kunkel SL, Walz A, et al. The role of cytokine networks in the local liver injury following hepatic ischemia/reperfusion in the rat. Hepatology. 1996;23(3):506–14.
12 Shirasugi N, Wakabayashi G, Shimazu M, et al. Up-regulation of oxygen-derived free radicals by interleukin-1 in hepatic ischemia/reperfusion injury. Transplantation. 1997;64(10):1398–1403.
13 Thornton AJ, Strieter RM, Lindley I, Baggiolini M, Kunkel SL. Cytokine-induced gene expression of a neutrophil chemotactic factor/IL-8 in human hepatocytes. J. Immunol. 1990;144(7):2609–13.

14 Shito M, Wakabayashi G, Ueda M, et al. Interleukin 1 receptor blockade reduces tumor necrosis factor production, tissue injury, and mortality after hepatic ischemia-reperfusion in the rat. Transplantation. 1997;63(1):143–8.

15 Suzuki S, Toledo-Pereyra LH. Interleukin 1 and tumor necrosis factor production as the initial stimulants of liver ischemia and reperfusion injury. J. Surg. Res. 1994;57(2):253–8.

16 Busuttil RW, Tanaka K. The utility of marginal donors in liver transplantation. Liver Transpl. 2003;9(7):651–63.

17 Casillas-Ramírez A, Mosbah IB, Ramalho F, Roselló-Catafau J, Peralta C. Past and future approaches to ischemia-reperfusion lesion associated with liver transplantation. Life Sci. 2006;79(20):1881–94.

18 Jaeschke H. Molecular mechanisms of hepatic ischemia-reperfusion injury and preconditioning. Am. J. Physiol. Gastrointest. Liver Physiol. 2003;284(1): G15–26.

19 Hashimoto K, Miller C. The use of marginal grafts in liver transplantation. J Hepatobiliary Pancreat Surg. 2008;15(2):92–101.

20 Ijaz S, Yang W, Winslet MC, Seifalian AM. Impairment of hepatic microcirculation in fatty liver. Microcirculation. 2003;10(6):447–56.

21 Fernández L, Carrasco-Chaumel E, Serafín A, et al. Is ischemic preconditioning a useful strategy in steatotic liver transplantation? Am. J. Transplant. 2004;4(6):888–899.

22 Ben Mosbah I, Alfany-Fernández I, Martel C, et al. Endoplasmic reticulum stress inhibition protects steatotic and non-steatotic livers in partial hepatectomy under ischemia-reperfusion. Cell Death Dis. 2010;1:e52.

23 Massip-Salcedo M, Roselló-Catafau J, Prieto J, Avíla MA, Peralta C. The response of the hepatocyte to ischemia. Liver Int. 2007;27(1):6–16.

24 Van Der Hoeven JA, Ter Horst GJ, Molema G, et al. Effects of brain death and hemodynamic status on function and immunologic activation of the potential donor liver in the rat. Ann. Surg. 2000;232(6):804–13.

25 Qing D-K. Prolonging warm ischemia reduces the cold preservation limits of liver grafts in swine. HBPD INT. 2006;5(4):515–20.

26 Ma Y, Wang G-D, Wu L-W, Hu R-D. Dynamical changing patterns of histological structure and ultrastructure of liver graft undergoing warm ischemia injury from non-heart-beating donor in rats. World J. Gastroenterol. 2006;12(30): 4902–5.

27 De Rougemont O, Lehmann K, Clavien P-A. Preconditioning, organ preservation, and postconditioning to prevent ischemia-reperfusion injury to the liver. Liver Transpl. 2009;15(10):1172–82.

28 Miyagi S, Ohkohchi N, Oikawa K, Satoh M, Tsukamoto S, Satomi S. Effects of anti-inflammatory cytokine agent (FR167653) and serine protease inhibitor on warm ischemia-reperfusion injury of the liver graft. Transplantation. 2004;77(10):1487–93.

29 Yamauchi JI, Richter S, Vollmar B, Menger MD, Minor T. Warm preflush with streptokinase improves microvascular procurement and tissue integrity in liver graft retrieval from non-heart-beating donors. Transplantation. 2000;69(9): 1780–84.

30 Oikawa K, Ohkohchi N, Sato M, Satomi S. The effects of the elimination of Kupffer cells in the isolated perfused liver from non-heart-beating rat. Transpl. Int. 2000;13 (Suppl 1):S573–9.

31 Liu Q, Bruns H, Schultze D, et al. HTK-N, a modified HTK solution, decreases preservation injury in a model of microsteatotic rat liver transplantation. Langenbecks Arch Surg. 2012;397(8):1323–31.

32 Zaouali MA, Padrissa-Altés S, Ben Mosbah I, et al. Improved rat steatotic and nonsteatotic liver preservation by the addition of epidermal growth factor and insulin-like growth factor-I to University of Wisconsin solution. Liver Transpl. 2010;16(9):1098–111.

33 Ramalho FS, Alfany-Fernandez I, Casillas-Ramirez A, et al. Are angiotensin II receptor antagonists useful strategies in steatotic and nonsteatotic livers in conditions of partial hepatectomy under ischemia-reperfusion? J. Pharmacol. Exp. Ther. 2009;329(1):130–40.

34 Casillas-Ramirez A, Amine-Zaouali M, Massip-Salcedo M, et al. Inhibition of angiotensin II action protects rat steatotic livers against ischemia-reperfusion injury. Crit. Care Med. 2008;36(4):1256–66.

35 Alfany-Fernandez I, Casillas-Ramirez A, Bintanel-Morcillo M, et al. Therapeutic targets in liver transplantation: angiotensin II in nonsteatotic grafts and angiotensin-(1-7) in steatotic grafts. Am. J. Transplant. 2009;9(3):439–51.

36 Hill GE, Alonso A, Spurzem JR, Stammers AH, Robbins RA. Aprotinin and methylprednisolone equally blunt cardiopulmonary bypass-induced inflammation in humans. J. Thorac. Cardiovasc. Surg. 1995;110(6):1658–62.

37 Wan S, DeSmet JM, Antoine M, Goldman M, Vincent JL, LeClerc JL. Steroid administration in heart and heart-lung transplantation: is the timing adequate? Ann. Thorac. Surg. 1996;61(2):674–8.

38 Jansen NJ, Van Oeveren W, Van den Broek L, et al. Inhibition by dexamethasone of the reperfusion phenomena in cardiopulmonary bypass. J. Thorac. Cardiovasc. Surg. 1991;102(4):515–25.

39 Figueroa I, Santiago-Delpín EA. Steroid protection of the liver during experimental eschemia. Surg Gynecol Obstet. 1975;140(3):368–70.

40 Sileri P, Schena S, Fukada J, et al. Corticosteroids enhance hepatic injury following ischemia-reperfusion. Transplant. Proc. 2001;33(7–8):3712.

41 Bilbao G, Contreras JL, Eckhoff DE, et al. Reduction of ischemia-reperfusion injury of the liver by in vivo adenovirus-mediated gene transfer of the antiapoptotic Bcl-2 gene. Ann. Surg. 1999;230(2):185–93.

42 Saidi RF, Chang J, Verb S, et al. The effect of methylprednisolone on warm ischemia-reperfusion injury in the liver. Am. J. Surg. 2007;193(3):345–7; discussion 347–8.

43 Frankenberg MV, Forman DT, Frey W, Bunzendahl H, Thurman RG. [Proteolysis but not ICAM-1 expression in fatty liver increased in tissue harvesting–role of Kupffer cells]. Langenbecks Arch Chir Suppl Kongressbd. 1998;115(Suppl I):575–9.

44 Moore C, Shen X-D, Gao F, Busuttil RW, Coito AJ. Fibronectin-alpha4beta1 integrin interactions regulate metalloproteinase-9 expression in steatotic liver ischemia and reperfusion injury. Am. J. Pathol. 2007;170(2):567–77.

45 Amersi F, Shen X-D, Moore C, et al. Fibronectin-alpha 4 beta 1 integrin-mediated blockade protects genetically fat Zucker rat livers from ischemia/reperfusion injury. Am. J. Pathol. 2003;162(4):1229–39.

46 Moore C, Shen XD, Fondevila C, Coito AJ. Fibronectin-alpha4beta1 integrin interactions modulate p42/44 MAPK phosphorylation in steatotic liver cold ischemia-reperfusion injury. Transplant. Proc. 2005;37(1):432–4.

47 Koti RS, Yang W, Dashwood MR, Davidson BR, Seifalian AM. Effect of ischemic preconditioning on hepatic microcirculation and function in a rat model of ischemia reperfusion injury. Liver Transpl. 2002;8(12):1182–91.

48 Serafín A, Roselló-Catafau J, Prats N, Gelpí E, Rodés J, Peralta C. Ischemic preconditioning affects interleukin release in fatty livers of rats undergoing ischemia/reperfusion. Hepatology. 2004;39(3):688–98.

49 Burke A, Lucey MR. Non-alcoholic fatty liver disease, non-alcoholic steatohepatitis and orthotopic liver transplantation. Am. J. Transplant. 2004;4(5):686–93.

50 Baldwin D, Chandrashekhar Y, McFalls E, et al. Ischemic preconditioning prior to aortic cross-clamping protects high-energy phosphate levels, glucose uptake, and myocyte contractility. J. Surg. Res. 2002;105(2):153–9.

51 Murry CE, Richard VJ, Reimer KA, Jennings RB. Ischemic preconditioning slows energy metabolism and delays ultrastructural damage during a sustained ischemic episode. Circ. Res. 1990;66(4):913–31.

52 Cavalieri B, Perrelli M-G, Aragno M, et al. Ischemic preconditioning attenuates the oxidant-dependent mechanisms of reperfusion cell damage and death in rat liver. Liver Transpl. 2002;8(11):990–9.

53 Koti RS, Yang W, Dashwood MR, Davidson BR, Seifalian AM. Effect of ischemic preconditioning on hepatic microcirculation and function in a rat model of ischemia reperfusion injury. Liver Transpl. 2002;8(12):1182–91.

54 Clavien PA, Yadav S, Sindram D, Bentley RC. Protective effects of ischemic preconditioning for liver resection performed under inflow occlusion in humans. Ann. Surg. 2000;232(2):155–62.

55 Hardy KJ, Tancheroen S, Shulkes A. Comparison of continuous versus intermittent ischaemia-reperfusion during liver resection in an experimental model. Br J Surg. 1995;82(6):833–6.

56 Hardy KJ, Tancheroen S, Shulkes A. Comparison of continuous versus intermittent ischaemia-reperfusion during liver resection in an experimental model. Br J Surg. 1995;82(6):833–6.

57 Isozaki H, Adam R, Gigou M, Szekely AM, Shen M, Bismuth H. Experimental study of the protective effect of intermittent hepatic pedicle clamping in the rat. Br J Surg. 1992;79(4):310–13.

58 Horiuchi T, Muraoka R, Tabo T, Uchinami M, Kimura N, Tanigawa N. Optimal cycles of hepatic ischemia and reperfusion for intermittent pedicle clamping during liver surgery. Arch Surg. 1995;130(7):754–8.

59 White BD, Martin RJ. Evidence for a central mechanism of obesity in the Zucker rat: role of neuropeptide Y and leptin. Proc. Soc. Exp. Biol. Med. 1997;214(3):222–32.

60 Amersi F, Farmer DG, Shaw GD, et al. P-selectin glycoprotein ligand-1 (rPSGL-Ig)-mediated blockade of CD62 selectin molecules protects rat steatotic

liver grafts from ischemia/reperfusion injury. Am. J. Transplant. 2002;2(7): 600–8.

61 Coito AJ, Buelow R, Shen X-D, et al. Heme oxygenase-1 gene transfer inhibits inducible nitric oxide synthase expression and protects genetically fat Zucker rat livers from ischemia-reperfusion injury. Transplantation. 2002;74(1):96–102.

62 Saidi RF, Chang J, Brooks S, Nalbantoglu I, Adsay V, Jacobs MJ. Ischemic precon-ditioning and intermittent clamping increase the tolerance of fatty liver to hepatic ischemia-reperfusion injury in the rat. Transplant. Proc. 2007;39(10):3010–14.

63 El-Badry AM, Moritz W, Contaldo C, Tian Y, Graf R, Clavien P-A. Prevention of reperfusion injury and microcirculatory failure in macrosteatotic mouse liver by omega-3 fatty acids. Hepatology. 2007;45(4):855–63.

64 McCormack L, Dutkowski P, El-Badry AM, Clavien P-A. Liver transplantation using fatty livers: always feasible? J. Hepatol. 2011;54(5):1055–62.

65 Chavin KD, Fiorini RN, Shafizadeh S, et al. Fatty acid synthase blockade protects steatotic livers from warm ischemia reperfusion injury and transplantation. Am. J. Transplant. 2004;4(9):1440–7.

66 Net M, Valero R, Almenara R, et al. The effect of normothermic recirculation is mediated by ischemic preconditioning in NHBD liver transplantation. Am. J. Transplant. 2005;5(10):2385–92.

67 Minor T, Akbar S, Yamamoto Y. Adenosine A2 receptor stimulation protects the predamaged liver from cold preservation through activation of cyclic adenosine monophosphate-protein kinase A pathway. Liver Transpl. 2000;6(2):196–200.

68 Horstick G, Berg O, Heimann A, et al. Application of C1-esterase inhibitor during reperfusion of ischemic myocardium: dose-related beneficial versus detrimental effects. Circulation. 2001;104(25):3125–31.

69 Fu J, Lin G, Wu Z, et al. Anti-apoptotic role for C1 inhibitor in ischemia/ reperfusion-induced myocardial cell injury. Biochem. Biophys. Res. Commun. 2006;349(2):504–12.

70 Hill J, Lindsay TF, Ortiz F, Yeh CG, Hechtman HB, Moore FD Jr. Soluble comple-ment receptor type 1 ameliorates the local and remote organ injury after intestinal ischemia-reperfusion in the rat. J. Immunol. 1992;149(5):1723–8.

71 Heijnen BHM, Straatsburg IH, Padilla ND, Van Mierlo GJ, Hack CE, Van Gulik TM. Inhibition of classical complement activation attenuates liver ischaemia and reperfusion injury in a rat model. Clin. Exp. Immunol. 2006;143(1):15–23.

72 Lehmann TG, Heger M, Münch S, Kirschfink M, Klar E. In vivo microscopy reveals that complement inhibition by C1-esterase inhibitor reduces ischemia/ reperfusion injury in the liver. Transpl. Int. 2000;13 Suppl 1:S547–50.

73 Chan RK, Ibrahim SI, Verna N, Carroll M, Moore FD Jr, Hechtman HB. Ischaemia-reperfusion is an event triggered by immune complexes and comple-ment. Br J Surg. 2003;90(12):1470–8.

74 Inderbitzin D, Beldi G, Avital I, Vinci G, Candinas D. Local and remote ischemia-reperfusion injury is mitigated in mice overexpressing human C1 inhibitor. Eur Surg Res. 2004;36(3):142–7.

75 Straatsburg IH, Boermeester MA, Wolbink GJ, et al. Complement activation induced by ischemia-reperfusion in humans: a study in patients undergoing par-tial hepatectomy. J. Hepatol. 2000;32(5):783–91.

76 Meyer zu Vilsendorf A, Link C, Jörns A, Nagel E, Köhl J. Preconditioning with the prostacyclin analog epoprostenol and cobra venom factor prevents reperfusion injury and hyperacute rejection in discordant liver xenotransplantation. Xenotransplantation. 2001;8(1):41–7.

77 Bergamaschini L, Gobbo G, Gatti S, et al. Endothelial targeting with C1-inhibitor reduces complement activation in vitro and during ex vivo reperfusion of pig liver. Clin. Exp. Immunol. 2001;126(3):412–20.

78 Caliezi C, Wuillemin WA, Zeerleder S, Redondo M, Eisele B, Hack CE. C1-Esterase inhibitor: an anti-inflammatory agent and its potential use in the treatment of diseases other than hereditary angioedema. Pharmacol. Rev. 2000;52(1): 91–112.

79 Suzuki S, Nakamura S, Koizumi T, et al. The beneficial effect of a prostaglandin I2 analog on ischemic rat liver. Transplantation. 1991;52(6):979–83.

80 Davis AE 3rd, Mejia P, Lu F. Biological activities of C1 inhibitor. Mol. Immunol. 2008;45(16):4057–63.

81 Fausto N. Liver regeneration. J. Hepatol. 2000;32(1 Suppl):19–31.

82 Michalopoulos GK, DeFrances MC. Liver regeneration. Science. 1997;276(5309): 60–6.

83 Guo JT, Zhou H, Liu C, et al. Apoptosis and regeneration of hepatocytes during recovery from transient hepadnavirus infections. J. Virol. 2000;74(3):1495–1505.

84 Schieferdecker HL, Schlaf G, Koleva M, Götze O, Jungermann K. Induction of functional anaphylatoxin C5a receptors on hepatocytes by in vivo treatment of rats with IL-6. J. Immunol. 2000;164(10):5453–8.

85 Mastellos D, Papadimitriou JC, Franchini S, Tsonis PA, Lambris JD. A novel role of complement: mice deficient in the fifth component of complement (C5) exhibit impaired liver regeneration. J. Immunol. 2001;166(4):2479–86.

86 Almeida-Porada G, Zanjani ED, Porada CD. Bone marrow stem cells and liver regeneration. Exp. Hematol. 2010;38(7):574–80.

87 Ishikawa T, Banas A, Hagiwara K, Iwaguro H, Ochiya T. Stem cells for hepatic regeneration: the role of adipose tissue derived mesenchymal stem cells. Curr Stem Cell Res Ther. 2010;5(2):182–9.

88 Di Bonzo LV, Ferrero I, Cravanzola C, et al. Human mesenchymal stem cells as a two-edged sword in hepatic regenerative medicine: engraftment and hepatocyte differentiation versus profibrogenic potential. Gut. 2008;57(2):223–31.

89 Arias-Diaz J, Ildefonso JA, Muñoz JJ, Zapata A, Jiménez E. Both tacrolimus and sirolimus decrease Th1/Th2 ratio, and increase regulatory T lymphocytes in the liver after ischemia/reperfusion. Lab. Invest. 2009;89(4):433–45.

90 Kuboki S, Sakai N, Tschöp J, Edwards MJ, Lentsch AB, Caldwell CC. Distinct contributions of CD4+ T cell subsets in hepatic ischemia/reperfusion injury. Am. J. Physiol. Gastrointest. Liver Physiol. 2009;296(5):G1054–9.

91 Monbaliu D, Brassil J. Machine perfusion of the liver: past, present and future. Curr Opin Organ Transplant. 2010;15(2):160–6.

92 Starzl TE, Groth CG, Brettschneider L, et al. Extended survival in 3 cases of orthotopic homotransplantation of the human liver. Surgery. 1968;63(4):549–63.

93 Vogel T, Brockmann JG, Friend PJ. Ex-vivo normothermic liver perfusion: an update. Curr Opin Organ Transplant. 2010;15(2):167–72.

94 Imber CJ, St Peter SD, Lopez de Cenarruzabeitia I et al. Advantages of normothermic perfusion over cold storage in liver preservation. Transplantation. 2002;73(5):701–9.

95 Reddy S, Greenwood J, Maniakin N, et al. Non-heart-beating donor porcine livers: the adverse effect of cooling. Liver Transpl. 2005;11(1):35–8.

96 Schön MR, Kollmar O, Wolf S, et al. Liver transplantation after organ preservation with normothermic extracorporeal perfusion. Ann. Surg. 2001;233(1):114–23.

97 García-Valdecasas JC, Fondevila C. In-vivo normothermic recirculation: an update. Curr Opin Organ Transplant. 2010;15(2):173–6.

98 Valero R, García-Valdecasas JC, Net M, et al. L-arginine reduces liver and biliary tract damage after liver transplantation from non-heart-beating donor pigs. Transplantation. 2000;70(5):730–7.

99 Lee CY, Jain S, Duncan HM, et al. Survival transplantation of preserved non-heart-beating donor rat livers: preservation by hypothermic machine perfusion. Transplantation. 2003;76(10):1432–6.

100 Dutkowski P, Furrer K, Tian Y, Graf R, Clavien P-A. Novel short-term hypothermic oxygenated perfusion (HOPE) system prevents injury in rat liver graft from non-heart beating donor. Ann. Surg. 2006;244(6):968–76; discussion 976–7.

101 Bessems M, Doorschodt BM, Van Marle J, Vreeling H, Meijer AJ, Van Gulik TM. Improved machine perfusion preservation of the non-heart-beating donor rat liver using Polysol: a new machine perfusion preservation solution. Liver Transpl. 2005;11(11):1379–88.

102 Rojas A, Chen L, Bartlett RH, Arenas JD. Assessment of liver function during extracorporeal membrane oxygenation in the non-heart beating donor swine. Transplant. Proc. 2004;36(5):1268–70.

103 Wang C-C, Wang S-H, Lin C-C, et al. Liver transplantation from an uncontrolled non-heart-beating donor maintained on extracorporeal membrane oxygenation. Transplant. Proc. 2005;37(10):4331–3.

104 Vekemans K, Liu Q, Brassil J, Komuta M, Pirenne J, Monbaliu D. Influence of flow and addition of oxygen during porcine liver hypothermic machine perfusion. Transplant. Proc. 2007;39(8):2647–51.

105 Pringle JH. V. Notes on the Arrest of Hepatic Hemorrhage Due to Trauma. Ann. Surg. 1908;48(4):541–9.

106 Belghiti J, Noun R, Zante E, Ballet T, Sauvanet A. Portal triad clamping or hepatic vascular exclusion for major liver resection. A controlled study. Ann. Surg. 1996;224(2):155–161.

107 Man K, Fan ST, Ng IO, Lo CM, Liu CL, Wong J. Prospective evaluation of Pringle maneuver in hepatectomy for liver tumors by a randomized study. Ann. Surg. 1997;226(6):704–11; discussion 711–13.

108 Terblanche J, Krige JE, Bornman PC. Simplified hepatic resection with the use of prolonged vascular inflow occlusion. Arch Surg. 1991;126(3):298–301.

109 Cunningham JD, Fong Y, Shriver C, Melendez J, Marx WL, Blumgart LH. One hundred consecutive hepatic resections. Blood loss, transfusion, and operative technique. Arch Surg. 1994;129(10):1050–6.

110 Bismuth H, Castaing D, Garden OJ. Major hepatic resection under total vascular exclusion. Ann. Surg. 1989;210(1):13–19.

111 Belghiti J, Noun R, Malafosse R, et al. Continuous versus intermittent portal triad clamping for liver resection: a controlled study. Ann. Surg. 1999;229(3):369–75.

112 Makuuchi M, Mori T, Gunvén P, Yamazaki S, Hasegawa H. Safety of hemi-hepatic vascular occlusion during resection of the liver. Surg Gynecol Obstet. 1987;164(2):155–8.

113 Murry CE, Jennings RB, Reimer KA. Preconditioning with ischemia: a delay of lethal cell injury in ischemic myocardium. Circulation. 1986;74(5):1124–36.

114 Peralta C, Closa D, Hotter G, Gelpí E, Prats N, Roselló-Catafau J. Liver ischemic preconditioning is mediated by the inhibitory action of nitric oxide on endothelin. Biochem. Biophys. Res. Commun. 1996;229(1):264–70.

115 Hardy KJ, McClure DN, Subwongcharoen S. Ischaemic preconditioning of the liver: a preliminary study. Aust N Z J Surg. 1996;66(10):707–10.

CHAPTER 14

Legal and administrative issues related to transfusion-free medicine and surgery programs

Randy Henderson[1] and Nicolas Jabbour[2]

[1]Transfusion-Free Surgery and Patient Blood Management Program, Keck Medical Center and Keck Hospital of USC, Los Angeles, CA, USA
[2]Service de Chirurgie et transplantation abdominale, Cliniques universitaires Saint-Luc, Bruxelles, Belgium

Introduction

Few would argue that patient rights should be protected and respected. However, when this right involves a patient's refusal of potentially life-saving treatment, serious issues come to the fore. In this chapter we will discuss the rights of patients to refuse blood transfusion, and the right and duty of the physician assuming care for such patients. We will also review how the implementation and establishment of bloodless medicine and surgery programs evolved from Jehovah's Witnesses' position on blood, and the lessons that science has learned in the process.

History of Jehovah's Witnesses and blood

The issue involving Jehovah's Witnesses and blood transfusions became most prominent in the 1940s at the height of World War II [1]. Blood was liberally transfused into wounded soldiers, and this led to an increased demand for blood donors. Most individuals in the medical profession, as well as members of the lay community, regarded the practice of blood transfusion as an accepted therapeutic method. But those who were members of the religious organization known as Jehovah's Witnesses did not. And the passage of time has not changed their point of view.

The Witnesses' belief is that God, the Creator of life, views blood as sacred and holy, and therefore it should not be used for the purpose of transfusion, regardless of the consequences [2]. They cite several Bible passages found in both the Old and New Testaments. One such passage is found in Genesis, the first book of the Bible. Genesis Chapter 9 verses 3 and 4, says: "Every moving animal that is alive may serve as food for you. As in the case of green vegetation, I do give it all to you. Only flesh with its soul–its blood–you must not eat." The Bible book of Leviticus chapter 17 verse 10 says: "As for any man of the house of Israel or some alien resident who is residing as an alien in their midst *who eats any sort of blood*, I shall certainly set my face against the soul that is eating the blood, and *I shall indeed cut him off* from among his people." Furthermore, in the New Testament of the Bible, Acts chapter 15 verses 28 and 29 states: "The holy spirit and we ourselves have favored adding no further burden to you, except these necessary things, to keep *abstaining ... from ... blood.*" Although no mention is made of transfusing blood, Jehovah's Witnesses' view this directive to "not eat blood" or "to abstain from blood" as something that applies to both *oral* and *intravenous* feeding.

While it is true that Jehovah's Witnesses refuse blood, they are not averse to medical and surgical treatment. On the contrary, many of them are physicians, even surgeons. However, as already stated, their position on blood is unequivocal and absolute [3].

Acceptable products, treatments, and procedures

Although Jehovah's Witnesses do not accept blood transfusions, accepting products *derived* from red cells, white cells, platelets or plasma is viewed as a decision that individual Witness patients must make for themselves. In a recent issue of *The Watchtower*, the principal journal of Jehovah's Witnesses, a distinction is made between whole blood and its *primary components* (i.e. red cells, white cells, platelets, and plasma) and *fractions* [4]. These primary components are unacceptable to devout Jehovah's Witnesses. However, acceptable blood fractions may include plasma proteins such as immune globulins, albumin, and cryoprecipitate. Platelet-derived wound healing factors may also fall into this category of acceptable blood fractions. The rationale of Jehovah's Witnesses in regards to products fractionated from blood is partly based on the complexity of blood itself. Medical practitioners recognize that plasma, for example, consists of many substances such as hormones, inorganic salts, enzymes, and nutrients. Plasma also carries proteins such as albumin, clotting factors and antibodies. Jehovah's Witnesses believe that the Bible does not give details about these products that, medically speaking, are not typically defined as blood. Therefore, each individual Witness is instructed to use their conscience in making a decision to accept or refuse these products.

The availability of recombinant growth factors such as erythropoietin to stimulate hematopoiesis has been very helpful in minimizing or eliminating a patient's exposure to allogeneic blood. However, while the majority of Jehovah's Witnesses will accept recombinant erythropoietin, since all formulations of the product available in the United States are packaged with a stabilizer that includes trace amounts of human serum albumin, consent must be obtained prior to its use. There are some Witness patients who refuse to accept any blood-derived product, regardless of the amount. Therefore, health-care providers should utilize a specific form that allows patients to choose the products, treatments and procedures that are acceptable to them (see Figure 14.1).

Autologous procedures and equipment

Citing other Biblical statements that discuss the use of blood, Jehovah's Witnesses do not allow the preoperative collection and storage of their own blood for later infusion. For example, in the Old Testament book of Leviticus Chapter 17 verses 13 it says what a man should do if he killed an animal for good. It states: "He must in that case pour its blood out and cover it with dust." According to some Bible scholars, this act of pouring out blood is best understood as an act of reverence demonstrating respect for the life of the animal and, thus, respect for God who created and continues to care for that life [5]. Again, Jehovah's Witnesses' principal journal *The Watchtower* addressed the therapeutic and surgical use of procedures or equipment involving autologous blood. As with fractions of primary components of blood, this too is a matter for personal decision. If the intra-operative cell-saver machine is not primed with blood, and is set up in a closed circuit that is in constant contact with the patient's circulatory system, this is acceptable to many Witness patients. The same principle would apply to the use of dialysis and heart lung machines, as well as acute normovolemic hemodilution (ANH) (see Figure 14.1).

Organ transplantation

There has been a great deal of confusion over the fact that the doctrine of Jehovah's Witnesses prohibits them from receiving blood transfusions but not organ transplants. Blood itself is often viewed as a "liquid organ transplant." Why then do Jehovah's Witnesses view organ transplants differently than they do blood?

Some 24 years ago, *The Watchtower* briefly discussed this issue [6]. The principle guiding Jehovah's Witnesses' decision to accept organ

TRANSFUSION-FREE MEDICINE AND SURGERY PROGRAM
PRODUCT, TREATMENT AND PROCEDURE ACCEPTANCE

Patient: _____
  (Please Print)

1. Your attending physician is Dr. _____ and your supervising physician or surgeon is Dr. _____.

2. I request that no blood or primary components of blood (**including, without limitation, another person's blood, my own stored blood, platelets, or fresh frozen plasma**) be administered to me, or to the patient named below for whom I am legally authorized to give or withhold consent for medical treatment, no matter what consequences, and even if health care providers believe that only blood transfusion therapy will preserve my (or the patient's) life or health. I certify that the potential risks and consequences of this refusal have been fully described to me by my attending physician or health care provider and that I accept those risks and consequences.

3. *On behalf of myself, or on behalf of the Patient, if I am acting as a legal representative, I hereby fully and unconditionally release the Hospital, my physicians, and all other health care personnel, facilities or entities involved in my care, or the Patient's care, from any claim or liability related to this refusal to accept blood transfusions, despite their otherwise competent care.*

The following are my wishes and directions regarding procedures, treatments and **blood fractions** (initial appropriate boxes):

PRODUCT/TREATMENT//PROCEDURE	I Will Accept:	I Will NOT Accept:
Albumin (minor blood fraction)		
Erythropoietin, thrombolytic enzymes (contains albumin)		
Immune Globulins (minor blood fractions)		
Topical Procoagulants (Tisseel, fibrin glue, thrombin)		
Plasma Protein Fractions (Cryoprecipitate)		
Recombinant Factor VIII, IX and VIIa (may contain human albumin)		
Dialysis & Heart-Lung equipment (non-blood primed)		
Intraoperative Blood Salvage (Cell Saver) where extracorporeal circulation is a closed circuit without blood storage		
Hemodilution (closed circuit)		
Plasmapheresis (without fresh frozen plasma infusion, but does contain albumin)		

Date: _____   Time: _____ A.M./ P.M.

Signature: _____
  (Patient)

Patient's Legal Representative: _____

Witness: _____

Figure 14.1 Sample transfusion-free medicine & surgery program/product, treatment and procedure consent.

transplants or human tissue focuses on their view that while the Bible specifically forbids consuming blood, there is no Biblical command or injunction proscribing the "taking in" of other human tissue. They mention that meat is not prohibited for human consumption as long as it is properly bled, and therefore this principle can be applied to organ transplantation. However, each member of the Jehovah's Witness faith is instructed to weigh all relevant factors and make a personal, conscientious decision about accepting an organ transplant. In the main, if a human organ transplant does not involve blood or blood products, it is left up to each individual Witness to decide for themselves.

Overview of legal principles related to refusal of blood

A. Refusal of blood as life-sustaining treatment

Does a patient have the right to refuse blood transfusion at the risk of their life? Before we address that question, it's important to understand the legal rights of patients to refuse *any* type of medical or surgical treatment

The basic common law right of bodily self-determination establishes that every person of sound mind is master over his/her own body. Therefore, such an individual is free to prohibit surgery or medical treatment deemed by others as potentially life saving. Over 100 years ago, the United States Supreme Court upheld the notion of individual autonomy. They stated that "no right is held more sacred, or is more carefully guarded, by the common law, than the right of every individual to the possession and control of his own person, free from all restraint of interference of others, unless by unquestionable authority of law." [7]

This fundamental legal principle of bodily self-determination serves as the basis for the doctrine of informed consent. The right to privacy dovetails with informed consent. No doctor or hospital should subject patients to medical and/or surgical treatment without informed consent. The patient must be informed of the name, means, and likely consequences of the proposed treatment in order to "knowingly" determine what should or should not be done to their body.

Informed consent

Informed consent rests on two very important values: 1) the patient's own conception of his personal well being, and 2) the patient's right to self-determination. The principle of self-determination "is best understood as respecting people's right to define and pursue their own view of what is good." [7]

In Cobbs v. Grant, a landmark California Supreme Court decision, it was determined that physicians have had a duty to obtain the informed consent of patients before performing certain medical procedures [8]. Over 90 years ago, Justice Benjamin Cardozo stated: "Every human being of adult years and sound mind has a right to determine what shall be done with his own body; and a surgeon who performs an operation without his patient's consent, commits an assault, for which he is liable in damages." Justice Cardozo's statement was in response to the case of a woman who was admitted to the hospital with abdominal pain and a palpable lump. She gave her doctors consent to physical examination, but she refused surgical examination. However, while under general anesthetic (ether) for further physical examination, surgeons surgically removed a fibroid tumor. Subsequently, gangrene developed in her left arm, and two fingers were amputated. The physicians were held liable for negligence and battery [9, 10].

Therefore doctors who administer treatment or perform surgery without a patient's consent are liable for battery. Battery can be legally defined as an intentional, non-consented act causing harmful or offensive contact with the person of another. Put simply: it is any physical contact with another person to which that person has not consented. Battery is concerned with the right to have one's body left alone by others. A surgical operation on the body of a person is a technical battery or trespass unless he or some authorized person consented to it, regardless of the skill and care employed in the performance of the operation. In addition, a case of battery is established where a physician obtains consent to perform one type of treatment and thereafter performs a substantially different treatment for which consent was not obtained [9, 11].

In the precedent setting case of *Cruzan v. Missouri Dep't of Health*, 497 U.S. 261 (1990), the Supreme Court determined that "the logical corollary of the doctrine of informed consent is that the patient generally possesses the right not to consent, that is the right to refuse treatment." [7] Even if a patient refuses treatment that a physician views as life-sustaining, "the primacy of a patient's interest's in self-determination and in honoring the patient's own view of well-being warrant leaving with the patient the final authority to decide."

B. Specific issues related to refusal of blood in J.W.
1. Competent adults
In view of clearly established laws regarding informed consent, any competent adult has the right to refuse blood.

At least three high courts have found that the 1st Amendment Free Exercise Clause protects religion-based refusals of medical treatment from state interference [7, 12–14]. The fact that Jehovah's Witnesses' refusal of blood may be viewed as a non-act or refusal to act rather than a positive, affirmative act is a significant point to consider. Whereas some states have exercised their "law enforcement" authority to limit or prohibit religiously motivated action in order to protect public health, safety or welfare, there is no precedent for prohibiting action motivated by religion when there is no grave or pressingly imminent danger to the public [7, 15–18].

Example
In Re Brown: [9, 19]

Mrs. Brown was a Jehovah's Witness who was shot by her daughter and consequently required surgery. The doctors recommended a blood transfusion, to which she refused to consent. Thereafter, the state sought and obtained a court order to force a transfusion due to the fact that Mrs. Brown was the only eyewitness to the shooting, and if she died from lack of a blood transfusion, she would not be able to testify for the state in the prosecution. The surgery did take place and Mrs. Brown did receive blood transfusions.

Mrs. Brown required further surgery and again her surgeon recommended blood transfusions. She refused and made an appeal to the Court to stop the order. The decision of the court was that the order be vacated and Mrs. Brown not be required to submit to or receive a blood transfusion against her will. The Supreme Court made the following statement regarding her common law right to privacy:

"Each individual has a right to the inviability and integrity of the person, freedom to choose or bodily self-determination." The Supreme Court added: "The right to be left alone ... which is the most comprehensive of rights and the right most valued by civilized man. Violation of this rule constitutes a battery."

The court also stated that "the factual information available to us makes clear that Brown's position has been consistent throughout: that she wants to live, that she wants the benefits of all that medical science can do for her with the sole and only exception that she rejects any treatment proscribed by the tenets of her religious faith."

2. Emergency/incompetent adults (patients known to be J.W. refusing blood)

Generally speaking, the fundamental right of bodily self-determination does not vanish when a patient loses consciousness or becomes incompetent. That right remains intact even when the patient is no longer able to assert the right [9, 20, 21]. In addition, when a patient has religious views against certain forms of medical treatment that predate and are unaltered by their incapacity, physicians and health care providers are not justified in substituting their own judgment for the patients at the time of treatment.

When refusals of treatment are religiously-motivated they are "usually considered more thoroughly and less likely to change than non-religious ones because they are not dependent upon predictions of future circumstances, available medical treatment, or preferences." [9, 22]

In reality, the main question is whether there is evidence of the patient's previously expressed wishes or refusal, not whether incompetent or unconscious adults in general have the right to refuse treatment.

Example #1
In re Estate of Dorone: [7, 9, 23]

Mr. Dorone was a 22-year-old Jehovah's Witness man who was seriously injured in an automobile accident and thus rendered unconscious. After being taken to a New Jersey hospital, his medical alert card indicating that he wanted non-blood treatment was found. Thereafter, Mr. Dorone was transferred to a Pennsylvania hospital but his personal effects, including his medical alert card, were left behind. He required two more emergency surgeries, one for a subdural hematoma and another to remove a blood clot on his brain.

In each case, the hospital sought and received oral, telephonic court orders to allow blood transfusions against Mr. Dorone's previously expressed refusal and over the objections of his family. His family had been excluded from the judicial hearings. The Pennsylvania Supreme Court upheld the prior orders to allow blood transfusions for Mr. Dorone. The Supreme Court stated: "When evidence of this nature is measured against third party speculation as to what an unconscious patient would want, there can be no doubt that medical intervention is required. Indeed, in a situation like the present, where there is an emergency calling for an immediate decision, nothing less than a fully conscious contemporaneous decision by the patient will be sufficient to override evidence of medical necessity."

Example #2
Werth v. Taylor [7]

Mrs. Werth, a Jehovah's Witness and mother of two children, became pregnant with twins in 1985. In preparation for delivery, she filled out a "Refusal to Permit Blood Transfusion" form with the hospital. A few months later, she went into labor and upon admission to the hospital her husband filled out another "Refusal to Permit Blood Transfusion" form in her behalf.

Subsequent to the birth of her twins, Mrs. Werth required an emergency D & C due to bleeding. Prior to performing the procedure, the attending physician again confirmed her refusal of blood with Mr. Werth. The D & C was completed but after she continued to bleed and became hemodynamically unstable, Dr. Taylor, the anesthesiologist, believed that a transfusion should be given to save her life. Mrs. Werth remained unconscious. Despite being informed that Mrs. Werth was one of Jehovah's Witness, and therefore refused blood, Dr. Taylor proceeded with the order for transfusion. In his opinion, this was a life-threatening emergency.

Mrs. Werth and her husband did file a medical malpractice and battery suit against Dr. Taylor but the trial court accepted his defense that her refusal was not binding. His argument was similar to the Dorone case; he argued that Mrs. Werth's refusal was not a conscious, competent, contemporaneous, fully informed refusal made in contemplation of the life-threatening situation that arose. In July 1991, Mrs. Werth appealed the trial court's decision to the Michigan Court of Appeals but they upheld the decision in favor of Dr. Taylor. The court of appeals did acknowledge that competent adults can refuse medical treatment, but they determined that a life-threatening emergency was different from a routine elective surgery. Applying the Dorone case to Mrs. Werth's condition, they believed that the lack of a fully informed, contemporaneous decision was sufficient to override evidence of medical necessity.

These cases raise several legal/ethical questions. Is the requirement of a contemporaneous, fully informed or fully conscious refusal truly practical and realistic? How can an unconscious or non-communicative patient be able to satisfy this standard?

Example #3
In re Hughes [7]

Mrs. Hughes was scheduled for an elective hysterectomy. Before consenting to the surgery, she spoke to her doctor, Dr. Ances, about her refusal of blood transfusions due to her religious beliefs. He agreed to perform the surgery without blood. On the morning that Mrs. Hughes was admitted to the hospital, she filled out the hospital's standard refusal of blood form. The form released the doctor and the hospital from liability for respecting her wishes that no blood products be used. It also stated that she "fully understood the possible consequences" of her refusal of blood–a key phrase.

Unfortunately the surgery was not uneventful and Mrs. Hughes experienced massive bleeding. Despite the conversation she had with Dr. Ances before the surgery, and the refusal form she filled out at the hospital, he felt that a blood transfusion was necessary. Mrs. Hughes' husband was contacted and after being told that his wife would likely die if she did not receive a blood transfusion he gave permission. Mr. Hughes was not a

Jehovah's Witness. Mrs. Hughes' sister (who was a Jehovah's Witness) was at the hospital and she eventually discovered that a transfusion had been recommended for her sister. She objected to the use of blood and decided to contact the Philadelphia Hospital Liaison Committee for Jehovah's Witnesses. This conflict came to the attention of hospital administration and therefore a court hearing was arranged.

Dr. Ances testified that Mrs. Hughes' discussion with him regarding her refusal of blood, though clear and competent, was not in anticipation of such complications that led to massive blood loss. Although Mrs. Hughes' husband agreed to the use of blood for his wife after being called by the doctor, he stated in court that he knew his wife would not want blood. Mrs. Hughes' sister and teenage daughter, testifying on behalf of Mrs. Hughes, said that she would not want blood under any circumstances.

The trial court's decision was to grant the hospital authority to transfuse until Mrs. Hughes regained consciousness and could again speak for herself. Mrs. Hughes was transfused and after regaining consciousness she reiterated her refusal of blood. As stipulated by the terms of the court, the order for transfusion was then terminated.

Mrs. Hughes did appeal to the New Jersey Superior Court but the earlier decision of the trial court was upheld. The appellate court did not base their decision on the requirement of a contemporaneous, fully informed or fully conscious refusal. Rather, they ruled that in an emergency involving a refusal of allegedly life-saving treatment, the refusal will be honored only if there is "clear, convincing, unequivocal evidence" that the patient's refusal was "fully informed." Furthermore, they stated that such a refusal can be established by the patient's "oral directives, actions or writings." They also indicated that if there exists even a "glimmer of uncertainty" about the patient's wishes, the refusal would not be honored.

Indirectly, the court criticized Dr. Ances and the hospital. Dr. Ances failed to thoroughly discuss with Mrs. Hughes all the possible consequences of the surgery. And the hospital's refusal form was lacking in that it did not accomplish its intended purpose.

Example #4
In re Duran [7]

In 1996 Maria Duran was diagnosed with liver failure. As one of Jehovah's Witnesses, Ms. Duran sought treatment at the University of Pittsburgh Medical Center since they were known to have successfully performed "bloodless" liver transplants on Jehovah's Witnesses. Ms. Duran and her husband (who was not one of Jehovah's Witnesses) traveled to Pittsburgh in early 1997 to be evaluated for liver transplantation. The transplant team accepted her as a candidate with the stipulation that blood transfusions would not be given under any circumstances.

To ensure that her wishes would be respected, Ms. Duran executed a health-care durable power of attorney (DPA) form and appointed an elder from a Pittsburgh area congregation of Jehovah's Witnesses to be her health-care agent. Ms. Duran and her husband moved to Pittsburgh in 1999 after being informed that a liver would soon become available. She was transplanted in July 1999. Just a few days later, however, she experienced an episode of organ rejection. Since she was still unconscious, the doctors sought and gained consent for another transplant from her health-care agent. One week later she was re-transplanted. However, her body once again rejected the liver organ.

Ms. Duran remained unconscious and despite the poor prognosis for recovery, her doctors recommended blood transfusions as a means to improve her chances of survival. A court hearing was quickly arranged in order to appoint her husband as emergency guardian for the purpose of granting consent for blood to be given. Her health-care agent was not informed. The court heard testimony from Ms. Duran's attending physician, her husband, and her adult sister who was in favor of giving her blood transfusions. Mr. Duran was granted authority as her emergency guardian and over a period of three weeks multiple blood transfusions were given. Ms. Duran died having never regained consciousness.

Ms. Duran's health-care agent was eventually informed about what transpired and he filed an appeal with the Pennsylvania Superior Court. He challenged the trial court's order on several grounds, namely: (1) overriding Ms. Duran's oral and written refusals of blood, (2) circumventing her personally appointed health-care agent and appointing a guardian with authority to consent to blood, and (3) failing to notify the health-care agent of the guardianship petition and trial court hearing. The Superior Court's decision was to uphold the agent's challenges and it unanimously reversed the trial court's order.

In commenting on its decision, the superior court noted that the right of a patient to "refuse medical treatment is deeply rooted" in common law. They further explained that Ms. Duran's Durable Power of Attorney (DPA) was unequivocal in its pointed refusal of blood transfusions under any circumstance. Furthermore, in regards to the appointment of her husband as emergency guardian, the superior court agreed that since Ms. Duran had already appointed a health care representative when she executed her DPA, her husband "should not have been appointed emergency guardian for the express purpose of consenting to a blood transfusion because his beliefs conflicted with [his wife's] regarding blood transfusion therapy." They also stated that the trial court should have taken into consideration her unequivocal directions when the very situation contemplated by her DPA arose. Regarding the failure of the trial court to notify her self-appointed health-care agent, the superior court ruled that in view of the fact that both Ms. Duran's husband and the hospital staff knew where to find her health-care agent in an emergency situation, it was "reasonable under these circumstances" to afford the agent notice of the hearing.

The above case illustrates that despite a patient's right to refuse blood transfusions, certain situations put physicians in hesitation mode, especially when confronted by other family members. This enforces the necessity of clear policies and procedures within a transfusion-free program to clearly delineate such possibilities in advance. This is mostly true when electively treating adult patients undergoing high-risk procedures. The refusal of blood in such situations should equate with any other consent between physician and patient prior to initiating therapy. Refusal of blood transfusions should not be different from any other directive given by the patient. The consent form developed in a transfusion-free program should clearly stipulate that the patient's wishes should not be questioned, even if the patient becomes incapacitated and even if their life is endangered due to lack of transfusion. (see Figure 14.1 and 14.2).

In the case of an emergency, health care providers should do their best to ascertain whether or not the patient has previously expressed their position either verbally or in writing. Exercising such due-diligence can greatly reduce, if not eliminate liability and possible legal action.

3. Emergency/incompetent adults (no information available)

What is the responsibility or duty of the physician/hospital staff when there is no information available?

No physician or hospital is subject to liability based solely on failure to obtain consent in rendering emergency medical, surgical, hospital, or health services, to any patient regardless of age if 1) the patient is unable to consent, 2) no other person is reasonably available to legally authorize consent, and 3) the hospital and medical staff have acted in good faith and without any knowledge of facts that would negate the consent [7]. However, if it is discovered that a patient's religious status is Jehovah's Witness, reasonable efforts should be made to abort a transfusion and to proceed in a manner that accords with the patient's religious beliefs.

REFUSAL TO PERMIT BLOOD TRANSFUSION

I request that no blood or blood derivatives be administered to (name of patient) _____
_____ during this hospitalization. I hereby release the hospital, its personnel, the attending physician, and any other person participating in my care from any responsibility whatsoever for unfavorable reactions or any untoward results due to my refusal to permit the use of blood or its derivatives. The possible risks and consequences of such refusal on my part have been fully explained to me by my attending physician and I fully understand that such risks and consequences may occur as a result of my refusal.

I understand that my attending physician and other doctors who provide services to me are not employees or agents of the hospital. They are independent contractors.

The undersigned certifies that he/she has read the foregoing, received a copy thereof, and is the patient, the patient's legal representative, or is duly authorized by the patient as the patient's general agent to execute the above and accept its terms.

_____ _____ am / pm   Signature _____
     Date   Time   Patient/Parent/Guardian/Conservator/Responsible Party
_____ / _____   _____
   Witness signature / Witness print name   If signed by other than patient, indicate relationship

Translator I have accurately and completely read the foregoing document to _____
(*name of patient/person legally authorized to give consent*) in _____, the patient's or patient's representative's primary language. He/she understood all the terms and conditions and acknowledged his/her agreement thereto by signing this document in my presence.

_____ _____ am / pm   _____ / _____
     Date   Time   Translator signature / Translator print name

TRC1080 (7/04)

REFUSAL TO PERMIT BLOOD TRANSFUSION

PATIENT ID

FACE

WHITE - MEDICAL RECORD   CANARY - PATIENT

Figure 14.2 Refusal to permit blood transfusion.

What can be done when a patient who is one of Jehovah's Witnesses is incapacitated or unconscious?

Most Witness patients carry a wallet-sized advance medical directive/medical durable power of attorney that documents their refusal of blood. However, due to negligence or perhaps unforeseen circumstances, some Jehovah's Witness patients may not always have this document with them. In cases where the patient was previously a patient at the hospital, chart notes can be checked [7, 9]. There may also be a family member or friend previously appointed by the patient as health care agent or surrogate decision-maker. In regards to adults who are viewed as incompetent, if they never had decision-making capacity the law views them the same as minor children lacking capacity. However, the law is different for those who have had such capacity but are currently incapacitated.

If prior to losing capacity the adult was rational and capable of expressing their views and opinions regarding unacceptable treatment, a doctor or hospital is obligated to honor the patient's decision even if they are incapable of speaking for themselves. This applies especially in cases where the incapacitated patient's treatment preferences are based on deeply held religious beliefs. The basic standard for dealing with incompetent or unconscious adults is: What would the patient choose if able to communicate his/her choice? Acceptable evidence of their previously expressed refusal would be: (1) prior written or oral direction; (2) advance medical directive/medical durable power of attorney; (3) living will and medical power-of attorney; (4) chart notes; and (5) testimonial evidence from others, that is, surrogate decision makers. While the rest may be questioned, a medical DPA is the best legal document to outline the incapacitated patient's treatment preferences [7, 9].

If a physician is faced for the first time with an incapacitated patient or emergency situation, this could pose a dilemma for the physician regardless of any available information from a third party or family members that the patient is one of Jehovah's Witnesses. If the patient has a medical directive or DPA in which the patient refuses blood transfusion, the patient's wishes should be upheld. Having verbal information from family members or friends does not completely satisfy the physician's decision to transfuse or not, since people may change their mind regarding issues related to consent or refusal of blood. Therefore a policy should be in place to prepare for this dilemma if and when it arises.

Disagreeing family members
One of the most challenging scenarios arises when a patient's spouse, family member, relative, or friend disagrees with their refusal of blood. As previously mentioned in this chapter, every competent adult has the constitutional right and freedom to determine what shall be done to their bodies. Therefore, courts have uniformly upheld that competent persons have the legal right to accept or refuse medical treatment absent of consent from their spouse or other relatives [7]. It is viewed as a natural corollary

to an individual's rights of self-determination and personal autonomy to honor a patient's choice of treatment regardless of the views of their family.

For example, regarding a non-Witness husband's "consent" to blood transfusion for his Witness wife, a Florida Supreme Court stated: "marriage does not destroy one's constitutional right to personal autonomy." [7, 24]. The basic rule on spousal consent is that patients who are conscious, mentally capable of consent, and who give their consent do not require consent from their spouse, nor is it otherwise material [7, 25]. Another reason for the uniformity of case law that supports a patient's choice of treatment despite the disapproval of family or relatives is that family members may have a bias against the patient's interest due to conflicting interests [7, 26]. In addition, some family members may base their actions on their own religious beliefs. This may cause them to request treatment that contradicts the patient's wishes or desires [7, 27].

In summary, the patient's decision should control their medical treatment. The fundamental rights of personal privacy, bodily self-determination (informed consent) and, for Witness patients, religious freedom would be rendered void if respect for a patient's health-care decisions were contingent upon the unanimous agreement of the patient's spouse or relatives. Health-care providers should not be unduly concerned about litigation whenever these rights are upheld [7].

Minors

Generally, a minor is a person under the age of 18 and is not legally able to consent to medical treatment unless the law designates them as an emancipated minor [28]. In most cases, a minor's parents have the legal authority to consent to treatment for their child and consent must be obtained prior to treatment. There is a caveat, however, to such consent. If the minor objects to the treatment, the case should be referred to the hospital attorney if doubt exists about proceeding with treatment. For instance, if the objection is by a minor who is 14-years-old or older, it may be appropriate to seek legal advice if the parents consent to a procedure that involves significant risk of severe adverse consequences.

Most Witness families recognize the delicate balance between their rights and the legal obligations of the physicians. The U.S. Constitution protects the fundamental right of parents to make decisions concerning the care, custody, and control of their children. Therefore, with the exception of an emergency, if a surgeon operates on a child without the parent's consent, they will be liable for assault [7, 9].

Issues arise when the State seeks to interfere with the parent's right to make decisions regarding their child's medical treatment due to the state's interest in protecting those who are disabled or who are unable to protect themselves. If the state perceives that a minor child's life or health is in danger because of a parent's refusal to consent to a blood transfusion, they may grant a court order for the transfusion. However, such an order should only be granted if the State's interest in the protection of the minor child is "compelling." For the State's interest to be compelling it must be proven that there are no reasonable alternative non-blood treatments available. When the State's interest is viewed as compelling and there is risk of imminent harm or death, the court will order that blood be given. The physician or hospital may otherwise be held liable.

Mature and emancipated minors

An exception is sometimes made in the case of a mature minor. A mature minor is one who is able to understand the nature and extent of their condition. They should also understand the recommended alternatives to blood and they should be able to appreciate the consequences of their blood refusal. Their decision is not solely dependent on their parents but is based on their clear understanding of the facts.

California Legislature has enacted a series of statutes that authorize particular classes of minors to consent to various medical services [28]. However, a minor who would otherwise have the legal authority to consent to medical treatment may not be permitted to do so if they do not fully understand and appreciate the nature and consequences of the proposed health care, including its significant benefits, risks, and alternatives. In a scenario such as this, consultation with legal counsel should be arranged to eliminate any doubt that may exist.

According to the California Family Code, when a minor is at least 14 years of age, willingly lives separate or apart from his or her parent(s) or guardian with the consent or acquiescence of the minor's parents or guardian, manages his or her own financial affairs, and the source of his or her income is not from any illegal activity, that minor can petition a court to be emancipated [29]. Once emancipated, that minor is capable of giving a valid consent or withholding consent for medical or dental care without parental guardian consent, involvement, or financial liability. "Medical care" means "X-ray examination, anesthetic, medical or surgical diagnosis or treatment, and hospital care" under the supervision and upon the advice of a licensed physician.

When dealing with emancipated or mature minors who are Jehovah's Witnesses, physicians do well to have a clear understanding of the laws pertaining to their rights and to proceed in a manner that accords them with the same respect and dignity as they would give to an adult patient. However, decisions made by mature minors should be followed by the hospital only after a court decision is rendered regarding their ability to refuse treatment such as blood transfusion. This will protect health care providers from any potential liability.

Evolution of bloodless programs

Initially Jehovah's Witnesses' adamant refusal of blood and blood products was met with much controversy and frustration by members of both the medical and legal community. Many doctors viewed Jehovah's Witnesses position as one that "tied their hands" and prevented them from rendering adequate care under circumstances where profound anemia or significant surgical blood loss might compromise their patient's life. However, due to the continued growth of the Witness community, others recognized that this issue was not going away anytime soon, and a few physicians saw a unique opportunity in caring for these patients.

Early pioneers of bloodless medicine and surgery

Suffice it to say everyone wants effective medical care of the highest quality. To that end, a few members of the medical community began to ask the question: "Are there legitimate and effective ways to manage serious medical problems without using blood?" Fortunately for Jehovah's Witnesses, the answer was yes.

As early as the 1950s, a handful of physicians began to view the Witnesses' refusal of blood not as "tying their hands", but as just one more complication challenging their skill. Noteworthy among this group of pioneers was Dr. Denton Cooley of the Texas Heart Institute. In 1957, Cooley pioneered open-heart surgery without blood support [30, 31–34]. Dr. Cooley led a team of cardiovascular surgeons who performed thousands of cardiovascular operations on adults and children. In those days, most open-heart surgeries required 20 to 30 units of blood. In fact, as many as 12 units of blood were used just to prime the heart–lung bypass machine. However, Dr. Cooley and his colleagues used innovative methods to prime the bypass machine with non-blood fluids. In time other techniques were developed to obviate the need for blood. Dr. Cooley's experience revealed that "the risk of surgery in patients of the Jehovah's Witness group was not substantially higher than for others." This was indeed the genesis of "bloodless surgery."

In 1995, Dr. Hiram C. Polk Jr., editor-in-chief of the *American Journal of Surgery*, recognized Dr. Cooley's outstanding accomplishments [35]. He commented on the trailblazing efforts of Dr. Cooley in performing some 1 250 "bloodless" open-heart surgeries on patients who requested it due to their religious beliefs. He stated that "Dr. Cooley's blood conservation techniques are applicable to every operation and, therefore, meaningful to all 17 000 readers of *The American Journal of Surgery*."

Transfusion free "bloodless" program implementation

As more and more physicians began to respect Jehovah's Witnesses' position on blood, the atmosphere became less adversarial and much more cooperative. In fact, doctors and hospital administrators learned that the key to managing patients without blood transfusion required proper planning and good coordination between all members of the hospital staff, including nursing, laboratory, pharmacy, and social services. Although there are more doctors and hospitals willing to cooperate with patients who choose not to accept blood transfusion, a *promise* not to give blood is often not good enough to satisfy some patients. Thus the concept of a structured, formalized "bloodless" program was born! A bloodless or transfusion-free program offers a group of experienced and skilled physicians, surgeons, anesthesiologists and nurses who are dedicated and committed to "quality" medical care, without the use of blood.

As key "stakeholders" of a successful program, hospital administrators in concert with a core group of physician "champions" should elicit support from other members of the medical faculty. Since the Jehovah's Witness community is the main target audience, it would be helpful to perform a feasibility study or analysis to obtain information about the population of Witnesses residing in the hospital's primary and secondary service areas. One way to accomplish this is by arranging to meet with members of the local Hospital Liaison Committee for Jehovah's Witnesses (HLC).

Working under the direction of the Hospital Information Services of Jehovah's Witnesses (HIS), headquartered in Brooklyn, New York, the HLC's role is to seek out physicians and hospitals that will offer non-blood management to the Witness community. Presentations about Jehovah's Witnesses' position on healthcare, specifically blood and blood products, should be given to members of hospital administration and the medical faculty.

Subsequently, personal contact should be made with individual physicians to determine their willingness to treat Witness patients without blood. The goal of these one-on-one interviews is to ascertain each doctors comfort level, experience and clinical outcomes in providing elective and emergent treatment to adults and minors without blood product support. In-services for nursing and ancillary staff should also be arranged in order to facilitate good communication, proper identification and effective patient care management.

Legal structure of bloodless program

Consent: liability of physician and hospital

The Paul Gann Blood Safety Act, Health & Safety Code puts the onus on the physician to talk with patients facing the possibility of receiving allogeneic blood, and explain to them the risks, benefits, and alternatives. The Paul Gann Act emphasizes alternatives such as pre-operative autologous donation, directed donor blood, intra-operative cell-salvage and hemodilution. The physician must note in the patient's medical record that a standardized written summary produced by the State Department of Health Services is given to the patient (see Figures 14.3 and 14.4). No other pamphlet, other than the DHS pamphlet, will satisfy the physician's obligation under the law.

Upon admission to many hospitals, patients are asked to sign a release of liability form that clearly documents their refusal of blood and releases the physician from any untoward consequences of such refusal (see Figure 14.2). When patients do sign this release, there is little if any need to be concerned about litigation arising from a patient whose refusal of blood caused morbidity or mortality. Note that such a release would not include a general release of liability from medical malpractice.

Confirming a patient's decision to refuse blood

On occasion, a physician may feel compelled to "confirm" or "verify" a patient's decision to refuse blood transfusion. Their personal conscience may dictate that they *privately* discuss the matter with the patient without any input from family members. Such a discussion is appropriate and usually welcomed. However, a physician should be careful not to use this session as an opportunity to pressure the patient to revisit their refusal of blood. How far should he or she go in "confirming" the patient's choice of non-blood management without it being viewed as "badgering" or coercion? Often this can be a very subtle thing. The goal of this discussion is to give a physician the confidence and peace of mind that withholding blood products is the absolute decision of the patient. On the other hand, if a family member or friend is present to give advice or moral support to the patient (especially in the case of Jehovah's Witnesses), the medical staff should have it clear in mind that the decision being made is the patient's and not the other person(s). If the patient is looking to another person to answer questions being posed to him or her, it can make a physician quite uneasy, and understandably so. This sort of input should be given to the patient during pre-op or some other more appropriate time.

abg advance business graphics (909) 361-7100

- PERF -

TRANSFUSION INFORMATION AND CONSENT
PAUL GANN BLOOD SAFETY ACT, (HEALTH AND SAFETY CODE 1645)

Your signature below indicates that: (1) you have received a copy of the brochure *If You Need Blood: A Patient's Guide to Blood Transfusions*, (2) you have received information concerning the risks and benefits of blood transfusion and of any alternative therapies, (3) you have had the opportunity to discuss this matter with your physician, including predonation if applicable, and (4) subject to any special instructions listed below, you consent to such blood transfusion as your physician may order.

Special Instructions _____
(Describe here any specific instructions for patient's blood transfusion, e.g. predonation, directed donation,etc.)

The undersigned certifies that he/she has read the foregoing, received a copy thereof, and is the patient, the patient's legal representative, or is duly authorized by the patient as the patient's general agent to execute the above and accept its terms.

_____ _____ am / pm   Signature_____
Date   Time   Patient/Parent/Guardian/Conservator/Responsible Party
_____/_____ _____
Witness signature / Witness print name   If signed by other than patient, indicate relationship

Translator I have accurately and completely read the foregoing document to _____
(*name of patient/person legally authorized to give consent*) in _____, the patient's or patient's representative's primary language. He/she understood all the terms and conditions and acknowledged his/her agreement thereto by signing this document in my presence.

_____ _____ am / pm   _____/_____
Date   Time   Translator signature / Translator print name

PHYSICIAN VERIFICATION OF INFORMED CONSENT I, the undersigned physician, hereby certify that I have discussed with the patient and / or person legally authorized to give consent on behalf of the patient, the risks, benefits, alternative therapies, and any adverse reactions that may be reasonably expected to occur to any blood transfusion that I believe may be necessary or advisable.

The undersigned further certifies that the patient and / or legally responsible person was encouraged to ask questions and that all questions were answered.

_____ _____ am / pm   _____
Date   Time   Physician Signature

TRC1014E (2/04)   IMMS # 59158

BLOOD TRANSFUSION
INFORMATION AND CONSENT
(WITH PHYSICIAN VERIFICATION)

P
A
T
I
E
N
T

I D

FACE

Figure 14.3 DHS Pamphlet: Transfusion Information and Consent (Paul Gann Blood Safety Act).

The methods of using your own blood can be used independently or together to eliminate or minimize the need for donor blood, as well as virtually eliminate transfusion risks of infection and allergic reaction.

■ **AUTOLOGOUS BLOOD** - Using Your Own Blood

Option	Explanation	Advantages	Disadvantages
PRE-OPERATIVE DONATION Donating Your Own Blood Before Surgery	The blood bank draws your blood and stores it until you need it, during or after surgery. For elective surgery only.	✓ Eliminates or minimizes the need for someone else's blood during and after surgery.	• Requires advance planning. • May delay surgery. • Medical conditions may prevent pre-operative donation.
INTRA-OPERATIVE AUTOLOGOUS TRANSFUSION Recycling Your Blood During Surgery	Instead of being discarded, blood lost during surgery is filtered, and put back into your body during surgery. For elective and emergency surgery.	✓ Eliminates or minimizes the need for someone else's blood during surgery. Large amounts of blood can be recycled.	• Not for use if cancer or infection is present.
POST-OPERATIVE AUTOLOGOUS TRANSFUSION Recycling Your Blood After Surgery	Blood lost after surgery is collected, filtered and returned. For elective and emergency surgery.	✓ Eliminates or minimizes the need for someone else's blood after surgery.	• Not for use if cancer or infection is present.
HEMODILUTION Donating Your Own Blood During Surgery	Immediately before surgery, some of your blood is taken and replaced with I.V. fluids. After surgery, your blood is filtered and returned to you. For elective surgery.	✓ Eliminates or minimizes the need for someone else's blood during and after surgery. Dilutes your blood so you lose less concentrated blood during surgery.	• Limited number or units can be drawn. • Medical conditions may prevent hemodilution.
APHERESIS Donating Your Own Platelets and Plasma	Before surgery, your platelets and plasma, which help stop bleeding, are withdrawn, filtered, and returned to you when you need it. For elective surgery.	✓ May eliminate the need for donor platelets and plasma, especially in high blood-loss procedures.	• Medical conditions may prevent apheresis. • Procedure has limited application.

In some cases, you may require more blood than anticipated. If this happens and you receive blood other then your own, there is a possibility of complications, such as hepatitis or AIDS.

■ **DONOR BLOOD** - Using Someone Else's Blood

Donor blood and blood products can never be absolutely 100% safe, even though testing makes the risk very small.

Option	Explanation	Advantages	Disadvantages
VOLUNTEER BLOOD From the Community Blood Supply	Blood and blood products donated by volunteer donors to a community blood bank.	✓ Readily available. Can be life-saving when your own blood is not available.	• Risk of disease transmission (such as hepatitis or AIDS), and allergic reactions.
Note You may wish to check whether donors are paid or volunteer, since blood from commercial (paid) donors may not, in some cases, be as safe as blood from volunteers.			
DESIGNATED DONOR BLOOD From Donors You Select	Blood and blood donors you select who must meet the same requirements as volunteer donors.	✓ You can select people with your own blood type who you feel are safe donors.	• Risk of disease transmission (such as hepatitis or AIDS), and allergic reactions. • May require several days of advanced donation. • Not necessarily as safe, nor safer, than volunteer donor blood.
Note Care should be taken in selecting donors. Donors should never be pressured into donating. Donations from certain family members may require irradiation of blood			

Figure 14.4 DHS Pamphlet: Transfusion Information and Consent (Paul Gann Blood Safety Act).

Policies and procedures

An essential step to ensuring the success of a bloodless program is to develop well-defined policies and procedures that are legally, ethically, and clinically sound. They should make absolutely clear the role of every member of the medical and hospital staffs who have direct contact with patients refusing blood or blood products. Distinct methods of identifying patients should be implemented, e.g. colored armbands, computer codes/symbols and chart stickers. A mechanism should be in place to monitor orders to type and cross-match blood for patients enrolled in the bloodless program. In addition, laboratory draws for blood testing should be ordered judiciously, not routinely.

Future expansion of transfusion-free programs

When most people hear the words "bloodless" or "transfusion-free", they immediately think of Jehovah's Witnesses. Yes, historically Jehovah's Witnesses have been the largest users of bloodless and/or transfusion-free medicine and surgery. However, in recent years, this novel approach has expanded to a much larger population. A growing number of hospital organizations are seeing the advantage of implementing blood management strategies and protocols to address supply cost issues as well as patient safety. Religious, ethical and legal issues aside, one must take a hard look at whether or not blood avoidance offers benefits for the community at large.

One cannot deny that there are many modalities that have been heavily relied upon in the past, even as it relates to the use of blood, that are now considered archaic and unscientific.

With ongoing progress in the area of oxygen carrying products, autologous blood recovery systems, and synthetic clotting factors such as Factor VIIa, the future looks brighter in providing a safe and effective alternative to blood transfusions.

References

1 Bloodless Medicine and Surgery – The Growing Demand. Awake. Vol. 81: 3–6; 2000 Jan 8.
2 Jehovah's Witnesses and The Question of Blood. Watchtower Bible and Tract Society of Pennsylvania; 1977.
3 How Can Blood Save Your Life? Watchtower Bible and Tract Society of Pennsylvania, 1990.
4 Questions From Readers. The Watchtower. Vol. 121 (12) 29–31; 2000 Jun 15.
5 Questions From Readers. The Watchtower. Vol. 121 (20) 29–31; 2000 Oct 15.

6 Questions From Readers. The Watchtower. Vol. 101, No. 6; 31; 1980 Mar 15.

7 Legally Defending Jehovah's Witnesses View of Blood. Patterson, New York; 2001.

8 California Physician's Legal Handbook. California Medical Association 1997.

9 Legal Considerations for Balancing Patients' Rights and The Bloodless Medicine and Surgery Program. Ralph A. Leaf, Attorney at Law; 1997.

10 Schloendorff v. Society of New York Hospital, 105 N.E. 92, 93 (N.Y. 1914).

11 61 Am. Jur. 2d Physicians, Surgeons, and Other Healers 197 (1981).

12 In re Milton, 505 N.E.2d 255 (Ohio 1987).

13 In re Osborne, 294 A.2d 372 (D.C. 1972).

14 In re Estate of Brooks, 205 N.E.2d 435 (Ill. 1965).

15 Reynolds v. United States, 98 U.S. 145, 167 (1878).

16 Harden v. State, 216 S.W.2d 708 (Tenn. 1948).

17 The Refused Blood Transfusion, 10 Nat. L.F. 202, 207–9 (1965).

18 The Right to Die, 9 Utah L. Rev. 161, 163–8 (1964).

19 In re Brown 478 So.2d 1033, 1039 (Miss. 1985).

20 In re Conroy, 486 A.2d 1209, 1229 (N.J. 1985).

21 Winters v. Miller, 446 F.2d 65,69 (2d. Cir. 1971).

22 Developments in the Law-Medical Technology and the Law, 103 Harv. L. Rev. 1519, 1670 (1990).

23 535 A.2d 452 (Pa. 1987): Informed Refusal: Legal Befuddlement.

24 In re Dubreuil, 629 So. 2d 819, 827 n.13 (Fla. 1993).

25 2 Health Law Center, Hospital Law Manual 180 (P. Young 3d 1989).

26 President's Commission for the Study of Ethical Problems, Making Health Care Decisions 183 (1982).

27 Developments in the Law – Medical Technology and the Law, 103 Harv. L. Rev. 1519, 1651 (1990).

28 Consent Manual. California Healthcare Association 2001, 28th Edition.

29 California Family Code Section 7120.

30 Farmer S, Webb D, Your Body, Your Choice, Singapore: Media Masters; 2000, 14–15.

31 Cooley DA, Crawford ES, Howell JF, Beall AC Jr., Open Heart Surgery in Jehovah's Witnesses. Am J Cardiology. 1964;13:779–81.

32 Ott DA, Cooley DA. Cardiovascular Surgery in Jehovah's Witnesses: Report of 542 Operations Without Blood Transfusion. JAMA. 1977;238:1256–8.

33 Henling CE, Carmichael MJ, Keats AS, Cooley DA. Cardiac operation for congenital heart disease in children of Jehovah's Witnesses. J Thorac Cardiovasc Surg. 1985;89:914–20.

34 Carmichael MJ, Cooley DA, Kuykendall RC, Walker WE. Cardiac Surgery in Children of Jehovah's Witnesses. Texas Heart Institute Journal. 1985;12(1):57–63.

35 Cooley DA. Conservation of Blood During Cardiovascular Surgery. Am J Surg. 1995;170 (suppl 6A):53S–9S.

CHAPTER 15

Basic principles of bloodless medicine and surgery

Nicolas Jabbour

Service de Chirurgie et transplantation abdominale Cliniques universitaires Saint-Luc Bruxelles, Belgium

Questionnaire

Choose the correct statement(s) for each question (one or more are possible).

1 **Blood utilization in the USA:**
   (a) Over 12 million units of blood are used annually
   (b) Over 40% of blood used is prescribed by surgeons
   (c) Over 50% of blood is used in patients over 60 years of age
   (d) Blood utilization is expected to increase in the future

2 **Blood donors:**
   (a) In the USA, blood donors can be paid in order to increase the donor pool
   (b) The donor pool is increasing on a consistent basis due to the awareness of blood shortages
   (c) Donors may be excluded if they spend significant time in certain countries
   (d) The safest blood donation is from a directed-donor, i.e. family members or friends

3 **Cost of blood products:**
   (a) Currently the average cost of packed red blood cells (PRBCs) is approximately $200–250
   (b) This cost does not include costs related to type and crossmatching, blood administration and banking
   (c) Indirect costs of blood products should include the costs of its complications, i.e. fever or viral transmission

Transfusion-Free Medicine and Surgery, Second Edition. Edited by Nicolas Jabbour.
© 2014 John Wiley & Sons, Ltd. Published 2014 by John Wiley & Sons, Ltd.

4 **Potential risks of blood transfusion:**
 (a) The risk of hepatitis C transmission is less than 1 per 100 000 units
 (b) Some clinical studies have shown that blood transfusion may increase the risk of tumor recurrence
 (c) Blood transfusion may increase the risk of postoperative infection
 (d) As many as 1% of patients may experience fever as a result of blood transfusion

5 **Preoperative autologous donation (PAD):**
 (a) May decrease the need for homologous blood transfusion
 (b) Requires one or more preoperative visits to the blood bank
 (c) Does not decrease the risk of clerical error associated with blood transfusions
 (d) Significant amount of blood collected is not used perioperatively

6 **Acute normovolemic hemodilution (ANH):**
 (a) Does not eliminate the risk of clerical error when the blood is given to the patient
 (b) Can be used even in severely anemic patients
 (c) Unlike banked blood, the blood collected during ANH contains normal platelets and clotting factors
 (d) ANH has no effect on blood conservation

7 **Intraoperative cell salvage (cell saver):**
 (a) Cell saver is contraindicated in patients with gross contamination in the surgical field
 (b) Can be used in trauma with major bleeding such as hemothorax or major vascular injury
 (c) Blood saved is depleted from platelets and coagulation factors
 (d) May cause severe coagulopathy in patients with large amounts of blood loss
 (e) Can be performed without heparinization
 (f) May cause disseminated intravascular coagulation (DIC) or air embolism if not set up appropriately

8 **Erythropoietin (Procrit, Epogen):**
 (a) Erythropoietin is a recombinant factor available as an intravenous (IV) or subcutaneous (SC) injection
 (b) It stimulates the bone marrow to produce more RBCs
 (c) Requires the use of therapeutic doses of iron to be more effective
 (d) May yield up to 3 units of blood within 3 weeks of administration

(e) Although it was originally used in patients with chronic renal failure (CRF), erythropoietin is currently approved in selective patients pre-operatively

9 **Legal aspects of blood transfusion in Jehovah's Witness (JW) patients:**
   (a) In the USA, adult JW patients have the right to refuse blood transfusion at the risk of their life
   (b) If the patient is unknown to be a JW and is seen in a trauma or emergency situation, physicians must administer blood, if necessary, without consent
   (c) Pediatric patients of JW families should be transfused, if medically necessary, with or without court order depending on the urgency of the situation
   (d) In adult patients, if appropriate consent is signed prior to surgery, transfusions cannot be administered even if the patient became incapacitated postoperatively
   (e) If standard of care is applied appropriately when treating adult JW patients, the physician and the institution are not liable in case of patient demise from severe anemia

10 **The following are some of the contraindications to ANH:**
   (a) Hemodynamic instability
   (b) Low hematocrit
   (c) Underlying severe cardiovascular disease
   (d) Older than 75 years of age

11 **Activated factor VII (NovoSeven):**
   (a) Is a recombinant protein produced from hamster renal cells
   (b) Enhances coagulation cascade at the site of vascular injury
   (c) Its only FDA approved indication is for the treatment of hemophilia with inhibitors
   (d) Has proven beneficial in conditions such as severe trauma, liver disease and transplantation in off-label use

12 **Bleeding disorders in surgical patients:**
   (a) History of prior bleeding during minor surgery or minor trauma is one of the most important details regarding underlying bleeding disorders
   (b) Normal platelet count, prothrombin time (PT) and activated partial thromboplastin time (APTT) do not eliminate the potential risks for medical bleeding

(c) Platelets may need to be transfused even with normal platelet counts in patients treated with nonsteroidal anti-inflammatory drugs (NSAIDs) who have medical bleeding

(d) Thromboelastogram offers information regarding the quality of the clotting system

13 The following products may have some value in limiting surgical bleeding:
(a) Aprotinin in cardiac surgery, orthopedic surgery and liver transplantation
(b) Epsilon-aminocaproic acid (Amicar) in the face of fibrinolysis
(c) Desmopressin (DDAVP), especially in patients with chronic kidney disease
(d) NovoSeven (factor VIIa) in patients with severe coagulopathy from massive blood transfusion

14 These anesthetic techniques may decrease surgical blood loss:
(a) Controlled hypotension in surgeries such as liver resection
(b) The use of thromboelastogram to evaluate the coagulation system, especially in liver transplantation
(c) The use of ANH
(d) The use of cell saver

15 Blood transfusion in the intensive care unit (ICU):
(a) A significant percentage of blood transfusions given in the ICU is due to excessive blood testing
(b) Randomized clinical trials have shown that a higher hematocrit enhances patient survival
(c) Erythropoietin is very effective in ICU patients even in the presence of underlying sepsis
(d) Maintaining a high level of hematocrit is more important than maintaining normal intravascular volume status

16 Pathophysiology of acute anemia:
(a) Decreasing the hematocrit to a level of 20% is well tolerated in healthy patients
(b) Perioperative mortality is significantly increased in severely anemic patients with underlying vascular disease
(c) Oxygen delivery is maintained in moderate anemia as long as the patient has normal intravascular volume

(d) The physiologic response to acute anemia consists of decreased peripheral vascular resistance, increased heart rate and increased oxygen extraction

17 **Tissue oxygen consumption/need:**
   (a) Increases significantly with fever
   (b) Decreases in patients on artificial ventilation and paralyzed
   (c) Increases with shivering
   (d) May be decreased in hypothermic patients

18 **Oxygen delivery:**
   (a) Is directly proportional to hemoglobin concentration
   (b) Is directly proportional to cardiac output and heart rate
   (c) Can be maintained in anemic patients by increased cardiac output
   (d) Mechanical ventilation and increased inhaled oxygen concentration may increase oxygen delivery

19 **Severely anemic patients may benefit from the following:**
   (a) Increased oxygen delivery by increasing inhaled oxygen delivery and/or mechanical ventilation
   (b) Decreased oxygen consumption by artificial ventilation
   (c) Decreased oxygen consumption by the use of paralytics to avoid shivering in patients on the ventilator
   (d) Maintaining euvolemia
   (e) Potential benefits with hypothermia

20 **Artificial blood products:**
   (a) They are derived from hemoglobin, old blood or perfluorocarbon molecules
   (b) They have a long shelf life
   (c) They do not require refrigeration for banking
   (d) They have small-sized particles that can potentially deliver oxygen beyond critical obstruction such as in cardiac or cerebrovascular disease

21 **The pitfalls of artificial blood product usage:**
   (a) Has a high affinity for oxygen
   (b) Requires high FiO_2 to deliver significant oxygen to the tissues
   (c) Has shorter half-life in comparison to autologous blood once transfused
   (d) Requires the infusion of large volume to adequately increase oxygen delivery

22 **The potential benefits of artificial blood products:**
   (a) Can be used on site in trauma and in the military
   (b) Its use in the operating room increases the safety of ANH by maintaining close-to-normal oxygen delivery in the presence of severe anemia
   (c) May be used in JW patients with severe anemia while the RBCs are being synthesized by the bone marrow

23 **Transfusion-free surgery in pediatric patients:**
   (a) Techniques used in adult patients cannot be applied to pediatric patients
   (b) Transfusion in children should be avoided since the transmission of some diseases manifests itself many years following blood product transfusion
   (c) Erythropoietin has been used successfully in pediatric patients

24 **Major surgery in JW patients:**
   (a) Major surgery can be done safely in JW patients without blood product transfusion
   (b) Liver transplantation in JW patients has been done successfully in specialized centers such as University of Southern California/USC University Hospital
   (c) Large studies have shown that severe anemia (hemoglobin < 6 g/dl) significantly affects postoperative mortality in patients with underlying cardiovascular disease
   (d) Techniques used in treating JW patients can be applied to non-JW patients to decrease overall blood utilization

25 **Refractory conditions to erythropoietin therapy:**
   (a) Patients with underlying inflammatory disease from cancer
   (b) Patients with severe sepsis
   (c) The presence of iron deficiency
   (d) Bone marrow disease

26 **Reasons for surgeons to initiate transfusion-free program:**
   (a) More than half of blood transfusions are prescribed by surgeons
   (b) Elective surgery cannot proceed without available blood products
   (c) Blood savings decrease the overall costs of surgical care
   (d) Blood loss is a reflection of the quality of surgeons

27 **These pathogens can be transmitted via blood transfusions:**
   (a) Human immunodeficiency virus (HIV)
   (b) Mad cow disease

(c) West Nile virus (WNV)

(d) Hepatitis B and C virus (HBV and HCV)

28 **Despite donor testing, disease transmission via blood transfusion is still possible due to the following reasons:**

(a) Most testing detects antibodies rather than antigens

(b) There are still potentially unknown pathogens that escape testing and can be transmitted through blood

(c) There is always a small window between infection and disease detection in potential donors

29 **The benefits of blood product transfusion:**

(a) Increases oxygen delivery to the tissues

(b) Enhances coagulation by transfusion of fresh frozen plasma and platelets

(c) Serves as intravascular volume expander similar to colloids or crystalloids

30 **These products can only be derived from human blood:**

(a) Factor VIII concentrate

(b) Factor IX concentrate

(c) Fresh frozen plasma

(d) Cryoprecipitate

(e) Factor VIIa

31 **Drugs that may affect platelet function:**

(a) Aspirin

(b) Dextran

(c) Steroids

(d) Cox II inhibitors

32 **The basics for successful transfusion-free surgery:**

(a) Starting the surgery at a higher hematocrit level by preoperative bone marrow stimulation

(b) Careful surgical technique

(c) Selective hypotensive anesthesia

(d) The use of cell saver and ANH during surgery

33 **Iron use along with erythropoietin:**

(a) Can enhance bone marrow production of RBCs

(b) Very well tolerated orally and almost completely absorbed

(c) Can be safely used intravenously in gluconate form

(d) If not used with erythropoietin, may decrease the bone marrow response or lead to the production of hypochromic RBCs

34 **Current shelf life of blood products:**
(a) Packed red cells = 42 days at 0–6 °C
(b) Platelets = 5 days at room temperature
(c) Fresh frozen plasma = 1 year at –18 °C
(d) Cryoprecipitate = 1 year at –18 °C
(e) Frozen red cells = over 1 year

35 **Potential perioperative complications that may lead to postoperative bleeding disorders:**
(a) Thrombotic thrombocytopenic purpura (TTP) induced by surgery
(b) Thrombocytopenia from use of heparin, even as a flush solution
(c) Sepsis
(d) The presence of large intra-abdominal clot with local fibrinolysis that promotes localized bleeding

36 **These interventions may decrease the side-effects of blood transfusion:**
(a) Pretreatment with benadryl and oral Acetaminophene
(b) The use of white cell filters that may eliminate or decrease the risk of febrile reaction to blood transfusion
(c) Careful verification by two persons of the crossmatch between the blood being transfused and the patient receiving the transfusion

37 **Signs and symptoms of potential transfusion reactions:**
(a) Hematuria
(b) Severe back pain
(c) Chills and fever
(d) Hypotension

38 **The optimal threshold for red cell transfusion:**
(a) Hematocrit level of 30% (hemoglobin of 10 g/dl) is the optimal accepted threshold
(b) A precise threshold cannot be used universally in any patient and in any situation
(c) Threshold is lower in younger, healthy patients
(d) The threshold of 30% or higher is appropriate in patients with underlying cardiovascular disease

39 **Absolute contraindications to cell saver:**
(a) Presence of amniotic fluid at the surgical site
(b) Presence of gastrointestinal (GI) fluid at the surgical site
(c) Cutting through tumor during the surgery

(d) The use of certain local hemostatic products that may lead to intravascular coagulopathy

40 **The following are local hemostatic agents used in surgery to decrease blood loss:**
(a) Fibrin glue (Tisseel, Floseal, etc.)
(b) Surgicel
(c) NovoSeven (factor VIIa)
(d) Avitene
(e) Amicar

41 **Indirect costs of blood transfusion include:**
(a) Type and screen testing
(b) Type and crossmatching
(c) Blood dispensing and administration
(d) Work-up for transfusion reaction

42 **The calculation of the increase in oxygen delivery as a result of blood transfusion should take into consideration the following:**
(a) Old RBCs may lose some elasticity with negative effect on tissue perfusion
(b) RBC affinity for oxygen increases with aging
(c) The rbc half-life is lower in banked blood than in native RBCs
(d) 1 unit of blood transfusion administered to an adult is expected to yield a 3% increase in the hematocrit level

43 **Contraindications to the use of erythropoietin:**
(a) Known sensitivity to antibiotics
(b) Recent coronary surgery
(c) Uncontrolled hypertension
(d) Anemia

Index

Transfusion-Free Medicine and Surgery, Second Edition. Edited by Nicolas Jabbour.
© 2014 John Wiley & Sons, Ltd. Published 2014 by John Wiley & Sons, Ltd.

anemia (*continued*)
    transfusion trigger/threshold
        defined by risk of transfusion
            vs risk of, 32–3, 62, 70–72, 78,
            207, 210, *345*
anesthesia, 93, 162, *341*
    controlled hypotensive
        see hypotensive anesthesia
anesthestic agents and normovolemic
    hemodilution, 169–70
angiotensin receptor antagonists in
    hepatic ischemia–reperfusion
    injury prevention, 294–5
animal blood transfusion, 5–7
antibodies (immunoglobulins)
    to erythropoietin, 258
    to red cells, 45, 46, 47
    see also autoantibodies
anticoagulants
    circulating (endogenous), 118
    use, 132–4
        autologous blood, 177, 178
        donated (allogeneic) blood, 8
antidiuretic hormone analog
    see desmopressin
anti-factor Xa activity assay, 121
antifibrinolytics, 130–131, 184–6
    in blood conservation, 184–6
    children, 227
    in topical products, 150
antiplatelet agents, 132–3, *344*
antithrombin, 113–14
antithrombotic drugs, 133–4
apheresis (pheresis), 29
    platelet, 38
apixaban, 134
aprotinin, 94, 130–131, 150
    in blood conservation, 94, 184
    children, 227
argatroban, 134
arterial thromboembolism risk with
    peripheral red blood cell
    transfusion, 260–261
artificial blood (carriers of
    oxygen), 271–88, *342–3*
    defining the need for, 274–6
    hemoglobin-based, 24–5, 97,
        216–17, 274–83

aspirin, 132
assent (child), 21
autoantibodies
    (autoimmunoglobulins),
    anticoagulant, 118
    to factor VIII, 187
autologous blood collection/
    donation, 164–82
    DHS pamphlet and consent
        issues, 335
    pre-operative, 92–3, 174–7, *339*
        collection technique, 175
        contraindications, 175–6
        cord blood, 226, 229–30
        criterion for, 175
        Jehovah's Witnesses, 317
        normovolemic hemodilution as
            alternative to, 174
autologous blood transfusion
    (autotransfusion), 89, 90, 159, 196
    children, 225–7, 231
    Jehovah's Witnesses and, 317
autologous intraoperative cell salvage
    see cell salvage
Avitene, 179

bacterial contamination, 49–50
Bioglue®, 144
bivalirudin, 134
bleeding *see* blood loss
bleeding disorders *see* coagulation
bleeding time, 119–20, 121
blood
    artificial *see* artificial blood
    autologous *see* autologous blood
        collection; autologous blood
        transfusion
    conservation, intra-operative,
        88–95, 164–91
        children, 227–8
        pharmacological agents for,
            182–91
        see also specific methods
    donation *see* donation
    early beliefs and practices, 2–4
    loss *see* bleeding
    microparticles, 111–12
    oxygen transportation, 272–4